T0315033

Why People Smoke

Why People Smoke

An Innovative Approach to Treating Tobacco Dependence

Frank T. Leone and Sarah Evers-Casey

With illustrations by Joey Leone

PENN

University of Pennsylvania Press
Philadelphia

Copyright © 2024 University of Pennsylvania Press

Published by
University of Pennsylvania Press
Philadelphia, Pennsylvania 19104-4112
www.pennpress.edu

Printed in the United States of America on acid-free paper
10 9 8 7 6 5 4 3 2 1

Hardcover ISBN: 978-1-5128-2477-3
Paperback ISBN: 978-1-5128-2478-0
eBook ISBN: 978-1-5128-2479-7

A Cataloging-in-Publication record is available from the Library of Congress

To our families …
Thank you for your endless support and patience.

Contents

Part IV. **Knowing "More"**

Part IV. Knowing "More?"

Introduction
Thinking About Tobacco Treatment

"Okay, how?" a patient asked one day twenty-five years ago during a routine pulmonary appointment. Those two simple words had a profound impact. The answer to that question hadn't really been the subject of a lot of deep discussion within medicine. This patient had a serious lung problem, one that would probably take her life in a miserable, protracted way. Her problem was the legacy of forty years of smoking a pack of cigarettes every day. She had received the advice to stop smoking from her doctors, her family, and her friends. So when she heard it one more time from her brand-new lung doctor, she'd had enough. She was directly challenging us to do something about it. With two short words and a look that said "if you're so smart . . . " she was really asking, "What are you going to do to help me?"

None of our training to that point had prepared us to fully answer that question. We had always been taught that the absence of smoking was the result of a decision to switch off the bad behavior. Although the addictive potential of nicotine was well established by that point, it was not yet treated the same as other addictions. Clinicians expected patients to tolerate headaches and mood swings for a few days—because it was clearly worth the trouble. It was expected that the patient would take responsibility for making it happen. Every time clinicians pointed out that a smoking-related disease was preventable, the implication was that the addicted person was the one who needed to prevent it.

By asking her question, our patient had suddenly turned the tables. She was saying that "un-smoking" is not simple. Quitting is not just the absence of smoking. She was saying that un-smoking was a new skill, one that needed to be learned, and one that she needed help learning. She was saying it was our responsibility to help her.

For twenty years now, we have been caring for patients with tobacco dependence. We've learned so much from our patients over the years, and every day they teach us new ways of seeing the problem and making a difference. A decade ago, we started an effort we called Project 430K. The U.S. surgeon general had just published a report estimating that 430,000 people died each year in the United States from smoking-related illness and disability. The catastrophic price paid for failing to recognize the true nature of nicotine's effect motivated us to begin sharing what we had learned about treating tobacco dependence in a more meaningful way. Like every problem that faces a healthcare professional, the nature of tobacco dependence started off as a mystery—our understanding clouded by misconceptions and well-meaning common sense. But we soon found ourselves at a professional tipping point. Our nagging uneasiness over whether we were doing the very best job we could for our patients kept us searching for deeper answers. We have been fortunate in finding many generous colleagues outside the biomedical sciences who graciously shared insights from their own disciplines so that we could more fully understand the problem. There are lots of answers out there, but we all need to keep asking the correct questions to find them.

Smoking is not just the antecedent to disease; it is the cardinal sign of a distortion in the brain's wiring. Despite its enormous death toll, this problem is the product of a predictable exposure, which means it's also a problem where a single responsible professional can make a major difference. One of the goals of Project 430K is to shift the responsibility for addressing the problem of tobacco dependence off the shoulders of those afflicted and onto the shoulders of expert professionals. Over the past ten years, we have taught hundreds of people to think about tobacco differently—people just like you who have gone on to help thousands of patients stop smoking. In the process, we keep learning. This book is a product of that effort. While the insights into practice we present should never substitute for sound clinical judgment, we hope you find this peek into the foundations of tobacco dependence as awesome and as empowering as we do.

One of the biggest challenges we had to face writing this book was accepting the incompleteness of our own frame of reference. For any problem as complicated as the problem of tobacco dependence, the way a person approaches the problem depends on the initial category of thinking. For example, a psychologist might focus on describing specific behaviors and their effect on emotional well-being. A cognitive neuroscientist, with a perspective rooted in the function of the nervous system, might focus on the mechanics of neurons and circuits. An evolutionary biologist might think about how the millennia have shaped the probabilities of some behaviors based on their impact on survival.

We are clinicians, so this book discusses nicotine and tobacco from a clinical treatment perspective. We worked to distill important information from a host of other perspectives into a clinically meaningful model, but there are two unfortunate consequences of our emphasis on the clinic. First, we had to exclude some very cool experiments and insights within related fields because they have not quite worked their way into the clinic just yet. Even when included, we had to take some liberty paraphrasing amazing ideas that have taken decades of intense research to illuminate in order to make them relevant to the day-to-day concerns of patient interactions. Our hope is that this book serves as a starting point for your exploration, generating questions in your head that will compel you to find your own answers. Second, the spread of the tobacco epidemic is contingent on a number of very interesting social, environmental, and cultural variables. They are critically important, but you will not find them discussed here. We focused strictly on the role healthcare providers can play in directly helping addicted people overcome their burden and left those other topics for authors with more expertise in those fields.

We also recognize that people outside of healthcare may have an interest in the topic. Maybe you elected to study the clinical perspective to help stimulate new research questions, to gain lived insight perspective into a policy choice you are facing, or to help a loved one better understand their behaviors. The best way to use this book may vary a bit depending on what you would like to get out of it. You will notice early on that the process of relating the material to your needs is very likely to be nonlinear. The concepts presented in the book aren't just cumulative; they are interrelated. For this reason, we have included a series of exercises in Chapter 15 that can help you identify the connections between concepts that appear in various places throughout the book. Whatever your perspective, going through these exercises after reading once through the material can be a very useful way of identifying chapters or topics that may be worth a second look or a deeper dive into the bibliography reading list.

Keep in mind that the way the brain works is really complicated. The one universal message within these pages is that none of us are finished figuring out the answers to the problem of tobacco dependence. What makes perfect sense today might not make sense tomorrow. What has yet to be imagined might someday become a fundamental truth. But the first step in achieving your goal is taking a moment to respect your goal: by reading this book, it is clear that you are trying to rethink everything you have ever heard about helping people control their nicotine addiction. Sometimes, that will be hard. You will be asked to reassess all your prior assumptions and evaluate them against the science. Sometimes, those two things won't square up on the first pass. Richard Dawkins, an esteemed evolutionary biologist and author, was famously quoted as saying, "Science does violence to common sense." What you think you know, you might not; what you assume is true might just be orthodoxy. And orthodoxy prevents progress. Just because an idea has been considered not-wrong for a long time does not necessarily mean that it is right. In this book, we do our best to present what we have found to be correct over the years of doing this work. Some of it will be familiar; some of it will seem to contradict established common sense. In either case, our hope is that the information we present will spark a clinical curiosity within you. The drive to learn beyond these pages will help us all do a better job in the future.

To make our points, we make use of quite a few of the very human stories we have heard from our patients over the years. Throughout the book, we will tell you about Helen, an addicted person, and David, one of her physicians. The narratives that Helen and David represent are archetypal, a compilation of actions, emotions, and thoughts that we have encountered in the clinic again and again. In that sense, the story of Helen and David is not fictional per se—everything that they experience happens every day—but we have taken the liberty of piecing bits together to form a story arc that is clearer and, we trust, more instructive. While the story of Helen and David runs throughout the book, we also use several specific case presentations to highlight clinically important points. In all cases, names and personal details have been changed to protect identities. Any similarities to someone you have met should be construed as proof of the universality of the core experience of tobacco dependence and any differences as proof of human uniqueness.

We'll leave you with this: There's only so much good the written word can do for you. Go out and live this thing. Don't be shy about experiencing it from Helen's perspective. Start by shelving the goal of encouraging people to quit for a minute and just go out and talk to someone who uses tobacco about the dependence itself. Ask questions instead of giving answers. Listen. Challenge yourself to have a conversation about smoking with Helen that she will enjoy. Your own answers are out there; you just have to do a little digging to uncover them.

Share them with someone after you do.

Good luck!

Part I

Knowing "What"

Chapter 1
Ambivalence

It's a trap. It's a trap you step in when you're ten, a trap you're not even aware you're trapped in, a trap you've been taught to feel guilty about being stuck in, and a trap you spend your money to stay in.

—Thomas J., 62 years old

Helen looks around the room. It is packed today, as usual. Every patient waiting room seems to her to have the same appearance—an old tweed rug, coffee stains on the chairs, and magazines on the tables. Her husband always hated the doctor's office. He would complain about the TV blaring in the background and the futility of trying to "fix" problems for which the path of destiny was already paved. She glances around the waiting room, unable to make eye contact with anyone. She looks down at her nails, and a familiar feeling of disgust envelops her. She forgot to paint her nails, and she can see the yellow stains. As she sighs, she gets a strong whiff of her own perfume, a clear sign that she had probably overdone it.

"Helen. Please come on back," the medical assistant (MA) calls.

She gathers her things and follows the MA. She feels a twinge of pain shoot from her hip down her leg, followed by her chronic cough. She hates this cough, and the hip pain was becoming a source of constant frustration. The past few months had been particularly difficult, and she is finding it hard to motivate to leave her home. She imagines the other patients watching her hobble away, coughing, unable to keep up with the MA. She sighs: "At least I'm not on oxygen."

After the MA takes her vitals, she waits for her doctor to knock on the door and tries to suppress the mounting anxiety. Her oxygen level was 94%, the lowest it had ever been. She knows the inevitable questions are coming. As much as she dreads the routine questions about her smoking and the disappointed look from her doctor, what she hates even more is the reality that she has not quit smoking. She is unable to reconcile these two opposing, yet equally controlling realities: she did not enjoy smoking, yet she could not imagine her life without it. Even the smell bothers her, so she tries perfumes and gum in an attempt to mask it. She knows that her cough is probably related to her smoking but is unclear what difference quitting would make at this point. Chaos surrounded smoking, and yet it was the only constant in her life.

She takes a deep breath as she hears her doctor outside the door. She knows that he is going to tell her that she really needs to put the cigarettes down. "What does he know anyway? Did he ever smoke? My life is too stressful to think about quitting," she tells herself.

"Good to see you, Helen," Dr. Smith says as he enters the room. Helen sits up a little taller in her seat and clears her throat. She tries to silence the nagging voice telling her change is coming. She knows that she is going to have to use her inhaler more, probably go to physical therapy, and quit smoking immediately, if not sooner. She does not see how she can accomplish any one of those things, let alone all of them.

Helen's reaction is simultaneously familiar and completely alien to most healthcare providers. Assuming that she wants to live, is afraid of breathlessness, and understands cigarettes are stealing her future, then what is missing?

Where a rational person might reasonably be scared straight, Helen seems to be stuck in a behavioral cul-de-sac, making tentative moves toward emergence, only to duck and cover over and over. What is it that Helen is experiencing differently?

One way to see the problem has been to imagine that Helen's stasis is due to a deficit in knowledge. Maybe her nascent symptoms lead her to underestimate the true probability of future disability. Or maybe optimism bias leads her to incorrectly imagine that disease couldn't possibly be in her future. Or maybe Helen doesn't recognize all the problems, beyond breathing, that are caused by smoking. In response to all of these possibilities, providers have been taught to educate, to fill the empty knowledge bucket, and to eventually convince.

Another way to see the problem has been to imagine that Helen's continued smoking comes down to a deficit in skill. Maybe if she understood the utility of a patch or a pill, knew the statistics about quit rates, or realized free counseling was a phone call away, something would change. Providers try offering ideas that are somehow both self-evident and impossible, like "take a walk instead," or "find some way to put it out of your mind," or "just stop." Unfortunately, Helen has heard them all a million times before, from everyone she knows and from every direction she turns.

The third and perhaps most dangerous conclusion for a heathcare provider is to imagine that Helen's problem comes down to simple selfishness and lack of intrinsic motivation. Perhaps she is a sybarite, single-mindedly focused on maintaining the sensuous luxury of smoking. Or perhaps she is self-indulgent, worried only about her own needs and desires and blind to the impact her decisions have on those around her. Maybe she is just plain lazy. The traditional antidotes to indolence are to amplify, cajole, beg, shame, and ultimately threaten. But rather than overcoming Helen's behavioral inertia, the pressure inevitably leads Helen to smoke more.

If attempting to resolve deficits in knowledge, skill, or motivation is the wrong way for a clinician to approach Helen's problem, what is the alternative? Is there a more productive approach?

———

David glances over Helen's chart before knocking. "Emphysema, chronic hip pain, hypertension, and it is flu season . . . not a quick visit," he mumbles. He moved quickly through his first five patients, but he knows that he has another twenty patients on his schedule and then the laborious notes to complete, labs to review, and phone calls to return. As much as he likes Helen, the thought of engaging her in another conversation regarding the importance of a flu shot makes his head hurt. Each year Helen reiterates her concern based on the experience of her friend who "became so sick after the flu shot." And each year he reiterates the importance of getting it.

David knows that Helen has been having a difficult time since her husband passed away. Both were his patients for twenty-five years, and David smiles remembering the way they would endlessly bicker throughout the appointment and then leave holding hands. He hears her coughing inside the room. Helen had reduced her smoking following her diagnosis of emphysema, but he is concerned that her smoking has increased over recent months. Knowing hip surgery is in her near future, he is reminded that she really needs to quit smoking. "Perfect, one more thing on the list that I do not have time for today," he thinks.

"Good to see you, Helen," he says as he enters the room. After his physical exam and conversation with Helen, he makes his recommendations. "You are going to need physical therapy and you really need to quit smoking," David tells Helen. The last time he recommended PT Helen resisted, explaining that she had transportation issues and did not have the money to cover the copay costs. Those were obstacles that were difficult for him to help her overcome during a routine visit. He had also recommended that she quit smoking on multiple occasions in the past, but his efforts were to no avail. "The surgeon will not operate on your hip if you are still smoking, and I do not want your emphysema to get worse," he warns. He mentions this to Helen, not intending it as a threat but as a reality. Helen responds defensively: "Have you ever smoked? You do not know how I feel. I desperately want to want to quit smoking." Slightly taken aback by her rather abrupt change in demeanor, David ignores her question, assuming it was rhetorical, and says, "We all want you to want to quit smoking." Helen reiterated many times during their visit that she was desperate to stop smoking, but he wondered if she was actually desperate to continue smoking.

The Triune Brain

The Greek philosopher Plato understood human nature as akin to a chariot being pulled forward by two wild, winged horses. In his model, the horses represented human passions, both good and evil. One horse directed the chariot upward, toward godlike status, inspiring people to do good and become their better selves. The other horse was imagined as dark, dragging the chariot down, closer to earthly desires and away from transcendent goals. The charioteer was the metaphorical equivalent of reason in Plato's model, controlling the opposing forces of nature, constantly working the reins and adjusting to stay on course. To Plato, logic was the force that prevented submission to the passions of animal spirits and was the gift that distinguished humanity from the rest of the natural world. Plato saw humans as thinking animals that can feel.

This classical emphasis on rationality continued into the late twentieth century, when American neuroscientist Dr. Paul MacLean introduced a theory of brain structural evolution that seems to account for similarities between some human behaviors and the instinctive behaviors seen in our animal cousins. He introduced the idea of a "triune brain"—one brain made up of three distinct brain types. Each type was reminiscent of important evolutionary epochs and refined over countless generations, hierarchically layered from the most primitive, which was instinctive, to the most developed, which was intellectual. With this theory, the notion of a lizard brain was born.

As a scheme for subdividing the brain neurophysiologically, the triune brain theory provides a simple model. Helen's mind is the product of her whole brain's concerted efforts rather than different parts functioning independently. But sometimes a model is useful because of its simplicity. Notwithstanding the fact that Helen's brain is performing a million different tasks, a clinician trying to make sense of her shifting motivations can start by imagining all those functions fitting within three brain types.

In this model, Helen's first brain houses the most basic machinery. The functions of the brain that are fundamental to life, such as feeding, fighting, and mating, are concentrated here. Helen's first, or "lizard," brain includes functions that are reflexive, automatic, immutable, and out of her direct control. Just as a lizard might scurry away reflexively when approached by an outstretched hand, so too does Helen's first brain react reflexively to send flee signals when she sees a spider. It is hard to teach the first brain a new trick.

When Helen thinks about her own mind, she is most aware of her third brain—the human brain. The functions of this brain include abstract ideas, language, math, and music. This is the part of the brain that makes Helen who she is, the part responsible for the voice in her head, telling her what to think, what to do, and how to do it. The job of the third brain is to learn new ideas. Learning and integrating come easily to the third brain. While humans are not the only species with third brain functions, these tend to be the most dominant, loud, and ostentatious components of the human mind.

Between the first and third brain sits Helen's second brain—the mammal brain. This brain type is primarily driven by automatic instinct, yet modifiable based on our interaction with the world. Dogs generally act like a second brain on four legs, chasing squirrels around the backyard. Yet with proper training and enough treats, a dog's skills can work in a productive way. Instincts are mutable in a way that machinery is not, but instinctive learning is not quite up to fancy cognitive tasks like abstraction and metaphor. Instincts are pointed at survival and are adjusted in response to external signals so that the second brain's owner might be more likely to thrive within its environment. The second brain's job is to increase the probability of adaptive survival behaviors while decreasing the likelihood of maladaptive behaviors.

Helen sees herself as all third brain. Like Plato, she sees herself as a thinking animal that feels. But because the third brain is loud, Helen does not necessarily notice that her second brain is constantly sending instinct signals. These signals are checking the survival relevance of the environment around her and creating the context within which logic and reason interact with the world. When things are safe and sound, Helen's third brain can chill and think about poetry if she wants. When the outside world has survival salience, Helen's third brain is forced to stop meandering and pay ATTENTION! to the survival issue at hand. Behind every successful third brain is a second brain, quietly laying down the operational ground rules of the moment.

David's mistake is that he is also thinking like Plato. David imagines Helen's chariot of the mind to be controlled by reason, and so he seeks to use logic and rationality as his lever for change. When it comes to tobacco, David has been conditioned to rely on educating, motivating, and threatening to get his message across. He would be better off if he listened to his own second brain when it tells him it does not feel right to make Helen feel bad. What David doesn't yet understand is that through the dark magic of nicotine, Helen is more like a feeling animal that also thinks.

Nicotine Is Soft Power

To understand the relationship between instinct and cognition, it sometimes helps to first consider the difference between hard and soft powers. Hard power is most familiar—and most obvious—and is forceful or coercive in nature. Hard power is evident when a request is followed by a consequence, as in a command or directive. We experience hard power when someone with authority over our work lives gives us direction. Irrespective of how well received the direction might be, it is accompanied by implicit consequences if the direction is ignored. We tend to imagine addiction as a form of hard power, forcing continued substance use under threat of severe repercussion if forgone.

On the other hand, soft power does not depend on force or consequence. Soft power works by shaping preferences, co-opting the full range of choices in favor of the single option most favorable to the party holding the power. We experience soft power when our unit manager indirectly motivates us to provide high-quality care by complimenting our professional ethic. Soft power works by making the desired outcome attractive or by constraining the possible choices by making alternative choices seem nonsensical. Nicotine exerts its soft power through instinct, guiding us to a choice by changing what we think.

When caring for Helen, cognition is in control. She's not a robot. Understanding tobacco dependence requires an appreciation for the relationship between cognition and instinct and the soft power nicotine can exert on decisions. Instinctive soft power will often co-opt the range of thoughts available to Helen's cognitive brain when she faces the possibility of putting the cigarettes down. Helen doesn't have to experience something dramatic, like "I must keep smoking or else." It can be subtle—like "I enjoy smoking," or "It's not the right time to quit"—no matter how much she would rationally prefer otherwise.

David may not have noticed that this dual-mindedness is a universal human experience. For example, ordering dessert after finishing a delicious meal is familiar to most. Despite feeling overstuffed, the second brain sends the AT-TENTION! signal the moment the waiter appears with the tray of desserts. In that instant, calorie concerns are discounted, and the third brain's conversation shifts to "I will work out in the morning," or "Maybe we can split it," or even "I deserve this." It may appear that the third brain is in charge, but the decisions have been seriously constrained by the second brain's input. Immediately following that first bite of chocolate cake, the third brain often says, "I don't even want this."

It's not uncommon for patients to ask empathy-check questions when they find their decision-making outcomes difficult to understand. When Helen asks David, "Have you ever smoked?" she is really asking, "Do you understand my experience?" Imagine what it is like to be Helen going through the chocolate cake phenomenon thirty times a day. Then magnify that feeling by imagining David's warnings of consequential death and disability. Then imagine disappointing friends and family because of the decision to eat the chocolate cake. How deeply connected to chocolate cake would a person have to be in order to put up with that for forty years?

Loss Salience

Mary was a 67-year-old woman, living alone in a single-family home in suburban Philadelphia. She spent most of her days alone, except for the occasional phone call from her family and the companionship of her dog, Rosie. Mary was very attached to Rosie; she saw her as her only friend. Rosie had become the focus of Mary's dwindling social interactions in the neighborhood, out on walks and down at the dog park. One day, Rosie developed acute renal failure and passed away shortly after, leaving Mary shocked, lonely, and depressed. During her grieving, Mary realized that she had spent a considerable amount of time apart from her ailing buddy in an ironic effort to protect her from tobacco smoke. Mary was aware that environmental smoke was unlikely to be a factor in Rosie's illness, but she felt helpless, and so she did what little she could to contribute. She felt the cigarettes had robbed her of Rosie's last days.

During her visit, Mary related being thunderstruck one afternoon when it occurred to her in a flash of regret that *she had been doing the same thing with her children and her new granddaughter.* She described herself as being despondent for the next two weeks: disappointed in herself for prioritizing smoking over her daughter's baby girl but feeling empty and tearful when she imagined life without cigarettes.

Nicotine does not work by creating euphoria or by creating withdrawal drama. Nicotine exerts its soft power by creating safety and security in the survival centers of the second brain. The threat of taking nicotine away results in a profound sense of loss that then colors decision-making in ways that can be hard for the rational third brain to understand. To the instinctive second brain, nicotine does not have to feel good; it simply is good.

Ambivalence

When Helen tells David "I desperately *want* to want to quit smoking," there could be no clearer expression of the duality of mind and the confusion it generates in Helen. It is hard to remember that Helen holds contradictory ideas—simultaneously. Providers have been taught to see Helen's readiness to quit as dichotomous, an either-or situation. Helen is either ready to quit, or she's not ready to quit.

In fact, the desire to quit smoking is much more complicated. Patients who smoke are simultaneously desperate to quit smoking and desperate not to quit smoking. It is not ready or not; it is ready *and* not. This ongoing, irreconcilable conflict between logic and instinct manifests as complex accommodations to try to resolve this struggle—at least temporarily. Helen ultimately says things like, "It is my only vice," or "I smoke fewer cigarettes now," or even "I sometimes use the vape thing instead of cigarettes."

Simultaneous conflicting beliefs and feelings toward smoking is termed ambivalence. Psychologists noticed that it is common for people to possess both positive and negative thoughts about the same thing. For example, people are often excited about taking a plane ride to their vacation destination while they are concurrently afraid of the flight. In lay terms, ambivalence is often used to describe situations in which people have mixed feelings or when they do not care either way. Clinically, however, subjective ambivalence refers to the state of mind wherein patients feel stuck in their duality, experience cognitive dissonance and internal conflict as a result, and find themselves in significant psychological distress. From David's perspective, Helen's ambivalence is experienced as an obvious desire for change that coexists with a considerable resistance to change. David could be more effective if he recognized Helen's ambivalence not as a state of simple indecision but rather as the cardinal sign of her addiction. It is futile to wait for the cardinal sign of a disease to resolve before attempting to manage that disease.

> *Helen's ambivalence is not a problem for David.*
> *It is the problem that David will work to resolve.*

Chapter 1 Learning Points

- Remember that patients only have one brain. But it helps them to construct this problem as the conflict between the logical third brain and the instinctive second brain.
- The traditional approach of turning up the heat by relying on increasing rational motivations can have the unintended effect of driving patients away.
- The struggle between brains results in mutually exclusive goals and is experienced as subjective ambivalence; your patients could be desperate for change and resistant to change at the same time.
- Ambivalence cannot always be acknowledged by the person experiencing it because it is difficult to articulate. Ambivalence feels bad.
- By understanding the manifestations of ambivalence, it is possible to develop an effective approach to overcoming resistance to change, not by increasing logical motivations to stop but by resolving instinctive obstacles to stopping.

Chapter 2
Structure

When I was in AA, they used to say one is too many but a thousand not enough. I feel the exact same way about my cigarettes.

—Kevin S., 56 years old

As Helen waits at the bus stop after her appointment, she looks around and wonders, "Why does that cigarette smell so good right now?" She reminds herself that she hates the smell of smoke as she watches a young mother trying to keep her child from running in the street while taking the last few drags off a cigarette. She instantly remembers that struggle with her own children—never enough space or time to enjoy a cigarette. Thinking about what she discussed with Dr. Smith, she begins to feel overwhelmed. She starts calculating the cost of physical therapy: three times per week, for six weeks, with a $20 copay each time. She racks her brain, thinking, "Where will I get that extra money? And how will I handle this additional stress without my cigarettes?" She remembers her husband telling her the adage, "It takes twenty-one days to break a habit." Twenty-one days without cigarettes feels like a lifetime right now. Except for during her two pregnancies, the most consecutive days she had gone without smoking was ten—and that was five years ago. She had also heard it could take thirty attempts to quit smoking before a person finally quits. Well, she started smoking at the age of 12 and is now 67, and she has tried to quit at least once per month for the past twenty years. That math was too depressing to compute, but she knew it was more than thirty attempts. "Where is the bus?" she groans. "This is too stressful to think about, and now I really need a cigarette."

———

Subjective ambivalence in the face of anticipated abstinence is the hallmark of the tobacco dependence syndrome and represents the fundamental problem that clinicians like David need to resolve. To understand Helen's behaviors fundamentally and to develop a framework for intervention, David needs to first understand how the various structures of the brain affected by nicotine relate to each other and how distortions in their biology might manifest as the observable syndrome we think of as dependence.

There are important differences between tobacco ambivalence and popular concepts about the nature of drug use. With other drugs of addiction, ambivalence might painfully resolve itself over time as people approach some personal "rock bottom" state wherein the perceived value of behavior change begins to exceed the value of continued use. Fractured relationships, a lost job, or a stay in the intensive care unit might qualify as hitting rock bottom. When the pain of personal destruction begins to outweigh the need to avoid the discomfiting prospect of withdrawal, behavior change becomes more likely. In this model, attempts to ameliorate withdrawal while keeping the patient safe may be seen as an opportunity to help rebalance the relative value of opposing goals, making change more likely.

This overly simplistic representation does not reflect the complexity of addiction psychology or the impact and professionalism of treatment providers. However, it does reflect a common lay narrative describing the outwardly apparent path to recovery. But there is a problem: the idea of a personal rock bottom does not hold when considering the natural history of tobacco dependence. Generally, people do not get divorced because they smoke or end up in the hospital because of nicotine withdrawal. With tobacco, there will be no crisis moment for Helen until she hears the words "you have cancer."

Clinicians and smokers often describe smoking as a bad habit. At first, the idea of a smoking habit may seem plausible. After all, smoking happens routinely, in response to predictable triggers and sometimes without even much conscious awareness. However, "habit" does not hold up to scrutiny. Suppose Helen was shown evidence that her habit of biting her nails somehow caused lung cancer. There is at least a good chance that Helen would find a way to stop biting her nails, even if it took a few tries and a little work. But that's not the whole story for most people who use tobacco. There must be something else.

Alternatively, persistent smoking in the face of threat is sometimes framed as the result of a physical need for nicotine. After all, it seems plausible that there must be a powerful physical requirement for nicotine if Helen is willing to smoke herself to death, despite the significant financial and social costs. The difficulty with this concept of "physical need" is that Helen has never actually experienced a sense of need (whatever that is) or the drama of withdrawal, even when she's had to go a few days without smoking.

> *Don't call it a habit.*
> *"Habit" trivializes the problem and makes Helen*
> *feel like it should be easier to change.*
>
> *Don't call it a physical need.*
> *"Physical need" makes Helen feel like nonsmokers*
> *cannot understand her situation.*

There has been an artificial distinction between the "psychological habit" that makes smoking automatic and the "physical addiction" to nicotine that makes it hard to stop. This distinction requires the psychology of the mind to be discrete from the biology of the brain. Of course, the brain is the seat of the mind. Smoking is habitual because it is a learned behavior that happens routinely and without much thought, but it becomes a learned behavior specifically because of the complex physical ways that nicotine affects the biology of the brain.

Survival Salience

The brain is constantly getting input from all the sensory organs of the body and from the outside world. The ears do not stop registering sound when reading the newspaper, but the brain does stop paying attention to the signals the ears are sending. With limited attentional capacity, the brain has to pick and choose which inputs to focus on, which to devote energy and attention to, and which to safely ignore. An input becomes salient to the brain when one characteristic or attribute forces the brain to ignore all other inputs in favor of paying close attention to that special one. A loud noise, the smell of smoke, the disorienting loop of the rollercoaster cannot be easily ignored because the brain recognizes them as important to survival. But of course, a person does not go running out of the movie theater every time there is a loud explosion on screen. Nor does a charred hamburger on the grill result in screaming and activation of emergency services. Survival systems have the ability to learn—and that is a useful gift.

Imagine a baby mouse, warm and cozy in the nest that mama mouse built. Life is good. Mama has been the source of nutrition and shelter, helping the mouse to grow up big and strong. But eventually that stops, and the baby mouse is forced to wander out and navigate a very dangerous world. Its desperate need to stay away from predators is counterbalanced by its growing need for food. What to do? The yin-yang opposing survival needs eventually lead it to take a few tentative steps away from the nest and out into the open, where the unknown is waiting to pounce. It has a lot to worry about—cats, foxes, hawks—but starving to death is not a pleasant prospect either. Scurrying quickly, randomly at first, it happens to find a hollow log on the ground. Ah, safety! Suddenly, the earthy feel of the loam and the cool dampness beneath its paws are no longer irrelevant inputs. Because of the circumstances, those inputs have distinguished themselves as salient to survival. Its heart rate can slow a notch, and it can take a deep breath. The next time it repeats the process, those same inputs now begin to predict safety and security, and the drive to move in their direction strengthens. The survival salience of these particular inputs increases as they are repeatedly associated with safety, and it becomes progressively more likely that the mouse will move toward the log on future trips, finding shelter in its hollow.

Imagine that on one of its expeditions the mouse discovers some cheese. The experience of cool loam is now not only associated with safety, but it has also begun to predict a future, very soon, when food will be available. Salient inputs essentially form a survival GPS system, guiding the animal toward a future adaptive circumstance in much the same way a treasure map guides the adventurer toward a valuable destination. In this manner, the mouse can begin to venture purposefully and increasingly farther afield, maximizing its chances of survival by increasing the drive toward survival-relevant directions and ignoring the rest. Eventually, arrival at the food source way down by the river is predicted by the increasingly loud sound of running water, which was itself predicted by the sight of yellow flowers earlier, predicted in turn by the smell of honeysuckle in the breeze encountered previously, predicted by the safety of the log, and so on. Should happenstance bring the mouse close to the cat, the same process in reverse applies: the baby mouse's drive mechanisms seek to avoid the honeysuckle because that's where it encountered the cat last time, and so that specific input now predicts threat. The mouse learns to instinctively move closer to things that are good for it while moving farther from things that are bad for it in order to maximize its chance of survival.

The Mesolimbic System

One of the first steps the brain takes in processing incoming sensory signals is to run them through a midbrain structure called the thalamus. The thalamus's job in this context is to act as a coordinating center, taking independently generated inputs from multiple senses and organizing them so that they can make sense to the rest of the brain as a singular experience of the world around it. The thalamus takes independent bits of information and creates relationships between them that are important to the brain's ability to get the full story. For example, the meaning of a visual image of a cat is enhanced dramatically when accompanied by the sound of its purr. It is no longer just a cat but a bigger story about a cat, with meaning and depth that could not be derived from the visual image alone. It is a different way of thinking about the notion of a "common sense."

The thalamus also acts like a distribution center, directing the incoming signals outward through two main pathways and connecting the advanced "conscious" parts of the brain to the more primitive midbrain and brainstem. A very special part of the brain adjacent to the thalamus, called the ventral tegmental area (VTA), is responsible for assigning survival salience to the most consequential inputs, whether adaptive or aversive. Essentially, the VTA will tag important safety-threat inputs with an ATTENTION! marker so that these particular signals cannot be ignored. A cat that is purring is different than a cat that is hissing, which again is different than a hissing cat that is moving toward its prey. The VTA keeps track of those differences and adjusts the gain on AT-TENTION! signaling so that attentional resources can be directed toward the inputs with the greatest relevance to survival.

Neural projections from the VTA fan out across the striatum and communicate with a few key structures that work together to ensure survival. The striatum acts as a physical bridge between the midbrain and the rest of the brain, but it is not simply a conduit for information. The striatum both acts and is acted upon by the traversing signals. First, the striatum is essentially "translating" sensory inputs into motor activation outputs. The striatum transduces variations in thalamic activity into motivational signals that will be used by other areas of the brain to produce the pressure to react. But perhaps equally as important, the striatum is highly plastic (that is, adaptable), allowing important connections to become more efficient with repetition and promoting the progressive automatization (that is, habitualization) of recurrent stimulus-response associations. In this way, the striatum participates in the brain's process of adjusting the practical reaction to environmental situations in a manner that progressively maximizes the survival probability of the brain's owner.

One of the important connections the VTA makes is to an area of the ventral striatum called the nucleus accumbens. On receipt of the transduced ATTENTION! signal from the VTA, the nucleus accumbens is triggered and produces motor activation signals that project directly onto the motor control structures of the brain. Once triggered, the nucleus accumbens creates a "generalized appetitive state" wherein the organism is in action mode—unsettled, goal-oriented, and primed to respond to environmental cues. It is important here to recognize that use of the word "appetitive" is not restricted to just food;

it is any state where the brain is directed toward achieving some survival goal. Appetitive behaviors, like foraging for food or shelter, are flexible and learned through experience, whereas consummatory behaviors, like the act of eating, tend to be reflexive and solidified early in development. Remember that appetitive motivations act in both directions. Like a magnet, it is a force that attracts or repels based on the demands of the external world. After enjoying a delicious meal at a nice restaurant, when the server brings out the beautiful dessert tray, predictable appetitive behaviors—activated, goal motivated, and unsettled—finally lead to a consummatory decision: "one piece of chocolate cake with two forks, please."

The nucleus accumbens is a special collection of nerve cells that increases internal motivational pressure, stimulates goal-directed behaviors, and is able to learn from repeated activation. If there is one thing survival systems are good at, it is learning from successes and (near) failures. When the nucleus accumbens receives the ATTENTION! signal, it turns on the motor control centers and creates pressure to act in a goal-oriented way, but it does not stop there. This makes sense from a survival perspective: suppose the cat happens to grab the mouse's tail in a near failure event: acquiescence is death. The mouse must panic and respond with vigor and determination in order to avoid going the way of a tasty snack. Here is where the particulars of physiology become important. The nucleus accumbens is organized a little like a Spanish olive, with a shell and a core, each made of material with distinctly different attributes but that work together to achieve a function that is greater than the sum of its parts. As the shell transduces VTA signals into pressure to respond, the core, which is composed primarily of neurons responsible for sensorimotor integration, watches over the very next sensory inputs in order to ensure that movement is being accomplished as directed. Once triggered, accumbal core cells begin to fire at increasing frequency and amplitude until the next incoming signal suggests alignment between the motivation and the result. In other words, the nucleus accumbens has an automatic way of ramping up motivational pressure until the goal is reached or the situation outside changes. The efficiency with which the core can ramp up these response signals will change with repeated exposure. The faster and more aggressively the mouse learns to respond to the cat's advances, the more likely it is to live another day.

The nucleus accumbens is important here because it activates motor control centers, creates goal-oriented motivation, and then ramps up the pressure if that goal is not reached. A different way to state this is to imagine that the nucleus accumbens has a teleologic purpose and that its most important survival function is to alert the brain when those survival goals are not being met.

It is common to focus attention on the ways the motivational pressure behaves in pursuit of a goal, but people pursue and achieve survival goals all the time. The real action is in what happens when those goals fail to materialize. How is a brain supposed to respond? Suppose the nucleus accumbens sends a signal to run, and for a variety of reasons the person does not run. The next set of inputs the nucleus accumbens receives will not reflect a sensory package consistent with movement toward the goal. This disconnect represents an obvious error in that prediction. Since the error is in the negative direction (as opposed to the positive "the person ran too far" direction), the nucleus accumbens experiences a negative prediction error. Negative prediction error signals extend outward from the nucleus accumbens to a few other key spots in survival and can produce results that are not exactly subtle. Negative prediction error signals are not to be trifled with.

Integrated Threat Response

Imagine there is a threat response system in the brain. What would that look like? There needs to be a tool to increase "aggressive" emotions, like fear and anger, and there also needs to be a mechanism for preferencing quick, thoughtless reactions rather than slow, logical deliberation. Finally, it would be nice to have a way to store the nature of this threat and the response to it in a manner that allows for quick retrieval next time, sort of as an insurance policy against future incursions. Thankfully, the negative prediction error signals project outward to just such a protective system. Negative prediction error signals activate the amygdala, a tiny, almond-shaped cluster of nerve cells that act as an interface between the sensory world and our emotions. The amygdala has the ability to ignore pleasant inputs and react solely to the disturbing ones—perfect qualities for a threat detection system. When the negative prediction error signals start screaming "something is not right!" to the amygdala, it responds with fear, anger, aggression, and anxiety: in other words, the negative affective dimensions.

So negative prediction error signals produce negative affect. The amygdala is responsible for emotional memory, facilitating the negative affective response the next time that same threat occurs. But those same negative prediction error signals are also reaching the hippocampus, a seahorse-shaped bundle that is involved in short-term memory. The precise way that the hippocampus works in processing memories is unknown, but one of its functions is to process short-term inputs about the situation at hand before they get solidified and stored elsewhere as long-term memory. The hippocampus is involved

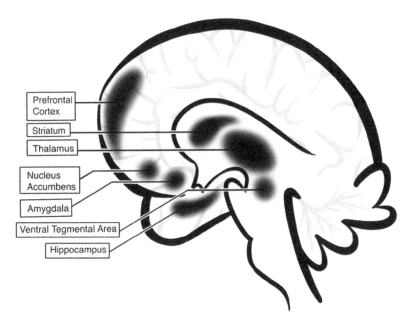

Figure 2.1. Major structures of the mesolimbic system involved in tobacco dependence.

in behavioral inhibition, environmental scanning, and obsessive thinking; it contains the ingredients for using recollection of past survival-related events in order to make a future approach to similar events more efficient. The negative prediction error signals also affect the function of the prefrontal cortex, an area of the brain that serves as the interface between the primitive emotional centers of the brain and the higher cognitive functions of the neocortex. The prefrontal cortex is involved in the emotional processing necessary for figuring out how things are going on the inside. It primes the higher cognitive centers, biasing their interpretation of otherwise ambiguous inputs from the outside world in a manner that is outside of conscious awareness. The prefrontal cortex forgoes logic and reshapes thinking based on emotion (Figure 2.1).

Let's review: (1) Sensory inputs go to the thalamus for coordination and processing; (2) the ventral tegmental area tags inputs that are survival salient, creating an ATTENTION! signal and causing the rest of the brain to focus; (3) the striatum begins the process of translating ATTENTION! into action, turning up the gain of connecting pathways that make future action more efficient; (4) the shell of the nucleus accumbens activates motor areas of the brain and creates a generalized appetitive state, motivating goal-directed behaviors; (5) motivated behaviors that are denied or forgone result in negative prediction error signals being delivered to the threat response system; and (6) the amygdala turns on the negative affective response, the hippocampus manages memories of how this was dealt with in the past, preferencing automatic and rapid responses, and the prefrontal cortex biases cognition so that thoughts and reactions are consistent with instinct.

Chapter 2 Learning Points

- An understanding of the structures involved in producing tobacco-dependence behaviors allows clinicians to reframe the problem as a matter of survival instinct rather than as habit or physical need.
- Tobacco dependence affects the survival centers in the brain, such that gratification of the resulting drive to smoke becomes the brain's prioritized objective, also known as a generalized appetitive state.
- The ventral tegmental area (VTA) tags important incoming sensory signals with an ATTENTION! marker so that these particular signals can no longer be ignored.
- Activation of the nucleus accumbens shell results in the internal pressure to respond to the environment. Accumbal core cells fire with increasing frequency and amplitude until subsequent inputs suggest alignment between motivation and result.
- An integrated threat response system—including the amygdala, hippocampus, and prefrontal cortex—preferences automatic and rapid responses while biasing cognition so that thoughts are consistent with instinctive inputs.

Chapter 3
Function

They say it's mind over matter. But smoking seems to matter to my mind a lot.

—Eric W., 65 years old

There is a certain bond that smokers share. "I can pick the smokers out in a room almost immediately," Helen frequently bragged to her nonsmoking friends. Recently, it had become harder and harder to find a fellow smoker, but that was fine because she always had Kathy. Throughout the years Helen shared many cigarettes with Kathy, her neighbor and good friend. They spent countless hours sitting outside, talking about everything: gossiping about the minutiae of neighborhood comings and goings, sharing the joy of their children getting married and the loneliness that follows as their children move away, and lamenting the heartache of losing a spouse. Through all of life's inevitable twists, there was no comfort quite like sitting together, unwinding with a cigarette and an occasional glass of wine. They joked that they would probably be buried with their pack of cigarettes. They made plans together to quit smoking more times than she could count, but it never seemed to be the right time for one of them. Kathy was going through a rough time, and Helen knew her friend needed those nightly chats, which meant not smoking was impossible. How could they sit outside in their favorite porch chairs and not smoke? They had tried that on numerous occasions, and it never felt right. As Helen walked into her home, she glanced over at the porch chairs and ashtray and felt sad and lonely.

———

The dominant neural system providing information to the ventral tegmental area is cholinergic, meaning it predominantly uses a neurotransmitter called acetylcholine for signaling. Human biology tends to express cholinergic receptors broadly and uses cholinergic signaling to control a bunch of different functions. From muscle contraction to heart rate control to central nervous system regulation, it can perform these widely divergent functions by virtue of small changes in the structure of the receptor to which it binds. Two distinct families of acetylcholine receptors, each with radically different signaling properties, have been identified based on their susceptibility to activation by foreign, or exogenous, signal chemicals. Nicotine is one of the exogenous ligands that can "trick" some of the cholinergic receptors into action. These nicotinic cholinergic receptors are ligand-gated ion channels. When they bind with nicotine, they respond in a manner similar to when they bind to acetylcholine, opening up a small hole in the cell's membrane and allowing electrically charged elements like sodium, potassium, and calcium to rush in and out of the cell. This change in relative charge across the cell's membrane sets into motion a series of events that control downstream release of neurotransmitters, a function necessary for communicating with other areas of the brain.

Nicotinic cholinergic receptors are pentameric, composed of five protein subunits in a ring. In the central nervous system, the dominant subunit proteins have been grouped into three families—alpha (α), beta (β), and delta (δ)—and each family has multiple members, numbered according to when they were identified. The specific combination of subunits provides the body with a straightforward way to change the function and sensitivity of these receptors to match their local requirements but also changes their susceptibility to being fooled by nicotine. The mesolimbic system is packed with nicotinic cholinergic receptors. The VTA is extensively equipped with the α4β2 variety—highly sensitive to the natural acetylcholine ligand and with a high affinity for its nicotine impostor.

What does this mean to Helen? When nicotine tickles the α4β2 receptors in the VTA, whatever sensory inputs are coming in at that moment begin to get imbued with survival salience, resulting in the following:

- Attentional resources get unfairly devoted to that sensory event.
- Future presentations of this sensory cluster result in motor activation and a generalized appetitive state.
- Pressure to act on the agitation builds until the drive is resolved.
- If action is forgone, negative prediction error signaling turns on negative affect.
- Facilitated recall makes resolution quick, easy, and direct.
- Thoughts and perceptions are influenced so that they are consistent with unsensed, unconscious survival signals.

It all happens instantaneously, even before the thought to smoke is fully formed in Helen's mind.

For many years, scientists debated whether nicotine was actually addictive. On one hand, they could see the types of behaviors in Helen that were very similar to the behaviors observed in those addicted to alcohol or other drugs. On the other hand, they had a really hard time reproducing the dependence phenomenon in the laboratory. When lab mice were given nicotine, the mice would not experience euphoria. Nicotine is anhedonic. When the mouse was administered nicotine for two weeks and then the nicotine was suddenly stopped, no significant withdrawal effects were observed. Sometimes the mouse could be taught to self-administer nicotine but not reproducibly. Then one day scientists began to realize that it was not just the drug involved in developing dependence; it was also the environment surrounding drug delivery that influenced addictive potential. If the circumstances of drug delivery kept changing, dependence was difficult to produce in the lab. But when the associated sensory inputs remained consistent, obvious behavior changes in the mouse could be engineered and investigated.

One important example of behavioral engineering is an experimental model called conditioned place preference. This model requires a cage with two distinct sides, separated from each other by some obvious but traversable barrier. The sensory characteristics of the two sides are differentiated by varying things, such as the texture of the floor or the color pattern of the walls. A sensor responds whenever the mouse is on the predetermined "right side," and small doses of nicotine are administered directly to the animal. At the beginning of the experiment, the mouse spends its time randomly moving about the cage, a fifty-fifty split between sides. But rather quickly, the association of nicotine with the sensory inputs on the "right side" of the cage changes how the mouse splits its time. By the end of the experiment, the mouse is spending 90% of its time on one side of the cage, which is no longer a random distribution of its time. Even when the nicotine administration is stopped, the mouse will continue to prefer the same side of the cage. It will still display a conditioned place preference. The mouse is not on the "right side" for the nicotine; it is there for the cage. Nicotine has dramatically influenced the survival salience of previously irrelevant sensory inputs, such that it has become important to survival. The mouse feels safe and sound when on the "right side" and activated, uneasy, threatened when it is not.

When Helen smokes, all the sensory inputs that she is experiencing at the time get tagged with survival relevance. That is true for the feel of the porch chair, the sight of the ashtray, and the sound of Kathy's voice, as well as the taste of tobacco on her tongue, the feel of the cigarette on her lips, and the warmth of smoke in her throat. All these sensory inputs get associated with one big survival-salient collection of senses. So the next time Helen sits in her porch chair, she is driven to complete the sensory package by smoking if she wants to feel safe and sound. Unlike the mouse that received the nicotine through direct administration, Helen's connection to the chair includes all the sensory inputs connected with the experience of smoking a cigarette. If she tries to sit in the porch chair while forgoing the smoking, the sensory package is incomplete: something is not right. It is like being on the wrong side of the cage. Helen is activated, uneasy, and threatened.

Distortions in Cellular Learning

Why does the mouse continue to prefer the "right side" of the cage, even after the nicotine is turned off? It can't be because it likes nicotine and is waiting for more. The mouse would have unlearned that trick, just like Helen might have unlearned to smoke after being away from it for a few months. Empirically, we know the converse to be true. It is all too easy to fall back into a priori smoking routines even after prolonged abstinence. The sensory package associations with VTA safety signals persist despite time away from nicotine. The impact of nicotine exposure lives on well after its chemical influence is gone. How does the brain translate an acute experience into a long-term understanding of the world?

Up until this point, the problem of tobacco dependence has been presented as a function of mesolimbic associations, with neurons sending and receiving information as neurotransmitters act on ion-gate receptors. However, there is also important hidden stuff that happens to the biology inside the cell after the receptors have been tickled. With repeated stimulation, charged calcium ions are making their way into the cell. The calcium has the ability to start a series of chemical reactions that result in recruitment of a special protein, referred to as CREB, to the nucleus of the cell. CREB turns out to be one of many transcription factors, which are proteins designed specifically to bind onto corresponding bits of genetic material and act as a genetic switch, activating and deactivating target genes as needed. In this case, the genes that get turned on happen to be responsible for growing and building new synapses in the sensory cell, physically strengthening the anatomy of connections—into long-term, committed relationships.

But that is not all. Nicotine also has the ability to block the action of an enzyme called HDAC, which the cell uses to pump the brakes on CREB activity. If nicotine blocks the brakes, it is "disinhibiting" CREB and creates an environment wherein CREB's activity is amplified. Another important downstream effect of CREB disinhibition is the expression of another transcription factor, called ΔFosB, within the motor activation structures of the brain. In both the striatum and the nucleus accumbens, ΔFosB works to increase expression of genes that code for a family of neurotransmitters in the brain's endogenous opioid system. Endogenous opioids, including endorphin, are used by the brain to regulate the strength of connections between cells. The presence of ΔFosB in the striatum results in more efficient connections, which results in more predictable firing, which in turn reinforces the pathways that were activated at the time the nicotine was administered.

Nicotine's ability to increase the presence of ΔFosB within the mesolimbic system is important for two reasons. First, ΔFosB is remarkably stable and doesn't go away easily. Most people have heard the old saying about once addicted, always addicted. ΔFosB is the reason why that's true. Even if the cell stops making the ΔFosB today, it is still going to be in the cell for a long time, sometimes for years, reinforcing dependence pathways and increasing the probability of returning to a priori behaviors. David isn't just trying to change Helen's behaviors; he's trying to find ways to reverse the impact of ΔFosB and prevent it from influencing Helen's dependence behaviors in the future—the long-term future. The transcription factor ΔFosB is why tobacco dependence is a chronic disease.

Second, similar accumulations of ΔFosB occur in the same mesolimbic system areas when people use drugs of abuse, struggle with obesity, run compulsively, gamble, or suffer obsessive compulsive disorder. The implications of this are dramatic. Smoking can no longer be viewed simply as the behavioral antecedent to illness in other organ systems. Instead, smoking should now be appreciated as the cardinal behavioral sign of a compulsion-producing distortion in brain structure and function; its genesis is in the most fundamental, molecular mechanisms of long-term learning.

> *Smoking is not a habit.*
> *Tobacco dependence is a chronic, relapsing disorder involving*
> *the functional building blocks of brain learning and memory.*

The "Pleasure" of Dopamine

The experience of smoking is unlike the experience of many other drugs of addiction. There is no euphoria, no trance-like ecstatic state at the end of the first cigarette, and no pain after a period of forced abstinence from smoking. While these reactions may be experienced by someone using opioids, they do not fit for nicotine users. So where did the notion of the pleasure of smoking come from?

It is true that cholinergic stimulation of the VTA excites dopaminergic neurons projecting onto the nucleus accumbens and that dopaminergic signaling then turns on the emotion and memory centers of the mesolimbic system. But the dopaminergic bits of the mesolimbic system aren't sensory in nature; they're activating and appetitive. In fact, it is possible to create mouse models that separate the sensory "like" from the appetitive "want." For example, mice depleted of dopaminergic inputs to the nucleus accumbens will still display pleasurable "like" behaviors when given sucrose water. Conversely, mice can be manipulated to "want" water treated to be unpleasant. Nicotine itself is anhedonic; it is an unsensed reinforcer. What smokers colloquially describe as the pleasure of smoking is actually the pleasurable experience derived from resolving the appetitive state produced by dopaminergic activation. It is the relief derived when a compulsive instinct has been fully realized. It is the gratification of completing a mission after having been called to ATTENTION!

In summary, smoking delivers nicotine to the VTA. After repeated exposure, the VTA improves communication with other areas of the mesolimbic system. The striatum gets better at translating VTA signals into motor activation, and the nucleus accumbens creates the internal push to act. If unresolved, the core of the nucleus accumbens is unleashed, sending negative prediction error signals up and out to emotion and memory parts of the brain. The prefrontal cortex produces an anxious-agitated context that then frames cognition, while the amygdala activates the negative and/or aggressive emotional responses, and the hippocampus quickly retrieves memories that give clues about how to resolve this unfortunate circumstance. The result? An ineluctable, compulsive instinct to smoke accompanied by invasive thoughts of smoking. Helen's problem is not about insufficient motivation to stop. It's about an incredibly efficient and overwhelming motivation not to stop. The balance between instinctive drive and cognitive control is broken, pushing Helen to find safety and security in smoking whenever her sensory inputs say it is the right thing to do. At that moment, it is not about a physical need, nor is it necessary that she enjoy smoking. It's only about pure, unchecked, untamed, amplified survival want.

Chapter 3 Learning Points

- Nicotine dependence is a result of distortion in the brain's molecular mechanisms of instinctive (not cognitive) learning and memory.
- Nicotine hijacks survival instincts by acting as an exogenous ligand. Amplified negative prediction error signals are the neural root of impulsive, maladaptive behaviors.
- CREB and ΔFosB are transcription factors that turn on genes in response to nicotine exposure, regulate the strength of long-term connections within motor-activation pathways, and lead to progressive automatization of recurrent stimulus-response patterns.
- The clinician's role is to help Helen stop smoking by controlling her compulsion to smoke and by managing amplified negative prediction error signaling until genetic switches like CREB and ΔFosB disengage, allowing the mesolimbic system to rebalance drive control mechanisms.
- Nicotine is anhedonic. It is an unsensed, yet powerful reinforcer that works by increasing the survival salience of otherwise inconsequential sensory inputs.

Chapter 4
Compulsion

People keep talking about "cravings." For me, they're not cravings. They're more like reminder calls that will not be ignored.

—Mary Ann B., 45 years old

Helen dreaded going to sleep since her husband passed away. For the thirty years that she shared a home with him, she never noticed all the noises at night. Tonight, the cars honking, babies crying, and the rattling of the heater all seemed to be surreptitiously conspiring to keep her awake. She thought about the many nights she went to bed vowing that tomorrow would be the day she puts the cigarettes down. But then tomorrow would come and go, and inevitably something or someone would interfere with her plan. "What plan?" she thought. The harsh reality was that it was more of a wish; she wished that she would simply wake up and no longer want to smoke. She would toss and turn for most of the night, and when she finally got up, she would look at her pack of cigarettes, succumb to the inevitable, and grab one in defeat. "Not today. I didn't sleep well. Tomorrow," she promised herself.

Helen wanted tomorrow to be different, but she was already tossing in bed. "I should have a cigarette right now," she thought. She did not smoke all evening, and if this was going to be her last cigarette, then why not? She could feel her heart racing and her chest becoming tighter when she heard herself say "last cigarette." Clang! The heater was relentless. As the minutes ticked by, her thoughts got darker. "My heart should not be racing this fast. This is too much stress. What if something happens to me and I am all alone in my apartment?" Honk! She jumped up. "Screw it. Where are my cigarettes?"

━━━

The occult magic of nicotine is its ability to take perfectly normal functions of the brain, balanced just right and fine-tuned to the sweet spot between the yin-yang opposing goals of survival, and mess with the strength of connections between structures in such a way as to throw the entire balance out of whack. Let's call this the prediction error model of dependence behaviors. Survival salience is amplified by nicotine. Motor activation is amplified by nicotine. Threat response is amplified by nicotine. And quick, noncognitive solutions to denied responses are amplified by nicotine. All of that occurs without a hedonic effect. Nicotine is the perfect stealth drug.

But none of that explains why Helen still finds it hard to exert some level of cognitive control over the impulse after she recognizes that instincts are keeping her from achieving her goal. After all, Helen might initially be rightfully disinclined to get into the deep end of the pool, but after a little training, we would expect her to be able to overcome those survival instincts. Humans do this all the time—fighting fires, parachute jumping. What makes these particular instincts so difficult to overcome? Why is it hard for Helen to find equivalent survival-salient inputs redirecting her in more adaptive directions? In the last chapter, the idea of compulsion was used colloquially, to describe the internal push to smoke. In this chapter, we are going to review the elements of compulsion as a disorder of behavior (as in obsessive-compulsive-related disorders) in an attempt to fully understand the obstacles Helen faces when thinking about change.

Impulsivity

An important effect of nicotine exposure is to make salient associations more efficient. This progressive automatization makes a lot of sense for a mouse responding to a cat. But as things get more complicated, automatization may not always be adaptive. There are many life examples wherein investing a moment or two of delayed gratification turns out to be worthwhile in the end. Financial advisers typically encourage investing in the stock market for the long-term gains, not the short-term returns. A 4-year-old participating in a psychology experiment can earn two marshmallows instead of one by simply waiting a few minutes longer. In any case, delaying gratification can have a beneficial effect on survival. Depending on the circumstances, more automatic is not always better. And yet, sometimes delaying action is easier said than done.

Disinhibited response automatization can lead to two different ways a brain can lose the potential advantage of delay. Let's call this first kind of automatization disadvantage response inaccuracy. Imagine confronting a forced choice with multiple options, but only one choice leads to the best possible outcome. Response disinhibition may prompt the brain to make a choice, any choice, quickly—sort of hoping the chosen path turns out to be the right one. It's a little like randomly choosing an answer to an exam question rather than investing effort into deducing the correct response. Controlling the motivational pressure to choose just long enough to ensure the most long-term beneficial action takes a little discipline and a proper balance between motivation and inhibition.

To measure response inaccuracy, there is a mouse model involving choice-making called a five-choice serial-reaction time task. In this model, the mouse is put in a cage that is equipped with five apertures in one end, through which the mouse can be trained to poke its nose. Each aperture is outfitted with a light that is controlled by the experimenter. When the light goes on, the mouse may or may not poke its nose through the lit-up aperture, as it wishes. But if it does poke the right aperture, the rig automatically reveals a sucrose pellet on the other side of the cage, reinforcing the behavior. With training, the mouse learns to wait for the light and poke at the right spot in response. If the light goes on and the mouse pokes at the wrong spot, that is an inaccurate response, and the proportion of total responses that are inaccurate are a well-validated representation of the mouse's impulsivity. If half of the mice are exposed to nicotine after training, the measured response inaccuracy goes up significantly. All the mice are accurate most of the time, but the nicotine mice are more likely to display this make-a-choice-any-choice response rather than hang back a second to ensure a correct choice.

The second way to lose the potential advantage of delay is to make the right decision but make it too early. Let's call this type of automatization error premature responding. Imagine making the decision to move into the right lane of traffic in anticipation of an approaching exit. The action may be easy to accomplish in the abstract, but rules of the road make timing an important variable to consider. A good (that is, long-term beneficial) choice is to slow down and wait to make the move until the car in the mirror passes. Imagine a musician with extraordinary technical skills who is able to play the most complicated pieces but who consistently returns from the pause a half-beat before her bandmates. Opportunities for stardom are lost without the capacity to delay the motivational impulse. In either case, the actions themselves might be correctly conceived, but motivations that are too efficient, too persuasive, lead to an impetuousness that is maladaptive in the end.

Measuring nicotine's effect on premature response rates requires a slightly different plan. It requires a cage that has a left and right lever. In between the levers is a pellet dispenser. When a light located above the left lever is turned on and the trained mouse presses the left lever, the dispenser gives it one sucrose pellet. But if the mouse waits a few seconds without touching the left, a light will go on over the right lever, indicating it is activated and ready to be pressed. The successful mouse waits a few seconds, touches the right lever, and three sucrose pellets are delivered. By alternating the side with the delayed super-reinforcer, the mouse learns to invest in waiting for the better option. Enter nicotine. Sure enough, the acute effects of exposing the mouse to nicotine are to increase impulsive choice-making in a dose-dependent fashion. Like the 4-year-old who cannot wait for a second marshmallow, the nicotine-treated mouse is more likely to sacrifice the opportunity for three pellets in favor of the immediate gratification of the single pellet. A pellet in the maw is better than three in the dispenser. The more nicotine, the more impulsive the mice become.

There are a couple of interesting experimental observations on impulsivity that are relevant to Helen's story. First, impulsivity remains increased after chronic administration of nicotine, even after nicotine exposure is discontinued. Second, using adolescent mice will reliably reproduce these results; animals that have reached adulthood are much less susceptible to the impulsivity effects of nicotine. Third, damaging the core cells of the mouse's nucleus accumbens will reproduce this effect, suggesting the mechanism of impulsivity has to do with disinhibition of negative prediction error signals. Finally, impulsivity can be measured in humans (no cages or sucrose pellets involved), and it is frequently increased in people who are about to relapse to smoking.

The "Screw it!" Phenomenon

Salvatore is a 49-year-old information technology engineer, working to keep data safe for a local military contractor. He lives in a center-city Philadelphia apartment with his wife and teenage daughter. His job keeps him busy, working at home late at night and over weekends to complete pressing tasks. He can sometimes put in as much as seventy hours in a week, and it limits his ability to be involved with his daughter's development. His wife has spoken to him on a few occasions about his tendency to sneak away to smoke during the infrequent times he has attended his daughter's school concerts. He doesn't want to seem disinterested, and he doesn't want to set a bad example. But sometimes, when the impulse comes, it is as though he can't talk himself out of sneaking away. It is not like he's craving, and he's definitely not withdrawing; he just wants to smoke. He feels embarrassed when he finally gives in and grabs a few puffs, and then he prepares himself to accept the disappointment in his wife's eyes.

Sal spends most of his workday alone, isolated in his office so he can concentrate on his work without interruption. He will occasionally take a smoke break outside in the parking lot, but since he can't really afford that much time away from his coding, he mostly just ignores the building rules and sneaks his cigarettes while at his desk. He's tried to use an electronic cigarette in an effort to keep the smell of smoke from escaping into the hallway, but that didn't seem to give him the kick he needed to stay focused on solving his computing problems. He compensates by exhaling the smoke toward a small fan he keeps in the window and using a lot of air freshener. Sal's boss has spoken to him about the smell on a few occasions, but each time he has the impulse to light up, he can almost *feel* himself go through the same process in his head: "I shouldn't . . . I won't . . . but I want to . . . but I shouldn't . . . but . . . screw it, I will." Most times, right after his first puff, he can also hear himself say, "I shouldn't have. Oh, well . . . next time." Sal gets disappointed in himself for risking his relationship with his boss, a future promotion, even his job, just to smoke a cigarette he didn't even really need in the first place.

He wonders how, if he cares as much as he does, could he possibly say "screw it" and smoke as much as he does, when he wants to quit smoking as much as he does.

Stress and Allostatic Load

At peace, the brain is in default mode, wherein processing functions are generally geared toward maintaining homeostasis. In response to a car horn blast slicing through the quiet, homeostasis is knocked off balance as the brain suddenly shifts to a state of alertness. This new work mode is energy intensive, uncomfortable, and unsustainable. Though it seems like restoring the balance ought to be as simple as shutting off the threat response system, the reset process is actually intensely active, requiring the investment of substantial resources. This active reset is referred to as allostasis. The brain's allostatic mechanisms bring processing back to default mode once the stressor has been resolved. The system works well when it is efficient, without a lot of resistance. But when that efficient switching is compromised in some way, the resulting inability to resolve the challenge quickly results in an allostatic load and can lead to serious consequences like receptor desensitization and structural damage within the involved cells.

Functional magnetic resonance imaging (fMRI) has helped us better understand exactly what happens to Helen during stressful circumstances. The fMRI scanner overlays information about the functional activity levels of various regions of the brain on an image of its anatomy. In that manner, it can allow for real-time assessment of the brain's functional responses to different challenges. Over time, scientists noticed that individual areas of the brain organize themselves into a variety of functional networks, such that a specific type of task would predictably "light up" the same set of structures. For example, the executive control network (ECN) is the set of structures involved in performing tasks that are dangerous or technically difficult or that require overcoming strong habitual response and resisting temptation. In other words, the ECN turns on when focus is demanded in response to the ATTENTION! salience signal sent by the VTA. In contrast, the default mode network (DMN) is most active during passive rest and daydreaming. When you lose focus on what you are reading and begin to drift, it is your DMN that's actively relaxing your mind. Stress takes us out of default mode and puts us in executive mode, and the allostatic mechanisms of the brain restore us to default mode. It is like shifting the brain from neutral into drive and back to neutral again as quickly as feasible.

A situation in which that shifting mechanism is not working as smoothly as it previously worked is likely to be uncomfortable, like things aren't quite working correctly. Responding more slowly to environmental threats is bad for business but so is staying on high alert longer than necessary. The efficiency with which salience signals can shift the brain from neutral to drive and back again can be expressed in terms of the degree of "coupling" between ECN-DMN function and the VTA salience signals controlling the shift. When Helen tries to remain abstinent from nicotine, the salience centers of the brain have a much harder time shifting the brain from neutral into drive and, just as importantly, from drive back to neutral. Nicotine exposure makes it harder for the allostatic mechanisms of the brain to resolve the consequences of stress.

To be most effective at protecting the integrity of the organism, it would help if the cells involved could get fast enough at responding to external clues that they essentially begin to predict stressors in the external environment rather than just respond to them. Remember that the hippocampus is the part of the threat response system that is involved in recalling quick, noncognitive responses to environmental threats. In essence, the hippocampus is working to recognize threat patterns and anticipate potential problems before they arise. It has to be a highly plastic region in order to maximize its ability to learn from past events. It turns out, one of the effects of sustained allostatic load is to upregulate expression of α7 nicotinic receptors in the hippocampus, making the hippocampus vulnerable to nicotine's influence on instinctive learning. Nicotine has not only become necessary for efficient (that is, effortless, comfortable, low-energy) allostasis; it has hijacked the hippocampus and progressively narrowed its repertoire such that smoking eventually becomes the only mechanism available for resolving stress.

For Helen, smoking has made her more susceptible to internal and external stressors, less likely to resolve stress the old-fashioned way, likely to spend more time under stress, and vulnerable to paying a higher price for unresolved stress. When she says stress makes her smoke, she is not kidding. Smoking does not sedate Helen or make her forget her problem, and it definitely does not make her problem go away. Smoking allows her brain to resolve stress normally.

> *Smoking is the ransom Helen's brain pays to allostasis.*

Anticipatory Anxiety

Understanding the mesolimbic infrastructure and appreciating the role played by emotion and memory in forming a response to negative prediction error signals make it easier to understand why Helen might get anxious and agitated when she's deprived of a cigarette. But why does Helen get anxious and agitated when she thinks about forgoing a future cigarette? Even if she's smoking at the time, the simple thought of never smoking again can cause her chest to tighten up and her heart rate to rise and produce a focused attention on resolving this quandary. Why?

The first thing to recognize is that the neuronal activity produced by positive survival rewards is soon enough also produced by signals that anticipate the delivery of the reward. The value of future reward is a function of just how strong a reinforcer the drug or behavior is, discounted for the probability the reward will not be delivered. To understand this, consider gambling: games with high payouts and favorable odds are likely to be highly reinforcing while games with high payouts but poor odds of winning are much less so.

Experimentally, this situation can be re-created by placing subjects in an fMRI scanner and watching which parts of the brain get activated when the subjects are given a chance to win money. In just such an experiment, subjects were first presented with a cueing image—an outdoor scene, for example, that preceded an upcoming monetary reward task. Correct completion of the task was accompanied by a green light, indicating the subject won fifty cents. As expected, once the association between financial gain and the green light was engineered, the green light gained the ability to activate the mesolimbic dopaminergic structures, demonstrating the light's salience and reinforcing value. Soon enough, the cue images of outdoor scenes, a cognitive construct that reliably preceded the possibility of green light, could elicit the same response. It was no longer necessary to get the money; just the promise of future reward was enough to activate the mesolimbic system. The same is true for threats, like anticipating a mild electric shock. The dopaminergic drive and threat response system lights up in advance of the actual threat and responds by generating negative emotions when a future threat is predicted based on precedent cognitive inputs.

The second thing to appreciate is that nicotine has an interesting bimodal effect on negative affect. Initially, nicotine acts a little like an anxiolytic, based on its effect on allostatic efficiency. It doesn't calm as much as resolve. After chronic exposure to nicotine, however, the brain's natural allostatic mechanisms get reset. The complex interactions between neurotransmitter systems, the body's stress hormone regulation, and learning are poorly understood, but there are a few interesting observations that provide some clues to nicotine's role in regulating anxiety circuits.

Norepinephrine input is important to training the amygdala to consolidate a global (all-hands-on-deck) fear response and helps the threat response system motivate avoidance behaviors when faced with a predicted danger. It turns out that $\alpha4\beta2$, $\alpha5\beta4$, and $\alpha7$ nicotinic receptors have a role in modulating norepinephrine's effect. Further, chronically unresolved allostatic load induces overexpression of corticotropin-releasing factor. This, in turn, results in chronic overproduction of cortisol, the body's stress-response hormone. Cortisol released during emotionally arousing experiences activates norepinephrine systems in the amygdala, resulting in a facilitated memory for those events. Cortisol overproduction also eventually leads to blunted cortisol production during stress and has been implicated as a possible contributor to the depression and dysphoria of nicotine withdrawal and relapse.

The bottom line: There is a situation where a prediction of abstinence from nicotine reliably leads to an anticipatory anxiety response. While access to nicotine resolves the anxiety in the short term, nicotine also distorts the system responsible for controlling the emotional response to abstinence, making it increasingly likely that predictions of abstinence will be met with avoidance behaviors and negative affect.

> *Helen smokes to avoid the anxiety of not smoking and becomes more anxious as a result.*

Persistence of Behavioral Effect

Transitioning from tobacco experimentation to dependence involves an evolution of sorts; discrete instances of tobacco use evolve into habitual patterns, and patterns plus anxiety coalesce into a compulsion to smoke. As it turns out, that transition doesn't take very long. Why then do people who abstain from smoking long term still find the drive to smoke and the emotional connection to smoking difficult to undo? If induction of tobacco dependence happens quickly, why doesn't undoing induction require an equally short process, albeit in the reverse? One of the theories implicates nicotine's ability to reorganize the orbitofrontal cortex, a part of the brain that lives next door to the prefrontal cortex. In lab animal experiments, damage to the orbitofrontal cortex results in resistance to extinction of reward-associated behaviors. Similarly, there's human evidence that orbitofrontal dysfunction limits behavioral flexibility and has become a central concept to the growing neurobiological understanding of obsessive-compulsive disorder. In fact, disordered orbitofrontal activity is associated with compulsive drug self-administration, even after the user has developed tolerance to the pleasurable effects and experienced distressing effects of drug use. In smokers, similar anatomic and functional patterns have been identified, with reduction in the gray matter volume and dysregulation of the orbitofrontal cortex similar to that observed among individuals addicted to other substances.

How can we study the relative persistence of nicotine's effect on the brain? Start with any of the experimental models described so far wherein nicotine was used to reinforce a target behavior, say, a lever press. Substitute a saline infusion each time the animal presses the lever, and watch to see how long it takes for the animal to get bored and passively "unlearn" the association. What is so striking about nicotine is that, despite a marked lack of hedonic effect, its ability to modify behavior is as, or more, persistent than many of the more well-recognized drugs of addiction. Start administering "blank" saline injections to squirrel monkeys that have been taught to press a lever for nicotine, and the monkeys will continue to work for their nicotine, even when up to 600 lever presses were needed to get it. That's an awful lot of blanks. What's even more striking, is that the same experiment was done in adult male (human) smokers; even though they experienced both positive and negative effects of nicotine administration, the subjects would tolerate as many as 1,600 blanks—the maximum number allowed by the protocol—to get to their next nicotine infusion.

Chapter 4 Learning Points

- Nicotine exposure leads to disinhibition of automatic responses, and Helen loses any potential advantage of delayed action.
- Disinhibition of automatic responses is experienced as the "screw it!" phenomenon—an instinctive release from the disincentives to smoking. "Screw it!" may be followed shortly after by disappointment and regret.
- Nicotine exposure makes it hard for the brain's allostatic mechanisms to return to a low-energy, comfortable, neutral homeostasis. Allostatic load creates an inefficiency in shifting the brain from neutral to drive and back again and can limit the body's response to stress in the long run. Helen smokes to relieve anxiety, and in return smoking makes Helen more anxious overall.
- The brain is designed to learn—to predict survival-salient circumstances before they happen based on clues in the environment. Helen's threat response system is designed to turn on and warn her in anticipation of threat. When faced with the future possibility of forgoing cigarettes, Helen experiences anticipatory anxiety.
- Compulsion is characterized by subjective distress caused when routine behaviors are forbidden or forgone. Returning to the ritual behavior is an attempt to neutralize the anxiety or distress produced by the obsessive thoughts.
- The behavioral effects of nicotine exposure accumulate quickly but dissipate slowly. Persistence of effect is thought to be mediated in part by the orbitofrontal cortex, where damage leads to resistance to extinction for reward-associated behaviors.

Chapter 5
Patterns

I went to the hospital with a stroke. They put me in a medically induced coma. That's what it took to get me to quit.

—Marilyn F., 60 years old

Every morning, at exactly 6:45 a.m., Helen's alarm clock rattles and starts her day off with a jolt. She often lies there, hitting the snooze button a few times, wondering why she puts up with that ugly noise. In fact, it is sometimes hard for her to understand why she uses an alarm at all, given that she hasn't worked a routine job in years. "I should just let myself wake up whenever," she tells herself. "It's not like I have somewhere special to go." Every morning the routine is the same; get up, brush teeth, comb hair, then bumble over to the coffee maker. "Nothing like that morning cup of coffee with a cigarette," she thinks. On occasion, Helen wonders exactly why those two things seem to go so well together—but only for a moment.

It occurs to her that there are multiple points in her day that seem to unfold in exactly the same manner, day after day, as though the plan was preconfigured by someone else. She sits in the same seat at the kitchen table to drink her coffee and smoke her cigarette. When her sons finally do call to say hello, she settles in for conversation by making sure her cigarettes, lighter, and ashtray are nearby. Just the thought of talking that long without a cigarette to smooth it out makes her uncomfortable. After the evening meal, Helen can't seem to motivate to wash the dishes before having a cigarette. Sometimes, she'll treat herself to a glass of wine with her meal, which almost always leads to an extra after-dinner cigarette.

"It's like someone is pulling my strings," she confides to Kathy one evening. "I don't even really want to do it, but I do it anyway. I don't understand why I don't just tell myself 'no' and keep going. What am I, some kind of robot? I have zero willpower."

Kathy just murmurs and nods her head knowingly, with nothing much else left to say.

———

Understanding Helen as the functional equivalent of a lab mouse has its limits. As a first step, it was important to be able to explain Helen's ability to discriminate safety versus threat, her ability to learn new information about her environment and to integrate it into an instinctive response. It was equally important to understand the genesis of her anticipatory anxiety in the face of impending abstinence and of her focused attention on resolving the problem. This book has described mechanisms that are involved in performing each of these component functions, but we still have some trouble trying to extend a mechanistic model into an understanding of Helen's conscious experience of nicotine dependence. Helen is clearly not a robot-zombie, with an instinctive brain responding to the environment and adjusting behaviors based on sensory inputs alone. She is also clearly not free to make up her mind in any way she chooses. If conscious beings are self-aware and volitional, why can't Helen's cognitive brain more easily exert its own influence over the activities of her instinctive brain to compensate for nicotine's effect? Why can't the third brain win more often?

Attention versus Awareness

One way to begin thinking about this problem is to recognize that the survival concept of attention is not strictly the same as the cognitive concept of awareness. It is true that under typical circumstances, attention and awareness go together. Sitting too close to an open flame and almost getting burned, for example, will focus the brain's attentional resources on resolving the threat and ensuring it is less likely to happen in the future. Alongside that response, however, the internal conversation will also instantly change to reflect the pain and fear experienced in that encounter. Predictions about future encounters with the stove will include strategies to avoid repeating the mistake. Often there is some judgment about culpability. Notice that the focus has shifted well beyond the person's hand to the second- and third-order implications of the event. It all happened so fast that it felt like attention and awareness were the same, but in fact, instinctive attention to the threat, along with resolution of the threatening situation, happened virtually instantly—perhaps even before all of the elements of awareness were fully formed. Reacting to the heat occurs before fully experiencing the heat.

Awareness is not simply a function of the mechanistic capacity of the brain to sense outer- and inner-world conditions and respond but rather a cognitive representation of "self" that is distinguishable from "other." People recognize their bodies, and their narratives, as their own. An infant is capable of paying attention to salient objects and circumstances but not capable of identifying "self" in a mirror until about 18 months of age. An intact attentional system is not the same as the ability to incorporate inputs into awareness. The conscious mind somehow models "self" as a player within a subjective, experiential world—the center of a personal narrative, which itself is the product of a lifetime of experiences.

So why is this important? It appears that consciousness is a distributed process involving the coordination of neural activity across several cortical regions; it is not something that happens in a single structure. Until now, the model of the brain has been reminiscent of a bunch of wires set up in series: a spark in A leads to a spark in B, which leads to a spark in C, and so on (Figure 5.1).

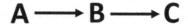

Figure 5.1. Linear model of neuronal interaction.

But the mind is a whole-of-brain application. Accurately understanding how nicotine affects the way Helen thinks requires a model that's more akin to the entire electrical grid. There are various electrical events that occur in the brain in various structures and at various times and affect each other's functioning in a manner that depends on how strongly those areas are networked. In this network model, a spark in A influences the response characteristics of both B and C, while B and C in turn simultaneously influence both A and each other. When an event happens in one area, it propagates and affects how the whole-of-brain responds to the event (Figure 5.2).

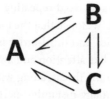

Figure 5.2. Network model of neuronal interaction.

Keep in mind that the brain has about nine billion cells in it, each with thousands of connections. When an event occurs, the pattern of cells activated in response translates information about the event into a format the brain can use in the future, a pattern known as the population code. The order and timing of cell firing, called the temporal code, and the frequency of cell firing, called the rate code, provide for the near-infinite number of coding permutations that the whole-of-brain can use to interpret, store, and retrieve the information it needs to coordinate the experience known as consciousness. Now imagine that the net effect of this coding is represented as numerical "relationship coefficients" between A, B, and C. The number—say, a decimal value between –1.0 and +1.0—could be used to indicate the strength and direction of influence one area of the brain has on another. A simple graphical representation of what happens when we learn would look something like Figure 5.3.

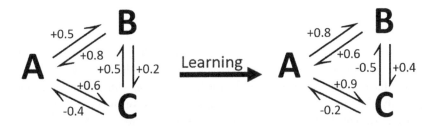

Figure 5.3. Neuronal relationships expressed as coefficients. Learning occurs when the strength of relationships is influenced by exposure.

When nicotine acts in its mechanistic way, strengthening some connections and trimming others, it alters the pattern of patterns that the brain uses to encode the full richness of our inner narrative. It doesn't just change the instinctive response to events; it shapes the interpretation of events, adjusts the working memory of events, and influences the management of the future probability of events.

> *Nicotine does not just change Helen's brain.*
> *It changes her mind.*

When Operant Becomes Classical

Ivan Pavlov's research focused on digestion, and he was intensely curious about saliva. In order to get a supply for his studies, he tried collecting it when his dogs started drooling in response to food. He noticed that the dogs also drooled when they saw or heard something that was related to the feeding. Since the dogs could predict when food was coming, he started ringing a bell every time the dogs were fed. Once the dogs were "conditioned" to associate the ringing with mealtime, he could trigger a physical reflex of saliva production and collect samples reliably by simply ringing the bell. A few decades later, B. F. Skinner noticed that the same conditioning paradigm could be used to get animals to perform behaviors that weren't reflexive but in fact voluntary, or "operational." Conditioning reflexive physiological responses came to be known as classical, while conditioning nonreflexive behaviors, such as teaching a dog to sit, came to be known as operant.

The network model of brain function explains conditioning as a way of altering the pattern of patterns by systematically strengthening some of the relationship coefficients in the model while allowing others to wither. Imagine a situation where the association between a stimulus and the consequent voluntary behavior becomes stronger and stronger over time, with a coefficient that is pretty close to +1.0. In that case, the involved areas of the brain have fired together so reliably that they have essentially become wired together. As a matter of degree, imagine that this progressive together-wiring eventually produces a voluntary response that is so reliable it is essentially reflexive. Another way to think about the implication of nicotine's effect on whole-of-brain awareness is to recognize that by strengthening some connections and trimming others, conditioned thoughts, emotions, reactions become so reliably reproducible that they essentially become reflexive. Operant has become classical.

> *What are the implications for Helen if volition becomes reflexive?*
> *What is volition if it isn't exactly volitional?*

The mind is somewhat like a prediction machine, designed to make millions of predictions per day and testing whether they are right. The mind is guided by the physical way the brain is organized and the rules under which it operates. When nicotine changes the relationship coefficients in the brain, it changes the circumstances under which the brain works; it does not change the way the brain works or the rules under which the brain functions. Nicotine simply progressively constricts the range of possible outcomes such that those same old brain mechanisms add up to fewer possible conscious responses.

> *Helen's brain knows what she will decide to do before Helen does.*
> *When she says she cannot imagine life*
> *without smoking, she means it.*

Plasticity

The brain is a dynamic organ, constantly reorganizing itself to better deal with circumstances in the world around it. The brain's capacity to change its structure and function in response to both internal and external influences is commonly referred to as neuronal plasticity. Adolescence is an important time in development when children are transitioning into adulthood. There is a remarkable amount of learning that goes on during this period of maturation, but not all areas of the brain are equally plastic at the same time. Anyone who has ever been a teenager remembers the emotional consequences; mood swings, impulsive risk-taking, and the all-important "what will my friends think?" social interactions come into full bloom well before the cortical areas of the brain responsible for cognitive control over behavior have a chance to catch up. Mesolimbic structures experience a major developmental boost around the onset of puberty, fueled by all those adolescent hormones, making the teenage years a supremely vulnerable time during which nicotine can exert its lifelong effects on the pattern of patterns.

The majority of adult smokers start smoking in adolescence. People who begin in adolescence smoke more and have a harder time quitting later in life. And dependence happens in adolescents more quickly than we imagine: the first symptoms of nicotine dependence can appear within a few weeks of initiating casual experimentation, usually before the young smoker progresses to daily use. That does not mean it is impossible for an adult brain to alter the pattern of patterns enough to alter cognition and behavior in response to nicotine exposure; it just means it is less likely. It is about probabilities. All brains are plastic, and the brain's plasticity allows for relationship coefficients in the network model to change in response to nicotine. But it is the same plasticity that makes the brain accessible to change in the clinic. All brain networks in all people cannot possibly adjust at the same rate. The pattern of patterns will change on its own timeline. The provider's job is to constantly nudge, prod, and influence the patterns, shifting probabilities such that Helen will one day roll the dice and experience a different outcome.

> *Smoking is not monolithic.*
> *Helen has a unique pattern of patterns, and it is*
> *the provider's job to see her uniqueness.*

When discussing with smokers the prospect of quitting, it is common to hear "Oh yeah? Well, what about . . . ?" questions. These questions come in many forms. What about my uncle who woke up one morning and just stopped smoking? What about my friend who only smokes on weekends? What about the fact that I can go sixteen hours straight without smoking? What about the last time I did not smoke for a month after my heart attack? All the "what about" questions stem from the same set of misconceptions about the impact of nicotine on the brain. Nicotine addiction does not produce robots, and it does not take away free will. Tobacco dependence isn't about what happens when a person can't smoke; it is about what happens when that person can smoke but would otherwise like not to. Nicotine is the perfect stealth drug, creating the impulsive drive to smoke at the same time it distorts and diminishes cognitive control mechanisms that might otherwise be able to get out of this trap. Nicotine tips the brain's balance between go and no-go, and constrains the possible outcomes following a trigger event. The scales are tipped.

> *A free will that is not completely free may not be free at all.*

Chapter 5 Learning Points

- Instinctive attention and conscious awareness are not the same thing. Nicotine affects both. By altering the inputs that form awareness, nicotine has the ability to change the internal narrative: how we incorporate, perceive, and judge our experiences.
- Understanding how nicotine affects the cognitive mind requires moving from a mechanistic "wiring" model to a whole-of-brain "network" model of function.
- Nicotine changes the pattern of patterns necessary for cognition by changing the relationship coefficients between networked areas of the brain.
- When associative learning is affected by nicotine, volitional (operant) responses essentially become reflexive (classical).
- By changing the pattern of patterns in the brain, nicotine does not change the way the brain works; it changes the range of possible outcomes that can follow a triggering event.
- A patient's pattern of patterns is unique, based on overall life experience. The clinician's job is not to treat the smoking but to find ways to change the probability that the patient can rebalance their pattern of patterns.

Chapter 6
Device

I tried the patch. It must be for people with a happy life because as soon as the stress hits, it sure as hell ain't a cigarette.

—Wilson V., 88 years old

Helen looks down at her cigarette and thinks, "How could something so little have such a hold over me?" She debates throwing it away, but she knows that she will regret wasting her money. Kathy told her about the corner store where she can buy loose cigarettes for $1 per cigarette, and Helen restricts herself to purchasing five cigarettes a day. She always saves one for the next morning so she can have it as soon as she wakes up. That cigarette has always been the perfect companion to her cup of coffee. A snowstorm was predicted in the forecast and that was making her nervous. "Should I buy a pack, just in case I can't get out tomorrow?" she ponders. It is 25 degrees Fahrenheit out, there is ice on the sidewalks, and her hip is really aching, but with a determined mind-set and tenuous gait, Helen walks to the store and buys a pack just to be safe. When she gets home, she notices that she still had some of her previous cigarette remaining in her ashtray. Since she started buying loosies and smoking fewer cigarettes, she would take a few drags, put the cigarette out, and then relight it later. Kathy always yelled at her, "You know stumping those cigarettes is more dangerous!" Helen thinks, "That seems unlikely to be true," as she takes a nice long drag and holds it an extra few seconds before exhaling.

On Sunday, January 31, 1971, Commander Alan Shepard, along with astronauts Stuart Roosa and Edgar Mitchell, sat atop a 50-ton roman candle and launched their nine-day Apollo 14 mission to the Moon, barely 8 months after a dramatic oxygen tank explosion forced the crew of Apollo 13 to use the lunar module as a lifeboat to bring them safely back to Earth. The world watched in real time as Shepard stood beside the landing module 239,000 miles away and famously hit golf balls across the lunar highlands. Grainy images fluttered across tiny screens everywhere in a breathtaking display of human potential.

Almost exactly one year later, twenty-five scientists from three western countries gathered on the island of St. Martin for an industry conference sponsored by the Council for Tobacco Research, USA. Their charge was to address one of the most nagging questions confusing the industry at the time: why do people actually smoke cigarettes? Was it a relaxing experience? A stimulating one? Could it be both? How? During the conference, William L. Dunn, chief of the Philip Morris Behavioral Research Group, laid out what he believed to be the personal characteristics that led people to smoke and described for his audience what was at the time a radically different way of thinking about cigarettes and smoking. Dunn stood beside the conference podium and famously explained:

> The primary incentive to cigarette smoking is the immediate salutary effect of inhaled smoke upon bodily function. The physiological effect serves as the primary incentive; all other incentives are secondary. Without nicotine, there would be no smoking. No one has ever become a cigarette smoker by smoking cigarettes without nicotine.

Okay, so nicotine is important. But why do people choose cigarettes as their favored means of getting it? He went on:

> The answer, and I feel quite strongly about this, is that the cigarette is in fact among the most awe-inspiring examples of the ingenuity of man. Let me explain my conviction. The cigarette should be conceived not as a product but as a package. The product is nicotine. The cigarette is but one of many package layers. There is the carton, which contains the pack, which contains the cigarette, which contains the smoke. The smoke is the final package. The smoker must strip off all these package layers to get to that which he seeks. . . . Think of a puff of smoke as the vehicle of nicotine. Smoke is beyond question the most optimized vehicle of nicotine and the cigarette the most optimized dispenser of smoke.

Up until then, it was routine to think about the cigarette as a paper tube surrounding a column of dried-up tobacco leaves. It was easy to imagine the evolution from farm to pack requiring only a few simple steps. Grow the plant, harvest, cure, and then chop it up into little bits and stuff it into a hollow paper cylinder. Instead, Dunn was hinting that there was more. Everyone knew the industry was experimenting with different materials for their filters, but the cigarette itself had ostensibly been unchanged since Buck Duke paid James Bonsack for the rights to his fateful machine nearly a hundred years earlier. Dunn was giving us a peek behind the curtain: if the cigarette was optimized, someone was doing the optimizing.

Targeting the VTA

In order to understand the idea of "optimization," consider first the goal of any enhancements. The net effect of optimization, of course, would be to create a product that more consumers will enjoy. But how? What are the mechanistic objectives of the optimization effort? Understanding the mechanisms by which nicotine affects the mesolimbic system provides insight into potential leverage points, but there must also be some insight into the manner of effect. In other words, if a specific delivery device can influence nicotine's effects, then the drug's effects can't simply be about its presence or absence in the brain. If that were the case, Dunn would expect any device delivering nicotine to have equivalent salutary effects. Instead, there must be something about the manner in which nicotine is delivered, the pattern of delivery, that has influence over degree of effect. There must be something unique to the cigarette that allows that particular device to access that optimized pattern.

The Pattern of Delivery

Given our brain's limited attention resources, survival advantage is a function of the ability both to focus our attention on cues that are important and to ignore the inputs that have proven themselves irrelevant. One method the brain uses to distinguish between the two types of input has to do with rate of change in signaling. For example, sudden, unexpected noises, like a creaking floor in the middle of the night, will reliably draw your attention and make you spring into action. On the other hand, you're likely to remain blissfully unaware of the noise your refrigerator makes while it is running—that is, until someone calls it to your attention. Try this: set up a chair in your kitchen when no one else is around, and see how long you can pay attention to your refrigerator noise. Force yourself to stay focused on the humming. How long does it take for your mind to wander off? How long before you have to remind yourself why you're sitting alone, in the dark, facing your refrigerator? Could you pay attention for thirty seconds? Maybe. It would be surprising if you could do it for a whole minute before your attention is drawn off to something else. Ask yourself if you could fall back asleep equally fast if your attention was suddenly drawn to the creaky floor noises coming from downstairs? As far as your mesolimbic system is concerned, one of the big differences between things that go bump in the night and your refrigerator hum is the periodicity of the stimulus. Bumps are occasional; hums are continuous. Bumps are phasic; hums are tonic.

Sensory inputs that evoke a tonic neural response produce a sustained cholinergic milieu in the VTA. Nicotinic cholinergic receptors desensitize and downregulate as a result, leading to a prolonged depression of evoked downstream dopaminergic response. But phasic stimulation amplifies dopaminergic activity in the mesolimbic system by allowing for a rapid rise in dopamine release. This has the effect of increasing the salience of the inciting sensory input, dramatically magnifying the alerting functions of the ventral forebrain and the anticipation of reward. In this manner, dopamine neurons involved in the development of dependence can encode reward-related information by switching from tonic to phasic (burst-like) activity. And in this manner, the addictive potential of nicotine, like that of cocaine and amphetamine, depends on developing a means of delivery that can maximize phasic, but not tonic, delivery to the VTA.

Optimization Rule #1: It is about the peaks, not the plateaus.

Maximizing Access to the Brain

In order to optimize a nicotine delivery system, the engineering needs to meet two criteria. First, the device needs to be capable of producing phasic firing across Helen's mesolimbic system. Second, the timing of that phasic burst needs to be closely associated with the sensory inputs that prompted them in order to maximize the rewarding potential of those exact inputs. Delivery of the drug now cannot reinforce a behavior that occurs later. After the nicotine leaves the device, it is Helen's blood that will carry it up to her brain. If the transposition from device to bloodstream is slow and steady, one might expect the device to present a similar pattern of nicotine concentration to the central nervous system neurons being affected. Tortoise-like absorption produces a (more or less) constant concentration of nicotine in the blood as it makes its way to the brain, with little second-to-second change, for as long as the nicotine remains in the blood. But if the nicotine is absorbed very rapidly, the blood will deliver the nicotine in a bolus pattern—from minimum to maximum concentration in the time it takes for a single heartbeat. Nothing, nothing, nothing, everything, nothing, nothing, nothing (Figures 6.1 and 6.2).

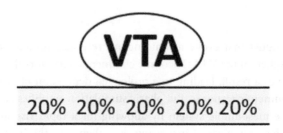

Figure 6.1. Venous drug delivery. Slowly absorbed nicotine results in a continuous low concentration delivered to VTA.

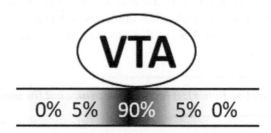

Figure 6.2. Arterial drug delivery. Rapidly absorbed nicotine produces a bolus effect, delivering nicotine in transiently high concentrations.

Pay attention to absorption. However, even super-fast absorption will not amount to optimization if the transport time from absorption site to target cells is long or interrupted. The delay between administration and effect needs to be as close to instantaneous as possible. Any delivery system that relies on the mouth, nose, gut, or skin as a point of entry has to contend with the fact that blood leaving those absorption sites will also mix together with venous blood returning from other parts of the body. This will severely dilute the nicotine content and ruin the bolus pattern.

Also, all blood returning to the heart from those sites will, by necessity, transit through the liver, where metabolic enzymes will soak up the nicotine and instantly begin the process of degrading it into waste products. Even if Dunn had found some hard-core volunteers to optimize on, he could not have gotten around these issues even by injecting nicotine directly into a vein. Sure, the size of the initial bolus would be bigger, but all that mixing and metabolizing would just end up leaving his volunteers with a higher plateau (tonic) blood level, which wouldn't be very reinforcing. It would probably just make them nauseated. Short of injecting nicotine directly into the brain, a paucity of options remains for achieving our goal of rapid, phasic nicotine delivery.

> *Then came the realization that the shortest distance*
> *from device to brain runs through the lungs.*

Because the lungs are responsible for exchanging oxygen and carbon dioxide with the air, they have by necessity some unique anatomical features. First of all, it is important to realize that our circulatory system isn't really a circle but more like a figure eight. Blood leaves the right side of the heart and enters the lungs as it prepares to make the gas exchange at the alveoli. Newly oxygen-rich blood returns from the lungs and enters the left side of the heart, where it gets pumped out to all the remaining parts of the body, including the brain. In the body, the blood delivers the oxygen, picks up carbon dioxide, and begins the return trip back to the right side of the heart, where the cycle starts all over again. Within Helen's lungs, compared to other organs, there's an enormous amount of blood dutifully getting ready to nourish her entire body with oxygen. To make sure that gas exchange happens without a hitch, the pulmonary capillaries are intimately juxtaposed to the air in the alveolar sacs, to within 3 microns, or 0.003 millimeters. Gas transfer times in this situation are extremely close to instantaneous. There is a bonus: blood returning from the lung doesn't mix with blood from any other organ system, so there is no dilution. And a double bonus: there is no need to worry about the liver because blood leaving from the left side of the heart doesn't pass through the liver on its way to the brain (Figure 6.3).

> *Instant absorption. No mixing. Bypass the liver. Eureka! All*
> *of Dunn's phasic delivery problems are solved. If we could just*
> *find a way to deliver nicotine to the alveolar capillaries.*
>
> *Optimization Rule #2:*
> *In order to get peaks, go through the lungs.*

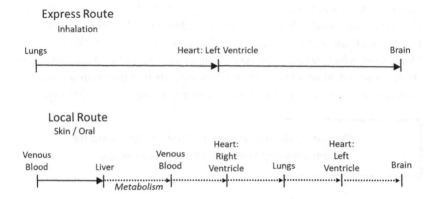

Figure 6.3. Distinctions in paths of nicotine delivery to the brain. Significant differences in concentration depend on the route of administration.

Smoke is an aerosol. That means that visible smoke is a fine mist of billions of tiny solid particles and liquid droplets, so small they can remain suspended in air. The lungs, in contrast, are built specifically to protect the body from stuff suspended in the air. The airways get progressively smaller, branching in all directions like the roots of a tree, until they terminate in alveolar clusters. A thin film of sticky mucus lines the airway walls, trapping smoke particles and aerosol droplets along the way. Any nicotine contained within the deposit may eventually be absorbed, but the same limitations plague Dunn here as elsewhere in or on the body. Absorption is not instantaneous from the airway itself. To be super rapid, absorption has to be at the level of the alveoli—which means it has to be a gas. Gas does not get trapped in the airway eddies. Fortunately, nicotine is a semivolatile compound, with temperatures required to release gas-phase nicotine from the tobacco leaf being quite reasonable and easy to attain. In fact, volatilization temperatures are several hundred degrees below the temperature produced by the burning coal at the tip of the cigarette. The burning tobacco coal serves as a heat source, facilitating gas transfer from the tobacco near it with relatively small variations in local temperature significantly affecting the relative proportion of nicotine that gets released as gas.

Now there is an extra bonus: additive composition, used to control combustion temperature and burn rate, can vary along the length of the tobacco rod, ensuring the smoker experiences a "front-end lift." This means the first puff has the greatest impact. Nicotine in the gas phase doesn't get measured by Federal Trade Commission methods, so as gas-phase portion goes up, "apparent" nicotine content of the smoke goes down. Now, Dunn's optimization problem comes down to finding just the right combination of water content and chemical additives to produce reliable control over combustion temperature.

Optimization Rule #3: More gas.

The Chemistry

Nicotine is an alkaloid. Under certain conditions, the molecule has the ability to act like a base. Remember that bases accept protons from other molecules, usually acids. In the tobacco plant, nicotine exists as a salt; the nicotine alkaloid binds to organic acids produced by the plant to form a stable salt compound that accumulates over time. When heated, nicotine salts dissociate into their two components: free nicotine plus the corresponding acid. It is the free, base form of nicotine that is volatilized to gas; the corresponding acids are dissolved in the droplet phase. Free-base nicotine reacts with water in the air and airway, accepts a hydrogen atom, and becomes "protonated." Free-base and protonated forms of nicotine exist in equilibrium within the airway, with the relative balance between the two forms depending on characteristics of the smoke. Understanding this reaction is important for a few reasons.

First, by alkalinizing the pH of the smoke, it is possible to alter the relative amount of nicotine that comes off the plant in the free-base form, offering at least one mechanism for controlling the proportion of nicotine in the gas phase of smoke. Second, protonated nicotine is a tiny molecule compared to its salt counterpart and as a result is both lipophilic and water soluble. This property makes it easy for the nicotine to cross the alveolar epithelium and enter the pulmonary capillaries by diffusion. Finally, once the nicotine gets to its destination, it has to cross the blood-brain barrier, a selectively permeable phospholipid protein bilayer separating the circulating blood from the brain's extracellular fluid. Crossing the blood-brain barrier is usually tricky, but the small size and lipophilicity of nicotine means it can diffuse across membranes readily. It also appears that nicotine may actively speed up its own delivery to the brain by (1) directly increasing the permeability of tight junctions between the endothelial cells that line the brain's microvasculature and (2) using an active transporter protein to carry it across cell membranes up to ten times faster than expected from simple diffusion.

> *Point of reference: These are the same chemical*
> *principles used to transform cocaine into crack.*
> *A "crack" form of nicotine is created.*

It is also important to note that there are dozens of different nicotine salts in tobacco and that in addition to maximizing availability of free-base nicotine, alkalinization also affects what happens to the acid portion of the salt. There are a few notable varieties of nicotine salt, including nicotine acetate and nicotine formate, that, when heated, produce discernibly repellent acids—namely, acetic (vinegar) and formic (fire ant) acids. These acids have the distinct potential to ruin the smoker's experience by creating an uncomfortable caustic sensation in the mouth and posterior pharynx. By adding an alternative base to the tobacco and adjusting the pH of the smoke, the sensory impact of the acids is mitigated, leading to a smoother taste and a less harsh smoking experience. One common base used to achieve this effect is ammonia. Ammonization was a technological breakthrough that allowed for a bigger central nervous system impact, better sensory experience of smoking, higher nicotine delivery with lower apparent nicotine content in the smoke, and less tobacco required per unit cigarette to produce the desired effect.

Ammonization was a chemistry breakthrough, but it was not the first. Menthol, a terpene alcohol component of peppermint, was first added to cigarettes in the 1920s in an attempt to make "stale" cigarettes taste better when smoked. Menthol has a strong mint-like, medicinal taste, capable of masking the unpleasant harshness of North American tobacco that has aged past its prime. Menthol is a volatile alcohol, evaporating quickly and producing a cooling sensation in the user's throat and airway. It would not be long before the majority of cigarette brands would be mentholated. Currently, almost all cigarettes contain some amount of menthol as an additive, though only the brands with menthol content high enough to be discernible by the palate are labeled as menthol cigarettes.

There are two reasons to invest money on a "flavor" additive that Helen might not even be able to taste. First, menthol has a mild anesthetic effect, numbing the lower airway and making the distal delivery of smoke less offensive to the lungs. Less coughing equals a smoother experience. Second, in some people, menthol has its own pharmacologic effect. In the presence of menthol, some of the brain's nicotinic cholinergic receptors have a harder time "resetting" after being activated. This closer-to-tonic stimulation of those receptors results in a degree of desensitization, as we might expect. It is believed that menthol's pharmacologic manipulation of nicotine's impact is, at least in part, responsible for the epidemiologic observations that menthol smokers are more severely dependent and find it harder to quit. The majority of young people who start smoking use menthol brands during initiation.

> **Optimization Rule #4: Make the crack nicotine minty fresh.**

The Minor Alkaloids

Robert is a 72-year-old retired physician with a complicated medical history. He smokes fifteen to twenty cigarettes every day, having achieved abstinence only for short periods during business trips. Robert has suffered the effects of poorly controlled hypertension for decades, including a stroke three years ago and a myocardial infarction ten years ago. His doctor has been monitoring a large, descending aortic aneurysm for a few years, but despite maximal blood pressure control, the aneurysm has recently worsened to the point where surgery has become unavoidable. It is a complicated procedure, and the surgeon has estimated a 5% intraoperative mortality. Robert is terrified; his older brother died four years ago at the age of 72, and the coincidence has really unsettled him. At the end of his visit with the surgeon, Robert resolved to quit smoking in an attempt to reduce his risk during and after the procedure. On his way home, he stopped at the pharmacy and bought a box of nicotine patches.

Six weeks later, on the morning of his procedure, Robert was proud of the fact that he had been able to successfully abstain from smoking in anticipation of his procedure, and he reported his accomplishment to the anesthesiologist during his preoperative evaluation. To assess Robert's adherence, the anesthesiologist ordered a urine cotinine level, which returned strongly positive. Surgery was canceled, and Robert was sent home.

Though nicotine is the overwhelmingly dominant alkaloid produced by the tobacco plant, there are several minor alkaloids produced that also contribute to the overall neuropharmacologic effect of tobacco smoke. There are four minor alkaloids with clinical significance: anabasine, anatabine, cotinine, and nornicotine. Together, these minor alkaloids, known to increase the activity of dopaminergic neurons in laboratory studies, are weakly reinforcing and can be used as substitutes for nicotine in conditioned place preference experiments. In humans, nicotine is very quickly metabolized to a variety of weakly reinforcing intermediate alkaloids, including nornicotine, with the major final metabolic product being cotinine. For this reason, though nicotine is difficult to detect in body fluids other than plasma, cotinine is detectable in generous supply within easily accessible fluids like urine and saliva. Cotinine levels are a reliable marker of exposure to nicotine. The problem is that cotinine is also the dominant metabolic product of nicotine delivered through the patch. For this reason, cotinine cannot distinguish between nicotine delivered through smoke and that administered via patch.

It is not the nicotine that confers surgical risk; it is the smoke. It is critically important to distinguish between the two sources. To do so, check for the presence of minor alkaloids that are produced by the plant *but are not significant metabolites* of nicotine replacement. A negative urine anabasine or anatabine result in the presence of a positive cotinine assay means the source of nicotine could not have been tobacco.

The Physics

The paper wrapping that holds the tobacco rod in place would usually never even get a second thought. In less ingenious applications, the paper might merely be conceived as a physical barrier, a container to hold the actual product in place. By carefully adjusting the physical characteristics of the cigarette paper, it is possible to alter the characteristics of the smoke and consequently fine-tune the delivery of nicotine to the lung. When Helen takes a drag off her cigarette, the burning coal at the tip brightens, an indication of air flow across the embers. What is also true, however, is that air is being pulled in through the sides of the cigarette column to dilute the smoke down to a more palatable concentration and temperature. The volume of diluent air drawn relative to the volume of smoke generated is a function of the porosity of the paper. With each puff, a less dense paper, with bigger spaces between fibers, will allow air to pass through it more easily than a denser paper wrap.

The problem is fewer fibers equal flimsier paper. So to solve this problem, one might start by using a paper with reasonable density and durability, then mechanically manipulate it to create microscopic pores big enough to get the desired airflow effects without compromising the structural integrity of the product. High-porosity paper contributes fewer combustion products to the tobacco smoke, and it is easy enough to treat the paper with additives that can control the rate and temperature of burning.

Pores can also be useful at the filter. Early filters were composed of a cellulose acetate that was crushed down to a prespecified "crimp ratio" to control the material's airflow characteristics and impregnated with a plasticizer to help it keep its form. More recently, filters are made of cheaper materials, like paper, and engineered to create a Venturi effect through premade channels. The material is covered with a "plug" wrap paper that is highly air permeable across its circumferential surface. The filter plug gets attached to the tobacco rod using "tipping" paper, which is sometimes colored or patterned to look like cork. The tipping paper usually has a circumferential embossment that helps produce a comfortable lip-release sensation and creates a slight gap between the tipping paper and the plug. The tipping paper is manipulated using static electricity or lasers to create microperforations that, when overlaid on the tiny gap produced by embossment, allow for filter ventilation to be increased from the side walls and dilute the smoke before it enters Helen's mouth.

Filter ventilation strategies work particularly well when the cigarettes are being evaluated by machines that do not apply pressure on the filter, creating a diluted apparent concentration of particulates in the measurement. But Helen, being human, is more likely to crush the embossment gap with her lips and cover the laser perforations with her fingers, ensuring that she gets the full, undiluted, gratifying smoke.

One last thing about filters: they do not do what most people think they do. Filters are designed to capture large particles aerosolized in the smoke, usually particles larger than 10 microns wide. But those particles were never destined to get to the lung anyway. Particles that big are nonrespirable, meaning they would get caught up in the water layer lining the oropharynx and upper airway. Respirable particles are much, much smaller—in the range of 0.1 to 3 microns. Particles that small go right through the filter. Sure, the filter gets dirty, and all that sludge it collected would have ended up in Helen's digestive tract. But filters do not do a thing to protect her from respiratory or cardiovascular illness or minimize the addictive impact of the gas.

> *Optimization Rule #5: Don't forget the physics.*

The User

An understanding of optimization would be incomplete without looking at the way the device interfaces with the user. Imagine a pill that carries 100 milligrams of drug X into Helen's system. The unit dose in this example is predetermined by the decisions made when engineering the pill. More milligrams equal a bigger dose of drug X. A single tablet will always reliably deliver the amount of drug that the manufacturer intended unless Helen purposefully alters the pill. After that point, it becomes a matter of absorption: the way the drug interacts with Helen's gut will determine the bioavailability of drug X. If bioavailability is high, more drug gets absorbed and delivered to the target organ. With poor bioavailability, most of those milligrams will end up in the municipal sewer system. It is the interplay between dose and bioavailability that determines the maximum amount of drug that can get to the target site. On the other side of the coin, drug X will also be subjected to the same sort of mixing and metabolizing described above, the body's mechanisms conspiring to reduce the amount of drug X that remains available to reach the target. The total amount of drug X the target "sees"—the total exposure—is a function of how much gets in minus how much goes out.

Things are a little different when the vehicle for the drug is smoke. Dunn may be the manufacturer, but Helen is in charge of engineering the administration of drug. She is in total control of how much drug ends up at the target site. How? Start with a simple, albeit ludicrous, example: assuming Helen smokes ten cigarettes over ten hours, the brain's exposure depends heavily on whether she has smoked one cigarette per hour or all ten in the first hour followed by a nine-hour break. Using another, slightly less ludicrous example and assuming the same ten cigarettes, exposure depends just as much on whether Helen takes ten or twenty puffs from each cigarette. And in a final example, which is extremely common and clinically relevant, total exposure depends on whether Helen takes ten tiny puffs from each cigarette or ten big, deep, luxurious puffs. The point is that Helen subtly controls her exposure, hour by hour, puff by puff, by unconsciously changing a few variables that are difficult to track without direct observation.

Variables like puff frequency, puff volume, depth of inhalation, and duration of breath hold all affect the degree of exposure Helen's alveoli have to gas-phase nicotine, and as a result, Helen holds a few important cards when determining how much nicotine makes it up to her brain. The term "smoking topography" has been used to describe the "shape," the peaks and valleys, of smoke exposure. The topographical characteristics of Helen's smoking behaviors are a better indicator of exposure, both to nicotine and toxicants, than a simple count of number of cigarettes. Topography changes as the measured nicotine metabolism rate changes; faster metabolism increases total smoke exposure. And as puff volumes go up and inter-puff interval goes down, biochemical markers of toxicant absorption, like blood levels of carbon monoxide, serum levels of cotinine, and urine concentrations of carcinogens, also rise. In fact, smokers who switch to low-yield cigarette brands may not change the number of cigarettes consumed daily, but they will alter topographic characteristics of their smoking in order to achieve similar blood levels of nicotine, a compensatory phenomenon responsible for the surgeon general's warning that light cigarettes are not to be considered less harmful. Topography also predicts response to nicotine replacement therapy in both adults and adolescents and appears to be related to a person's long-term risk for cardiac disease.

Even in the ludicrous thought experiment wherein there are two identical smokers, with exactly the same biology, exactly the same antecedent life experience, using the exact same brand of cigarettes exactly twenty times daily, it remains the unique manner in which each interacts with their cigarette that will influence their unique ability to abstain.

> *Optimization Rule #6: To keep them smoking,*
> *give them the ability to titrate smoke.*

Chapter 6 Learning Points

- The cigarette may look simple, but it is actually a highly engineered nicotine delivery device, maximized to produce the greatest and most reliable impact on the user.
- The cigarette is engineered to facilitate bolus delivery of nicotine. Phasic stimulation of cholinergic neurons results in amplified dopaminergic activity downstream. Tonic delivery results in receptor downregulation.
- The cigarette is designed to maximize the proportion of nicotine that is volatilized from tobacco in the gas phase. Gas allows delivery to the distal lung, where bioavailability is very high. More gas phase also decreases the "apparent" nicotine content of the aerosol.
- Ammonization (among other base additives) adjusts the pH of the smoke, increasing the proportion of nicotine released in the free-base form.
- Free-base nicotine becomes protonated when it interacts with water in the airway: its small size, effect on the permeability of tight junctions between cells, and affinity for active transporter proteins carry the molecule quickly across the otherwise impermeable blood-brain barrier.
- Check the urine for the minor alkaloid anabasine to determine whether the cotinine you found is there because of smoking or because of the pharmacologic management of tobacco dependence.

- Ventilation holes in the cigarette are engineered to dilute the smoke and produce a pleasant user experience. Don't forget that users cover up the ventilation holes to modify impact.
- The number of cigarettes consumed per day may not accurately reflect the total exposure to nicotine and toxicants. The topographic characteristics of smoking are related to severity of dependence and response to treatment.

Part II

Knowing "How"

Chapter 7
Approach

I asked my doctor if I could get the nicotine gum again because it worked in the past. She told me I wasn't quite ready yet. She told me not to worry because I would be ready in due time.

—Belinda C., 37 years old

David looks over his schedule for the day—twenty-eight patients and Helen is his first. When he enters the room, he notices that her appearance has changed markedly since her last appointment. Helen appears disheveled; her clothes are wrinkled, and she has dark circles under her eyes. As they begin talking, Helen tells him, "I have not able to arrange physical therapy. Between the bad weather and my hip, I am spending more time inside, so my days are long." But she was very happy to report that she has been smoking fewer cigarettes. Initially, David is happy to hear this and praises her: "That is great, Helen. Five cigarettes! You can get from five to zero." However, despite that encouraging news, something did not seem right with Helen. It occurred to David that his conversations with Helen about smoking were relatively limited to whether or not she was still smoking. The answer was always yes; therefore, he always reminded her how important it was for her to quit. Year after year he witnessed the harsh deterioration of her lungs as she continued to smoke, and nothing ever really changed. Before moving on to her next issue, he pauses to ask her how she was able to cut down. As Helen describes the local corner store and her ability to buy loose cigarettes, and the panic that sets in as she thinks about being without her cigarettes, David realizes there is a lot more to Helen's smoking story than he knew or had ever bothered to ask about.

———

Helen smokes because nicotine exposure created the conditions for a compulsive disorder. Ambivalence defines Helen's core experience; impulsivity and negative emotion make it hard for her to even have a conversation about stopping. It is hard for David to know how to proceed without undermining their relationship. Instinctively, David wants to motivate Helen to commit to quitting, but when he tries, he can almost feel her subtly moving further from his goal. It's like that magnet game he used to play as a child: the closer one magnet gets to touching the other, the stronger the invisible repellent force becomes, pushing the second magnet across the table in every which direction. When those two magnets are forced to come together, it is only a matter of time before one is released and goes skittering away, at a distance greater than at the start.

> *This happens until the magnets' polarities are reversed.*
> *At that point, the game changes.*

Meeting force with force is counterproductive. A smoker's addiction can't be wrestled to the ground; it has to be dealt with diplomatically. To be an effective clinician in the face of an intractable problem like this, it is necessary to find a way to curb the instinct to motivate, to avoid the lure of righteousness, and to withstand the trap of a dramatic ultimatum. It is worth repeating here: force against force is counterproductive.

> *Don't give them a mirror. Give them a magnet.*
> *Reverse the polarities.*

The easiest and most satisfying way to gain access to the part of patients that would like to quit smoking is to avoid focusing exclusively on the goal of quitting. That may initially sound counterintuitive. However, in the competition for Helen's attention, David's biggest competitor is Helen's threat detection system. It makes some sense to avoid triggering this significant obstacle right out of the starting gate. Helping Helen to stop smoking is always the objective, the destination David is always moving toward. But a focus on quitting simply may not be the best tactic when initiating work on the problem. Instead, focusing on understanding the nature of the patient's compulsion to smoke is much less threatening and often much more revealing. Separate the goal from the process, and work to find intermediate points of control available to each patient. But how?

Have a conversation with a smoker about their smoking, one that avoids discussing health consequences or ways to quit, a conversation in which the smoker has an opportunity to answer questions honestly, a conversation they enjoy.

Taking a Smoking History

In order to reverse the polarities, the clinician needs a robust picture of the depth and severity of the patient's tobacco dependence. Consequently, the history-taking repertoire has to go well beyond questions of "how much?" and "how long?" It is important to understand the patient's entire experience with dependence in order to begin to identify potential opportunities for helping and to note any significant obstacles to progress. A thorough smoking history serves not only as an inventory of tobacco-related facts but also as a peek at the patient's backstory. As in movies and literature, the backstory is the part of the patient's narrative that drives motives and decisions. The backstory—unlike the front story, which is often offered freely—is slowly revealed, usually in smaller chunks. Understanding the patient's backstory is critical to developing trust and avoiding recommendations that run counter to the patient's priorities.

Many providers will feel a strong incentive to interrupt the story the moment the patient reveals a previously held misconception or discloses a past success with some particular intervention. It is common to feel an impulse to interject and get right to the point in pursuit of the goal. Avoid this temptation. Ask questions, and leave the answers for later. Take some time to develop a fuller insight. Not only will the information be helpful at the moment, but it could prove critical to developing modifications to the plan later in the course of care. With practice, providers will develop their own rhythm, one that gives them the information they need in the manner they need it to be both efficient and effective. To start with, here is a simple mnemonic to give some structure. Remember the big brown truck and think, U*P*P*S*S, or Use, Past, Psych, Substance, Smokers.

Sample Questions

USE

Initial Use Questions

How old were you when you took your first puff? What was it like?

Who introduced you to smoking? What were the circumstances of your first cigarette?

What brand did you use when you started? Menthol? Do you use the same brand now?

How long did it take to become an everyday smoker?

Current Use Questions

How many cigarettes do you use in a day? Do you ever relight a cigarette?
How long after you wake up in the morning do you have your first ciga-
*   rette?*
What's the maximum smoked daily? Minimum?
Tell me about the times in the day that you smoke? What are your rou-
*   tines then?*
Who do you smoke with?
What brand do you use? Where do you get them?
Have you ever bought a loosie (individual, unpackaged cigarette)?
Have you ever done something embarrassing to get a smoke?

PAST

Past Quit Attempt Questions

Have you ever tried quitting? How long ago?
Have you ever gone more than a day without smoking? What were the
*   circumstances?*
What's the longest period you've gone without smoking?
When was your most recent quit attempt?
Tell me about what happened that brought you back to smoking.
Have you ever used anything to help you quit? Patches? Pills?
How did you feel while you weren't smoking? Did you feel sad? Angry?
Given your past experience, how confident are you that you can quit
*   smoking?*
What will keep you from quitting?
How does talking about quitting make you feel?
What worries you the most about quitting?

PSYCH

Potential Psychiatric Moderators

Any history of depression or anxiety? Panic disorder? Bipolar disorder?
Have you ever been treated with medication for any conditions like these?
How did you do in school?
Have you ever been tested for attention deficit disorder?
Would you say you're an impulsive person? Give me an example.

SUBSTANCE

Substance Use History

Have you ever used cocaine or methamphetamine?
Heroin or other narcotics? Alcohol? Marijuana?
Have you ever been treated for a substance use disorder?
How long ago was your last use?
Tell me about your recovery experience.
What did you learn in recovery that might seem applicable to smoking?
Describe your ability to stop smoking compared to your ability to stop using [other]?

SMOKERS

Household Smoking Questions

Do you smoke indoors? Where?
Does anyone else at home smoke? Who?
Do they know you're interested in quitting?
Do you smoke together? What are your shared routines?
Have you discussed how they might help you quit?
Do your friends smoke when they come to visit?
Do you think people are willing to move all the smoking to outside your house?

Affective Presence

The process of coming to a decision is intuitive and involves weighing the pros and cons of a particular choice. In a strictly utilitarian world, there's a balance between the price of a new car and functional metrics like anticipated miles per gallon, expected longevity, and the comprehensiveness of the warranty. However, emotion also plays a role in this decision. When the prospective buyer can imagine sitting behind the steering wheel on a beautiful day, sunglasses on, the window open and the radio playing, it is often enough to tip the balance in favor of purchase, even if utilitarian calculations do not align.

Given the complexity of the instinctive drive to smoke and the emotional efficiency of the threat detection system, the emotional context David creates during his visit with Helen becomes an important tool for reversing the polarities and bringing about change. The right emotions can amplify Helen's intrinsic motivations and reduce instinctive disincentives, while the wrong emotions can severely skew her decision balance in the opposite direction. Therefore, it becomes incumbent on providers to fastidiously tend to the positive emotions we are creating in the clinic the way a surgeon tends to maintain sterility in the operating room. To be clear, this is not an endorsement of gratuitous cheerleading or an accommodation of continued smoking, but rather an acknowledgment that David's effectiveness is not solely a function of his recommendations but equally a function of how they are presented.

> **It is not just what. It is also how.**

Clinicians are generally given the benefit of the doubt and are accorded a level of professional authority in recognition of their training and experience. It is the expertise heuristic. However, that privileged position is fragile. Just as our opportunities lie within the social norms of the clinic, our weakness is inherent to our custom of providing authoritative direction quickly. The initial evaluation represents a fleeting opportunity to solidify our relationship with the patient by paying attention to a few simple rules.

Approach Rule #1:
Interaction style builds trust. Trust is everything.

For a relationship between provider and patient to have inherent therapeutic value, both parties need to have agency during the interaction. From the patient's perspective, a natural power imbalance is already built into the relationship: they are the one with vulnerabilities, while the provider is the one with the potential solutions. This is particularly true for patients who smoke because they have often been made to feel marginalized by their community and harassed by previous healthcare providers. Minimizing this imbalance maximizes the therapeutic nature of the relationship. To do so, think about

- *Suspending moral judgment.* It is easy to conflate feelings about the person who smokes with feelings about smoking. As the smoking behavior has become increasingly delegitimized, the effects of that stigma can occasionally bleed into the clinic visit. When it presents itself, work to minimize the patient's shame. Adopt an advocacy stance and avoid falling into adversarial traps.
- *Demonstrating an appreciation of the suffering caused by nicotine.* Focus on the burdens of ambivalence, not simply on the health impact of smoking. From that perspective, it is possible to also demonstrate an understanding of our own contribution to the suffering. This is especially important when we are helping

patients who may have had uncomfortable interactions with other healthcare workers in the past.

- *Communicating an appreciation of the environmental context.* Continued smoking despite an interest in quitting is frequently thwarted by environmental factors that may lie just beyond the patient's control: an outdoor job surrounded by smoking colleagues, a store on the corner that sells "loosies." Recognizing these influences and validating their impact on continued smoking is an important prerequisite for agency.

Nonverbal communication is equally important. Remember that when what you say doesn't match how you say it, the nonverbal message will always land more persuasively.

- *Initial attachment.* Body position, touch, eye contact, and warmth of facial expression are examples of subtle but powerful indicators of your connection to the patient. Particularly in the era of electronic record keeping, it is common for clinicians to prioritize the burdensome practicalities of an encounter. Though intermittent pauses to take notes or refer to the record are certainly expected, be sure to turn toward your patients and engage them directly when they speak.
- *Genuineness.* Within medical practice, professionalism and constant positive regard for patients are the overarching principles of good clinical care. But within those parameters, remember that you should strive to be authentic. If humor is part of who you are, use it. If your patient's visit is unexpected, acknowledge it. If you are struggling to understand the message your patient is sending, ask about it. If an especially human moment presents itself, do not be afraid to express your humanity. Avoid adopting a manufactured demeanor or emulating a character that you've been led to believe you should be.

Approach Rule #2:
Boost your effectiveness with four magic words.

Struggling to find just the right turn of phrase to influence Helen's decision is a strategy too often based on the faulty assumption of motivational deficit and has the real potential to undermine the trust you've garnered so far. Instead, the clinician's soft power resides in communicating four important ideas that work together to reduce the disincentive to change.

- *Empathy.* Defined as the ability to place yourself in another person's shoes and show that you share their feelings, empathy is not the kind of thing you can easily express directly without undermining genuineness. Empathy is most appropriately expressed indirectly, through questioning, facial expression, reframing of the narrative, or relating previous experiences.

- *Joining.* At times, addressing tobacco dependence in the clinic can take on a well-intentioned but coercive character. David quite literally needs Helen to quit. The desire to stimulate change can be so intense that it may be tempting to try to convince your patient to stop smoking. Unfortunately, the obvious persuasive intent can easily become a source of dissatisfaction and loss of agency for both clinician and patient. Rather, by framing the effects of nicotine as the problem to be solved, it is easier to adopt the role of true advocate and join with your patient to sequentially solve problems. Once again, advocacy implies neither capitulation nor acceptance of smoking. In the clinic, it means accepting your patient with respect, as a person with a problem to be addressed. Effective joining means you're not getting anybody to do anything: you're just doing what you went to school to do.

- *Validation.* You can't be adversarial and therapeutic at the same time. Try to imagine the experience of subjective ambivalence, the implications of marginalization. It is conceivable that many smokers have been made to feel that their smoking is somehow a function of character flaw—that they, rather than their behavior, are somehow not quite acceptable. By validating their malposition, by suggesting that their predicament makes sense given what you understand about the effect of nicotine on the brain, you instantly create a positive, therapeutic dynamic. Validation alleviates shame. Validation denies purchase for blame. Validation emphasizes joint responsibility and deemphasizes justifications without accommodating continued smoking.

- *Hope.* The importance of this last magic word cannot be overstated. Tobacco dependence is a problem of learned hopelessness. Tobacco dependence is an entire lifetime of taking a step closer to quitting only to panic and step away. It is a problem of a thousand futile tomorrows, of trying a patch or a pill and having it not work, of coming to the conclusion that there is nothing new, nothing untried, and nothing that's going to help. To solve the problem, the problem must be solvable.

The "Framing" Paradox

Helen has a problem with breathing. David knows that's not a good sign: she's only going to get worse if she continues to smoke. There's a certain amount of urgency to quitting since David would like to preserve as much of Helen's lung function as possible. Imagine David says, "If you don't stop smoking, you will die a miserable death." Clearly, David is relying on the negative consequences of continued smoking to motivate Helen's decision to quit by focusing her attention on what she stands to lose. *Loss framing* depends on creating negative emotions to persuade toward a goal. He's hoping that by supplementing the unambiguous "will die" with the dramatic adjective miserable, he can increase the pressure to quit.

Imagine David recognizes negative emotions tend to repel an audience from a message, while positive messages are often more attractive. He may instead say, "Your breathing problem will get better if you stop smoking now." David has recognized that presenting the potential for "getting better" is likely to be attractive to Helen. *Gain framing* typically depends on highlighting the potential benefits of quitting as a persuasive mechanism. David is hoping that by supplementing the emphasis on health improvement with an encouraging smile, he can increase the attractiveness of change.

But because Helen is ambivalent, the notion of quitting is experienced *as both a gain and a loss.* Gain framing that relies exclusively on positive health benefits can be counterbalanced by the deep loss salience of abstinence. Helen remains stuck between the side of her that wants desperately to quit and the side of her that is desperate not to quit. To help Helen, gain framing in the clinic should also emphasize the benefits of resolving ambivalence. By focusing Helen's attention on relieving the subjective distress of ambivalence, she can escape the judgment of others, begin to mend her self respect and finally shrug off the weight of hesitancy.

The Way Adults Learn

In earlier chapters, an argument was made that abstinence from smoking is not simply the absence of smoking but rather gaining control of the compulsion to smoke, which may require developing a new set of skills. In contrast to didactic instruction, during which the transfer of information is generally unidirectional, adults often learn best when offered opportunities for experiential learning or through reflection on doing. Experiential learning is iterative, breaks down larger tasks into smaller components, and depends on building progressively more integrated, concrete experiences. It focuses learning on the process rather than the goal and depends on an instructional relationship between coach and learner. Isolating specific aspects of the smoking ritual presents opportunities for reflective thinking about ways to modify those routines. From there, the patient can more easily build an abstract conceptualization of how a typical day might proceed. Patients can be encouraged to actively experiment with some of these new concepts, which in turn generate more concrete experiences. The cycle never stops, with patients constantly encouraged to learn something new and do something a little different. In experiential learning, the learner is involved in the experience and is using analytical skills to solve problems. When clinicians serve as coach, focused on creating opportunities for experiential learning, the concept of success versus failure becomes anachronistic as the real question becomes, "Is my patient moving closer to the goal?"

Chapter 7 Learning Points

- Force on force is counterproductive. Instead, reverse the polarities, and rely on attractive pull to create change.
- Ask questions instead of giving answers. Let the backstory emerge.
- A full, robust smoking history offers unexpected insights into the balance between the patient's motivations and disincentives to change. This information is important to developing a stepwise plan and may help guide future management decisions.
- A structured approach to history taking allows for efficiency and reproducibility. The most effective questioning is conversational rather than rote. Remember the big brown truck, and think Use, Past, Psych, Substance, and Smokers (U*P*P*S*S).
- The clinician's affective presence is a therapeutic tool. Trust is everything: both verbal and nonverbal communication build (and undermine) trust.
- Empathy, Joining, Validation and Hope are the four magic words that reduce the disincentive to change. Patients will want to change for you, not because of you.
- Appropriate gain framing focuses on relieving the burden of subjective ambivalence.
- Adults learn best when clinicians create opportunities for experiential learning. Learning new skills is often iterative and sometimes relies on taking progressive intermediate steps toward the larger goal.

Chapter 8
Escape

I gave up giving up.

Cecilia S., 61 years old

"This is the most I've ever talked about my smoking with Dr. Smith," Helen thought. Kathy and Helen spent many nights analyzing their love-hate relationship with cigarettes, but Helen never really considered how much of her day revolved around smoking: planning her next cigarette, regretting her last cigarette, and the actual time smoking in between. As they continue talking, Dr. Smith suggests that she pick a quit day and start using the patch. Suddenly she feels a knot in her stomach. She reminds him, "I've tried everything. Patches, gum, that pill. Nothing works for me." Fighting back the tears, she says, "I am trying my best to cut down. This is the best I can do. I am not going to add more nicotine to my body when I have been working so hard to use less." She wishes that she never mentioned the five cigarettes. She thought he would be happy with her progress, but now she has to pick a day and the only day that seems remotely feasible is Monday, the 15th—of next year.

———

By establishing a positive affective presence, clinicians set the stage for patients to feel more comfortable taking relatively safe interpersonal risks. Maybe that means they will feel freer to discuss their anxieties in anticipation of quitting, or maybe it means they will test out a series of compromise positions in search of their clinician's blessing. Often, it simply means patients find it increasingly possible to engage their clinician with honesty and respect—and will voice their authentic reluctance to quit. When clinicians interpret reluctance as an unpalatable expression of autonomy rather than the natural and expected expression of ambivalence, they can find themselves acquiescing to the uncertainty or, worse, becoming personally disappointed in their patients.

There is an important misconception that warrants clarification at this juncture. Reluctance to quit is not an indication of being "precontemplative." In the transtheoretical model of behavior change, patients move through several distinct stages of change as they move toward their new behavioral goal. A person in the process of change begins as precontemplative, then becomes contemplative when considering the requirements for change. Contemplation gives way to preparation, which leads to action, which in turn leads to maintenance of the new target behavior. It is conceivable that patients exist who smoke but who have yet to consider the advantages of a status change to nonsmoker. Those individuals would be considered precontemplative. What is overwhelmingly more likely is that by reporting "I'm not ready to quit," those patients are actually paraphrasing a more complex articulation of ambivalence: "After careful consideration, my instincts have led me to believe this is a bad idea, and I suddenly feel anxious about the implications of this conversation. Therefore, I am reluctant to embark on an abstinence attempt at this time." In this situation, "I'm not ready" suggests that the patients have clearly thought through personal motivations and disincentives and have concluded that, on balance, they do not yet find themselves to be aligned with their clinician's point of view. In this case, it is egocentric to imagine that an opposing preference implies a lack of reflection on the matter. Stages of change are only relevant when change is at least possible. Until the conditions necessary for change are met, attention to stage is nonsensical.

When change does happen, human psychology tends to focus us most intently on the elements that are changing rather than emphasizing all that has stayed the same. Of course, it makes teleological sense for the brain's attentional mechanisms to design a system that focuses on the few blades of grass that are unexpectedly moving while ignoring all those that remain still. Unfortunately, humans are also exquisitely good at anticipating the impact of change that has not yet occurred. This has the counterproductive effect of focusing patients' attention entirely on the deficiencies expected with their future quit attempt, even before any actual change is undertaken. This overemphasis on the anticipated impact of abstinence results in undue magnification of the negative effects of quitting and significantly undervalues the fact that the majority of daily life will remain the same, despite the loss of nicotine. The tendency to succumb to impact bias leads patients to fall victim to affective forecasting errors—an overestimation of the future toll of quitting—which induces a pernicious retreat.

Approach-Avoidance

The ambivalence experience leads to a behavioral manifestation referred to as approach-avoidance. Imagine Helen's smoking behavior exists somewhere on a continuum between complete abstinence and uninhibited smoking (Figure 8.1).

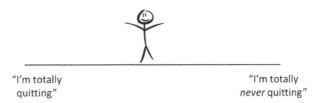

"I'm totally
quitting"

"I'm totally
never quitting"

Figure 8.1. Continuum representing opposing smoking goals.

In this situation, Helen obviously can't get closer to quitting without getting further from not quitting. As she takes steps closer to her quitting goal, the tension inherent to moving further from her not-quitting goal progressively increases, until Helen finds herself disengaging and getting pulled back toward her earlier behaviors. This is true regardless of which direction Helen seeks to move; Helen never fully commits to one side or the other because a commitment to abstinence is instinctively threatening while a forthright commitment to a lifetime of unrestrained smoking is daunting (Figure 8.2).

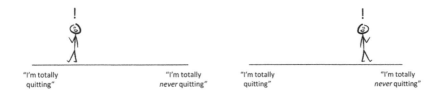

"I'm totally
quitting"

"I'm totally
never quitting"

"I'm totally
quitting"

"I'm totally
never quitting"

Figure 8.2. Representation of approach-avoidance behavior patterns. Movement toward either goal is simultaneous movement away from the opposing goal.

Approach-avoidance behaviors are the cardinal sign of dependence. When they remain unrecognized for what they represent, they can easily become a source of frustration for clinicians. Keep in mind that approach-avoidance behaviors are not the equivalent of indecision; patients cannot be motivated to get closer to their goal without increasing the pull from the other side. Rather, approach-avoidance is best conceived of as the cardinal sign of the duality of mind caused by nicotine's effects on the mesolimbic system (Table 8.1).

Table 8.1. Relationship between the underlying pathologic mechanism of tobacco dependence and the resulting cardinal manifestations in the clinic.

Pathology	Cardinal Symptom	Cardinal Sign	Chief Complaint
Mesolimbic distortion	Ambivalence	Approach-avoidance	Reluctance

Escape and Sabotage

There are typical behavioral derivatives of approach-avoidance that commonly manifest when discussing tobacco dependence. Escape is a behavioral strategy employed by dependent patients to help them resolve the otherwise irresolvable conflict between opposing goals. Escape takes many forms and is almost always structured as autonomous decision-making. It manifests both in anticipation and throughout the process of quit attempts (Table 8.2).

Table 8.2. Examples of commonly employed escape strategies—mechanisms for resolving the conflict between the rational and instinctive drives.

Anticipatory Escape	Example
Acquiesce	"Yes, I know. I already quit. This morning."
Delay	"I can't think about that now. I have too much going on."
Decline	"I'm fine quitting, but I'd rather do it without using any medications."
Past failure	"I've tried everything in the past. Nothing worked."
Health concern	"I can't afford to gain weight."
Compromise	"I'll switch to electronic cigarettes."

Transition Escape	Example
Alternative approach	"I always thought hypnosis would work for me."
Sudden stressor	"I did try to stop after you asked me, but then my nephew got on my nerves."
Home smoker	"I'll quit when he does."
Health concern	"I know people who develop lung cancer after they quit smoking."
Outside advice	"My neighbor said . . . "
Harm reduction	"I smoke less now than I did in the past. I'm happy here."

On occasion, the prospect of abstinence is so relentlessly threatening to the patient that escape takes on a particularly malignant quality, referred to as sabotage. In this case, the objective is not simply to find a means of resolving conflict but rather an attempt to shut down further conversation about the prospect of change. Like simple escape, sabotage may also be expressed as autonomous control. Sometimes, however, the patient projects the source of their anticipatory anxiety onto the provider, which can make for a tense exchange if misunderstood (Table 8.3).

Table 8.3. A framework for recognizing sabotage. Sabotage is a form of escape aimed at curtailing disquieting conversation.

Autonomous Sabotage	Example
Enjoyment	"I like smoking. I don't want to stop."
Indifference	"I don't care if it kills me. Everyone dies of something."
Expertise	"I quit before, and I'll do it again . . . when I want to."
Balance	"I'm in recovery and don't want to start craving again."
Last vice	"I've got nothing left."
Deflection	"I came here for advice on ___, not for my smoking."

(Table 8.3 continued)

Projection Sabotage	Example
Fallacy	"Doctors blame everything on smoking."
Déjà vu	"Everyone who walks in here says the same thing. I've heard it all before."
Alternative source	"I've done my research. Vaping is definitely safer than smoking."
Misadventure	"You tried to kill me with that stuff! I'm never doing that again."
Finance	"I can't. Do you know how much I spend on medicines already?"
Overprescription	"You people think everything is solved with medicine."
Aggression	"Stop pushing me!"
Control	"Here's one thing I can control. I can leave."

Benevolent Persuasion

Every nicotine-dependent person is reluctant to change. That is a given. Reluctance should not be experienced as a barrier to clinical intervention but instead as the chief complaint to be addressed through interventions. The process by which clinicians cognitively manage reluctance is most accurately characterized as benevolent persuasion and differs from clinical counseling and psychotherapy in that there is consistent, gentle direction toward a pre-specified goal. Benevolent persuasion is a social good in this context, ensuring patients retain agency and free choice within clinical visits, while clinicians' decision-making remains pointed exclusively at accruing benefit to the patients.

Benevolent persuasion requires that clinicians systematically

- anticipate and respond to escape,
- work to eliminate or resolve the patient's barriers to change, and
- minimize the impact of affective forecasting error by reminding patients of all that remains the same after quitting.

Benevolent persuasion is an iterative process within which clinicians may need to adjust their goals—sometimes accepting only baby steps toward abstinence—in order to best align their therapeutic objectives with the realities of the patient's dependence. Paradoxically, patients with the most severe manifestations of nicotine addiction may be exactly the ones who require the gentlest and most patient approach. Redefining success, away from the monolithic and imposing "quit," and finding a path forward through intermediate steps—repeated as often as necessary—may in fact be best suited to a patient's needs.

Every patient is unique. Sometimes benevolent persuasion brings the provider to a destination where a quit attempt is likely by the end of the visit. Other times, it can mean accepting a temporary compromise. Compromise is therapeutic if it creates a future advantage; compromise is abdication if, as a matter of expedience, it accommodates continued smoking. This distinction is important.

The Rhythm of Execution

When put all together, these ideas coalesce into a very simple, three-step clinical rhythm for engaging ambivalent patients. First, listen carefully to their concerns, remembering to ask questions instead of giving answers. As patients progressively reveal the nature of their reluctance to abstain, the clinician works to *validate* that concern. Again, validation does not mean accommodation or capitulation. It means finding a way to express empathy and understanding of the nature of the obstacle (Table 8.4).

Table 8.4. The difference between adversarial and validating responses to common sources of reluctance. Finding ways to validate the patient's concerns without aquiescing to continued smoking can be the difference between a visit that is productive and one that undermines trust and confidence.

Reluctance	Adversarial Response	Validating Response
"I already quit. This morning."	"You haven't quit until you've gone thirty days without smoking."	"Great! How did you get it done?"
"I have too much going on."	"Never too soon to quit."	"Yes, I see. That is quite a lot."

(Table 8.4 continued)

Reluctance	Adversarial Response	Validating Response
"I'd rather do it without using any medications."	"Medications make it more likely that you will quit."	"Lots of people feel the same way."
"I've tried everything in the past. Nothing worked."	"It takes eleven tries before a person quits."	"I imagine that's frustrating."
"I can't afford to gain weight."	"You can gain thirty pounds before it is as bad for you as smoking."	"I don't want you to gain weight."

Second, notice that the adversarial responses have the unintended effect of quickly transforming the conversation into a smoking standoff, where neither party can easily proceed or back away without ego injury or humiliation. Instead, harness the therapeutic value of the natural flow of communication by being prepared to *reframe* the conversation so that it directly addresses the source of reluctance the patient just expressed (Table 8.5).

Table 8.5. Reframing strategies employed in the face of common expressions of reluctance.

Reluctance	Step 1: Validate	Step 2: Reframe
"I already quit. This morning."	"Great! How did you get it done?"	"Now all we need is a way to help you keep doing so well."
"I have too much going on."	"Yes, I see. That is quite a lot."	"I have an idea that won't add to your burden."
"I'd rather do it without using any medications."	"Lots of people feel the same way."	"Let's think of some things we can do without starting meds."

"I've tried everything in the past. Nothing worked."	"I imagine that's frustrating."	"Sometimes it is about the way we use the medications. Let's review."
"I can't afford to gain weight."	"I don't want you to gain weight."	"We'll manage your weight, and make sure it is not going up."

Each time the clinician anticipates and eliminates an escape route, the goal of abstinence becomes increasingly likely to attain. The patient need not move closer to the goal; the goal gets closer to wherever the patient is located. The balance is shifted in favor of an abstinence attempt (Figure 8.3).

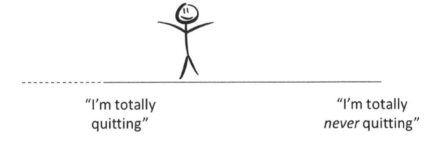

| "I'm totally quitting" | "I'm totally *never* quitting" |

Figure 8.3. Resolving ambivalence by addressing escape.

The third step recognizes that the tensions intrinsic to approach-avoidance are likely to increase as the patient moves ever closer to engaging the quitting goal. By *repeating* the first and second steps in an iterative fashion, clinicians begin to create the conditions for change and then facilitate the change as it tends to itself. Here is an example of a possible conversation:

CLINICIAN. I'd like to talk to you about tobacco dependence.

RELUCTANT PATIENT. Yes, I know. I already quit. This morning.

CLINICIAN. Hey! That's great! How did you get it done? I'm so proud of you. [Validate]
Now, all we need is a way to help you keep doing so well. [Reframe]

PATIENT. I'm actually fine quitting this time. I really want to do it without using any medications.

CLINICIAN. [Repeat] That's understandable. Lots of people feel the same way. [Validate]
Let's think of some things we can do without starting meds. [Reframe]

PATIENT. I can't think about that now. I have too much going on.

CLINICIAN. [Repeat] Yes, I can see that. Things have been quite difficult for you lately. [Validate]
I have some ideas that won't add to your burden. [Reframe]

PATIENT. I've tried everything in the past. Nothing worked.

CLINICIAN. [Repeat] I imagine that's frustrating. [Validate]
Sometimes it is about the way we use them. Let's review. [Reframe]

PATIENT. OK, but I really can't afford to gain weight. Last time I gained fifteen pounds.

CLINICIAN. [Repeat] I don't want you to gain weight. [Validate]
We'll watch over your weight together and make sure it doesn't go up. [Reframe]

PATIENT. What did you have in mind? [Contemplation]

Resistance Is Not Reluctance

The conversation could have had a much different feel if the patient began by sabotaging further conversation. This more dramatic version of the smoking standoff shows how clinicians have been traditionally taught to review the relevance of quitting to the patient's health and then wait for them to change their mind.

CLINICIAN. I'd like to talk to you about tobacco dependence.

RESISTANT PATIENT. I like smoking. I don't want to stop.

CLINICIAN. It is important that you quit smoking. Let me know when you are ready.

But how should clinicians respond when the patient doesn't want to talk about smoking? Remember that the responsibility for creating the conditions for change lies with clinicians, not dependent patients. If sabotage is recognized not as a disagreeable character flaw but as the manifestation of a visceral threat to survival, it is easier for clinicians to appreciate that today's resistance may be the product of cumulative pressures exerted during previous tobacco interactions. Smokers have heard it all before. Resistance is a fiercer expression of the threat response, whereas reluctance is a routine demonstration of anticipatory anxiety.

Consider resistance to be a function of interaction style. Imagine the impact of a lifetime of ineluctable, compulsive smoking in the face of predictable admonishment from every acquaintance. If true, then savvy clinicians can expect to create a counterbalancing impact by unexpectedly "flipping" the predicted interaction style 180 degrees. It becomes the clinician's job to avoid meeting resistance head-on and instead adjust to the resistance in order to create conditions in which change is less threatening. Adjusting to resistance is not the same as giving in or giving up. It is about rolling with that resistance while trying to understand why the resistance is there, keeping the conversation going long enough to find a "toehold."

In the face of resistance, a clinician's only momentary goal is to have a conversation that the patient enjoys. Remembering the four magic words and avoiding the temptation to monopolize the conversation are critical to bringing down the protective barriers the patient has erected. The goal is to create a discussion rather than forcing movement toward a particular behavioral goal. By first establishing an intrinsically therapeutic relationship with the patient, the clinician establishes basic trust and a respect for the patient's autonomy that will soon begin to facilitate change. It bears repeating: clinicians cannot meet force with force. Patients cannot be made to change through force of will. When managing a resistant patient, the only decisions that remain within the clinician's locus of control relate to interaction style. As the therapeutic relationship grows, so too grows the probability that change will come.

The rhythm for managing resistance involves the same three steps, repeated as needed until the conditions for change are created: validate, reframe, repeat. The content is the only thing that changes. With resistant patients, instead of validating their concerns about quitting, clinicians should focus on validating patients' autonomy. Finding ways to convey respect for their agency is critical. Reaffirming their intrinsic right to self-determination is a first step in reversing the cumulative effect of years of outside insistence.

After validating respect for autonomy, now what? Are clinicians to passively wait for autonomous change to happen? No. When facing resistance, the reframe step focuses on directing the conversation away from quitting and toward topics that allow the patient to speak about their autonomy in the context of previous experiences. As the conversation becomes less adversarial and the patient becomes more comfortable, at some point a conversational toehold will be offered. Like a rock-climbing toehold, a conversational toehold allows enough purchase to avoid "falling" while planning the next move. Patience is needed since the toehold may not reveal itself right away and doesn't guarantee success. But just like on the rock face, it can provide a temporary repose and dramatically increase the chance of eventual success.

After validating the patient's autonomy and reframing to nonthreatening conversation, the clinician can use the toehold to reinforce the patient's autonomy by offering to take a small step on the patient's behalf. That is, the clinician offers to help the patient meet self-imposed goals and is ready to repeat as necessary until a mutual agreement is achieved.

CLINICIAN. I'd like to talk to you about tobacco dependence.

RESISTANT PATIENT. I like smoking. I don't want to stop.

CLINICIAN. I don't blame you. Smoking smooths everything out.
[Validate]
Sometimes people don't recognize how important smoking can be in stressful situations. [Reframe]
I can help explain the connection to your spouse if that would help. What do you think? [Reinforce]

PATIENT. I think you people blame everything on smoking.

CLINICIAN. [Repeat] I've seen that happen. [Validate]
It's kind of a shame when people harp on that idea. [Reframe]

PATIENT. Everyone who walks in here says the same thing. I've heard it all before.

CLINICIAN. [Repeat] Ugh! How annoying that must be. [Validate]
Has it happened today? [Reframe]
I will talk to the staff and ask them to back off. OK? [Reinforce]

PATIENT. I don't care if it kills me. Everyone dies of something.

CLINICIAN. [Repeat] I can't deny that! But I don't want to see anything kill you except old age. [Validate]
Have you experimented with ways to reduce the harm to your body? [Reframe]

PATIENT. I've done my research. I'm vaping sometimes. Vaping is definitely safer than smoking. [Toehold]

CLINICIAN. [Repeat] Great that you looked into that. [Validate]
What do you like about vaping? [Reframe]

I think I can get you what you like about vaping without the stuff that hurts the lungs. [Reinforce]

PATIENT. What is it? [Contemplation]

Chapter 8 Learning Points

- Positive affective presence sets the stage. The clinician's intervention is aimed at specifically managing residual (inevitable) reluctance.
- Reluctance to quit is not the same as being precontemplative. Stages of change only become relevant when change becomes possible. The clinician tends to the conditions that promote change.
- Approach-avoidance behavior patterns are the cardinal sign of dependence.
- Escape and sabotage are the behavioral mechanisms that people use to resolve the otherwise irresolvable conflicts intrinsic to ambivalence.
- Benevolent persuasion is a strategic approach to approach-avoidance, wherein clinicians (1) anticipate escape, (2) resolve barriers to change, and (3) minimize affective forecasting error.
- A simple three-step rhythm helps manage reluctance and resistance without acquiescing to continued smoking: (1) validate, (2) reframe, and (3) repeat.
- Resistance stems from the cumulative impact of previous interactions. Benevolent persuasion in the face of resistance means shifting gears away from quitting and working to restore the patient's autonomous control in order to reestablish a therapeutic relationship.

Chapter 9
Medication

Every time I see someone else smoke, I want to smoke because I'm angry they get to smoke and I don't.

—Betty F., 59 years old

Helen sits by her phone waiting for Dr. Smith to call her back. She looks over at her arm and sees the red, irritated skin marking the spots where the patch had been placed. "I knew this would happen," she thinks. "Nothing ever works for me." She wore the patch for one week, and she did not notice any difference in her smoking. In fact, she wanted to smoke more. She took off the patch each night before she sat outside with Kathy. "I am not ready to give up our time together, and I am not taking any chances of having a heart attack if I smoke while wearing the patch," she tells Kathy. When Helen and David discussed side effects of the patch, he suggested changing the placement of the patch each morning. "Now my arm looks ridiculous, covered with these red blotches. I bet the dose was too high," she thinks. Dr. Smith recommended the 14-milligram patch, but now she wonders if she should have tried the 7-milligram patch instead. Finally, the phone rang, and it was Dr. Smith. After describing her weeklong tribulations with the patch, the conversation ended with Dr. Smith relenting: "You had better stop the patch."

———

"If smokers smoke for nicotine, why is nicotine replacement not 100% effective?" It is impossible to overstate how often some version of this question comes up in the clinic. Why? Why do patients and providers alike wonder about this sort of thing when it relates to tobacco dependence but not, for example, when prescribing medications in an asthma clinic? One possible explanation resides in the ways people have been taught to think about the mechanism of pharmacotherapy's action. For example:

- It replaces the source of nicotine so that the cigarette is no longer needed.
- It re-creates the experience of smoking.
- It alleviates the mounting pressure to smoke during abstinence.
- It keeps the smoker calm while they withdraw.
- It makes the cigarette taste bad.
- It makes the desire to smoke disappear.

In reality, none of these things are mechanisms. They are possible effects of tobacco-dependence medications. Most of these effects have been experienced and reported by patients in the past, but two observations call their value as a fundamental mechanism of action into question: (1) none of them have been universally experienced by all patients who achieve abstinence, and (2) it is not necessary for patients to experience any of them in order to achieve the clinical goal. So because they are neither necessary nor sufficient, these classical effects may be viewed as outward signs that a medication is working, but they do not in themselves explain the underlying mechanism of action. Take a look at Figure 9.1, and then review the familiar examples in Table 9.1 that illustrate the construct.

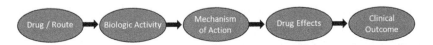

Figure 9.1. Links in chain between drug characteristics and anticipated clinical outcome.

Table 9.1. Examples of the typical framework relating biologic activity, mechanistic effects, and clinical outcomes of a medication.

	Drug/Route	Biologic Activity	Mechanism of Action	Drug Effects	Clinical Outcome
Asthma	Albuterol (inhaled)	Stimulates β-adrenergic receptors	Airway smooth muscle relaxation	Decreased resistance to airflow	Improved shortness of breath

(Table 9.1 continued)

	Drug/Route	Biologic Activity	Mechanism of Action	Drug Effects	Clinical Outcome
Hypertension	Lisinopril (oral)	Inhibits angiotensin-converting enzyme	Decreased vascular smooth muscle tone	Decreased resistance to blood flow	Reduction in blood pressure

When it comes to treating tobacco dependence, the distinction is more than semantic. Several medications have proven efficacy in controlling the compulsion to smoke, and a number of pharmacotherapeutic strategies have proven their effectiveness in achieving abstinence goals in the clinic. Yet many patients, along with a substantial portion of clinicians, continue to pursue abstinence without the assistance of pharmacotherapy. The reasons for this are complicated, but in our experience this phenomenon is at least partly explained by the conflation of these two pharmacologic concepts. Consider for a moment the patient who believes the patch should work by replacing the source of nicotine so that the cigarette is no longer necessary. When the patient continues to feel the connection to smoking, despite using the patch correctly, the utility of continuing the patch becomes less obvious. Consider what happens after David prescribes a pill, anticipating that it would alleviate Helen's pressure to smoke during abstinence. When she returns to smoking on impulse, both parties are likely to be convinced of the medication's ineffectiveness (or worse, Helen's lack of commitment). Finally, consider the insurer who imagines the mechanism of action to be synonymous with drug effect. Because the outward effects of the various drug classes and administration methods can substantially overlap, it is likely the insurer might erroneously assume all tobacco-dependence pharmacotherapies to be therapeutically interchangeable. All these misconceptions have conspired to limit the acceptability, utility, and availability of effective pharmacotherapy.

The role of tobacco-dependence pharmacotherapy is less about producing any particular effect and more about creating conditions within the brain's biochemistry that minimize the distortions in motivational control. It is about changing the pattern of patterns in such a way as to begin restoring the natural balance between drive and control mechanisms. It is not so much about directly creating any particular change but more about creating the conditions that allow change to happen. From this perspective, the mechanism of action common to the entire family of medications could more accurately be described as controlling the compulsion to smoke.

> *Pharmacotherapy is not a substitute for the work of change. Controlling the compulsion to smoke makes the work of change more efficient, with better results.*

By integrating the notion of controlling the compulsion to smoke into the understanding of tobacco-dependence pharmacotherapy, clinicians are better positioned to navigate concepts that might otherwise be difficult to explain. Such situations include

- the observed intra- and interpatient variability in drug effects;
- the need for pharmacotherapy in the absence of withdrawal symptoms;
- the importance of delivery kinetics when anticipating effects;
- the utility of combination pharmacotherapy;
- the observed variability in time to outcome;
- creative management strategies in the face of incomplete effect;
- appropriate—and inappropriate—therapeutic interchanges; and
- perhaps most important, the best ways to manage patient expectations.

Think Probabilistically, Not Linearly

The clinician's responsibility is to be attentive to the conditions necessary for change. Pharmacotherapy is not an answer to smoking but merely a preconditioner, rebalancing the distorted biochemical milieu of the mesolimbic system so that behavior change has a fighting chance. If this is the case, it becomes obvious that the management of tobacco dependence shouldn't be construed as a linear function; there are no "if this" interventions that can guarantee a given smoker any particular "then that" outcome. The clinicians' interventions aren't deterministic phenomena but rather a series of incremental nudges that alter probabilities in favor of quitting. This approach requires thinking probabilistically.

To understand the inherent power of probabilistic thinking, begin by imagining a process of quitting defined by several key steps, or "states." For example, imagine that a patient who becomes motivated to make an abstinence attempt has full freedom to decide the next step moving forward. That motivation may turn out to have been a passing inclination or may lead to taking a step in the direction of abstinence. If action is initiated, imagine that a period of early abstinence begins. Also imagine that for some patients a bit of iterative work is required before early abstinence is fully accomplished, during which the patient experiences momentary slips or lapses. A lapse is a fateful moment: patients who lapse may work to recover and keep moving forward toward abstinence, or the lapse quickly devolves into relapse back to their previous smoking routines. Figure 9.2 shows what the whole process may look like.

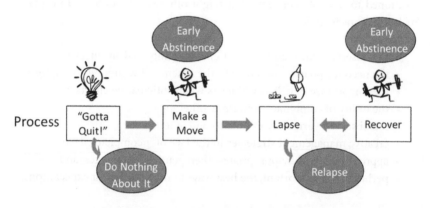

Figure 9.2. Basic model of tobacco abstinence attempts.

To understand the power of probabilities, imagine there are two distinct clinical scenarios applied to 1,000 patients each. In the first scenario, abstinence is pursued without the benefit of pharmacotherapy. In the second scenario, nothing is different except that pharmacotherapy is used to nudge the conditions for change in the direction of abstinence. For scenario 1 (Figure 9.3), assume that 50% of the group chooses the "Do nothing about it" option. Of the 500 patients who choose "Make a move," assume that 70% will experience "Lapse" and that 90% of people who lapse will relapse. After plugging in the numbers, scenario 1 would be expected to result in 185 of the initial 1,000 patients reaching early abstinence.

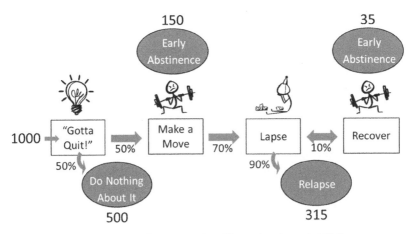

Figure 9.3. Baseline assumptions illustrating the probabilistic
nature of tobacco abstinence attempts.

Now consider scenario 2 (Figure 9.4). Assume that pharmacotherapy changes the probabilities only modestly. Maybe only 30% of patients who want to quit choose "Do nothing about it." Of the 700 patients who choose "Make a move," maybe only 60% go on to "Lapse," so that the risk of yielding to relapse drops to 75%.

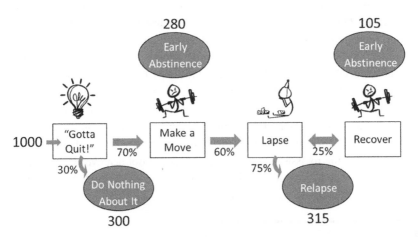

Figure 9.4. Impact of a probabilistic framework. Small changes in probabilities resulting from clinical tobacco interventions result in relatively large changes in overall outcomes.

Plug in the numbers, and scenario 2 leads to 385 of the 1,000 patients achieving early abstinence. That's over twice as many people who have a fighting chance at quitting, twice as many people who will experience the possibility of undoing the addictive power of nicotine, and twice as many people who can begin the process of healing the brain and body after years of smoking. That is a huge clinical impact, one that cannot be left off the table.

Notice a few important things:

- Pharmacotherapy did not change the process, only the patients' chances of transitioning through the process toward abstinence.
- The absolute change in transition probability between individual states need not be very large for there to be a large cumulative impact on outcome.
- Small changes in transition probabilities may be too small to be perceived when managing individual patients in the clinic.
- Though assumptions were used to illustrate the power of probabilistic thinking, the example generally reflects what providers might expect in the clinic. The calculated odds ratio for achieving abstinence in our example is 2.75; real-world odds ratios for pharmacotherapeutic interventions have been reported in the range of 1.5 to 3.85.

At this point, it is easy to imagine the clinician's job is done—at least for those lucky 385 people who found their way to early abstinence. However, it is important to remember that the change is not just about the behavior. It is also about facilitating an adjustment to the underlying pattern of patterns, including the intracellular biology that produced those patterns in the first place. The changes include turning off CREB translocation, allowing HDAC to get back to work, reducing the expression of ΔFosB transcription factor, and rebalancing the endogenous opioid reinforcement system (Chapter 3). Don't forget that ΔFosB is stable and can remain in the cell for years. Certainly, the clinician's job is to continue to assist the 615 people who did not achieve abstinence to find their way forward, but it is also to monitor the progress of the fortunate 385—because change is potentially bidirectional.

> *Relapse happens.*

From that perspective, it becomes important to examine how probabilistic thinking might affect a longitudinal approach. Similar to any other waxing and waning chronic illness, control over the compulsion to smoke should be thought of as dynamic, not static, as ongoing, not episodic. Once established, think of control over compulsion as something to be tended to and monitored periodically for signs of loosening, just as the person with asthma is evaluated for the reemergence of wheeze or the patient with hypertension for the gradual increase in blood pressure. From a chronic illness perspective, the goal of pharmacotherapy is not simply to help modify current behavior but to minimize the probability patients will return to that behavior in the future.

Think of it this way. At some point following birth, a person starts smoking. At some point before death, they stop (Figure 9.5). In a "smoking cessation" model, we imagine our intervention aims to help them stop earlier (Figure 9.6). Instead, like other chronic illnesses, notice that the experience of compulsion varies tremendously (Figure 9.7).

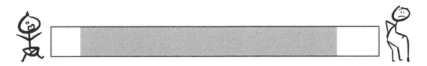

Figure 9.5. Baseline tobacco use experience.

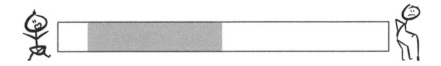

Figure 9.6. Imagined impact of the "cessation" intervention.

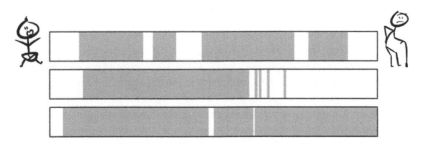

Figure 9.7. Observed population-level experience of smoking and abstinence.

In a probabilistic model of chronic tobacco-dependence management, the clinician's role is to control the compulsion to smoke over the long run: monitoring control, preempting threats to control, identifying loss of control, and re-exerting control as needed, in order to minimize the amount of time spent being compelled to smoke—over a lifetime (Figure 9.8).

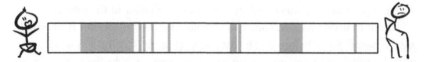

Figure 9.8. Clinical interventions over a lifetime.

"Ex? Really?"

On November 4, 2016, then U.S. president Barack Obama was interviewed by comedian Bill Maher, who covered a range of topics not often discussed in political contexts. During the conversation, the president mentioned his history of smoking. "Look, I'm an ex-smoker," the president explained. Maher pressed the issue, seeking confirmation from the president, not once but twice. "Ex? Really?" he asked, to which Mr. Obama replied, "Ex. Yep." The "yep" was accompanied by one of the most famous winks in broadcast television history. Mr. Obama delivered his fateful wink for Mr. Maher alongside a knowing grin and seemed to momentarily put viewers in the position of deciding for themselves whether or not he was being truthful. His reaffirmation came quickly, complete with an impish smile. "It's true," Mr. Obama explained. "I'm chewing the heck out of Nicorette."

The compulsion to smoke is not defined by the presence or absence of the smoking behavior but rather by the emotional contours of abstinence and the invasive qualities of the impulse to smoke. Patients who have not yet experienced complete resolution of their compulsion may still implicitly feel vulnerable to relapse and may warrant an extended period of treatment and counseling. A clinical overemphasis on the behavior rather than the symptoms runs the risk of ignoring the persistence of dependence. Patients' confidence in their ability to remain abstinent in the face of unexpected smoking triggers or emotional stress can be a useful measure of how well the pharmacotherapy is working, particularly in the absence of classical withdrawal symptoms. For clues, do not forget to watch their body language as much as you listen to their words.

Despite being the president of the United States, Mr. Obama was hesitant and bashful when admitting his persistent connection to nicotine.

Imagine the potential impact on Helen. Find a way to gently probe this with your patients, a way that does not involve double-checking their veracity or amplifying their shame.

Medication Basics

Understanding medication basics is important for all providers, regardless of their role in patient care or their prescriptive authority. A big part of patient education, counseling, and guidance involves correcting common sources of misinformation and misunderstanding and ensuring that the medications are used in a manner that takes full advantage of potential effectiveness. The following section is provided as a general clinical reference, addressing the key points of pharmacotherapy in practice. It is not intended to be a substitute for manufacturer instructions or good clinical judgment. When in doubt, refer to an online pharmacotherapy-specific database.

With all medications, pharmacokinetics matter. Tobacco-dependence medications are no different. There are seven first-line medications that have been shown to reliably increase long-term smoking abstinence. Of those seven, some have a pharmacokinetic delivery profile that makes them best suited for slower, more sustained-release applications, while others are better suited for acute or episodic uses. Clinicians can think of "controller medications" as those expected to have a delayed onset of effect, acting to reduce the frequency and

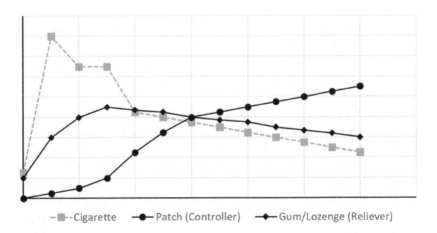

Figure 9.9. Pharmacokinetic profile of controller versus reliever nicotine medications.

intensity of the impulse to smoke, while "reliever medications" are expected to have more acute effects that could be especially useful in alleviating the distress of cue-induced cravings (Figure 9.9).

NICOTINE PATCH

The nicotine patch is a good example of a controller medication. It is not designed to be used in response to cue-induced cravings but instead delivers a reasonably constant level of nicotine to the bloodstream over a twenty-four-hour period. The clinical effect is to reduce impulsivity in the face of triggers and to reduce anticipatory anxiety associated with abstinence. It is easy to use, but the packaging can sometimes be difficult for the elderly to manage. The patient applies one patch to the skin daily—anywhere that is not too hairy or too sweaty. There is no truth to the rumor that patches should not be applied over the heart. Patients should be instructed to apply the patch as part of their morning hygiene routine and to leave it in place until the next morning. At that time, they should remove the old patch, clean the skin to remove residual vehicle and adhesive, and place a new patch on a different site. By rotating through a series of five or six different application sites, patients can avoid the skin irritation sometimes associated with chronic use.

The package insert recommends starting with a 21-milligram patch daily, or a 14-milligram patch for patients smoking ten or fewer cigarettes per day. However, in patients who report consuming only a few daily cigarettes, clinicians should consider several additional variables explored during the smoking history before deciding on dose. Important clues to severity of dependence, such as a bad experience with abstinence in the past, previous unresponsiveness to medication, or potential markers of compensatory smoking, might call for an upward adjustment of the initial dose recommendation. For example, a patient who smokes eight cigarettes daily but who suffered significant distress during past quit attempts, finds it difficult to change smoking routines, or relights each of the eight cigarettes multiple times may be better served by a 21-milligram patch.

The package insert also recommends a step-down dosing over a period of about twelve weeks. Unfortunately, this guidance can have the unintended effect of setting up unreasonable patient expectations that do not account for variability in treatment response. It may also create a time pressure that can exacerbate anticipatory anxiety. The step-down schedule frequently amplifies affective forecasting error and creates an opportunity for escape by focusing the patient's attention on reasons why it will not be possible to stop in three months. Clinicians should use the duration recommendations as a guideline but encourage flexibility in treatment duration based on the patient's symptomatic response and resolution of compulsion. Judgments on dose reduction should be shared decisions; patients should be instructed to discuss dose changes with the clinician in order to ensure that timing is based on effect, not on a self-imposed pressure to be done with the problem.

There are no absolute contraindications to using the nicotine patch. Before recommending the patch, however, clinicians should consider any history of adverse reaction to the patch in the past. While a simple history of essential hypertension does not preclude its use, patients with poorly controlled hypertension benefit from aggressive control of their blood pressure before initiating the patch. There are no drug-drug interactions that preclude the use of a nicotine patch. However, because the constituents of tobacco smoke compete for metabolic pathways in the liver, clinicians should be aware that medications metabolized by the cytochrome P450 enzyme system could theoretically require dose adjustments once the patient stops smoking.

Though patients often have a wide range of side-effect concerns, the only side effect of clinical significance is the potential for skin irritation. There are two possible causes for this reaction. By far, the most common relates to nicotine's ability to degranulate histamine-containing mast cells in the skin. Histamine in the skin leads to redness and swelling at the patch site, sometimes accompanied by local itching, muscle pain, or both. This is not a true allergic reaction and can be addressed by applying a small amount of topical corticosteroid to the area. Very rarely, some patients develop an allergy to the non-nicotine elements of the patch. In this case, the redness and swelling are more likely to have a wider distribution, up to and including a generalized pruritic rash. A true allergic reaction to the patch demands discontinuation.

Patch Pearls

1. There are data that indicate a six-month or longer treatment course can be more effective than a three-month course. Clinicians should consider setting the expectation of a six- to twelve-month treatment course early in the intervention to minimize affective forecasting error and to orient the patient toward a prolonged period of "brain healing." The data for twelve months of patch therapy is comparatively weaker than the data supporting a six-month course, but effectiveness seems to be mostly undermined by difficulties maintaining adherence that long. In situations where adherence is not an issue, up to twelve months of treatment could be useful for select patients experiencing prolonged recovery.

2. The majority of patients who attempt abstinence while wearing a patch will experience a lapse very early in their attempt. A common misconception is that

this defines treatment failure. This is not true. Instructing the patient to continue wearing the patch despite the lapse improves the probability of recovery from the lapse and reduces the potential for relapse.

3. Quit dates can be flexible, even when prescribing the patch. Sometimes patients with a strong anticipatory anxiety will be reluctant to start the patch because of the aversive prospect of abrupt, "forced" abstinence from cigarettes. In this situation, it is feasible to begin the patch before the patient is ready to abstain, allowing flexibility in timing the transition to the "Make a move" state.

4. Though the patch is available for over-the-counter purchase, prescribers should consider writing a prescription for the patch since many insurance plans will cover some or all the cost of the medication when prescribed but not when purchased over the counter. Check local plan formularies to identify any documentation requirements necessary for prior authorization.

BUPROPION SR

Initially identified for its efficacy as a tetracyclic antidepressant medication, bupropion was found to have the fortunate side effect of helping patients stop smoking. It appears to work by improving the efficiency of dopaminergic signaling in the nucleus accumbens. The clinical effect is to reduce impulsivity and improve cognitive control. There is no effect on mood when used in patients without preexisting depression.

The typical dose for tobacco dependence is 150-milligrams of the sustained-release (SR) formulation administered twice daily. Bupropion takes several weeks to reach peak effectiveness; clinicians should start bupropion well before the anticipated abstinence attempt. Start the medication at least four weeks before guiding the patient toward an abstinence experiment, adjusting variables like dose and timing of drug accordingly to minimize any side effects. Like the patch, the labeled duration of treatment is three months, but longer durations of six to twelve months, based on the patient's progress, are often preferable.

Bupropion should not be used in patients who are already using one of the several psychotropic medication brands containing bupropion (for example, Aplenzin, Buproban, Forfivo XL, Wellbutrin, or Zyban) or in patients being treated with tricyclic antidepressants (such as amitriptyline, nortriptyline, desipramine, and doxepin). Bupropion should also be avoided in patients treated with the monoamine oxidase inhibitor class of medications but is appropriate for combination with newer-generation antidepressants under close monitoring. Bupropion has the potential to lower the seizure threshold, so patients with an established seizure disorder, those likely to abruptly withdraw from chronic alcohol use, and those with metabolic disturbances from anorexia or bulimia should not be treated with bupropion.

The main side effect of bupropion is agitation and sleep disturbance. Agitation may paradoxically be experienced as anxiety, depression, or another mood disorder. Sleep disturbance is often experienced as vivid dreams—not necessarily nightmares but dreams the patient is more likely to remember in the morning. In rare cases, more significant sleep disturbances such as somnambulation have been reported. One way to avoid these symptoms is to direct the patient to take the evening dose of bupropion with dinner rather than at bedtime. If symptoms persist for more than a few days, clinicians should try discontinuing the evening dose and reevaluating the patient after one week rather than taking the more definitive step of discontinuing the medication altogether.

Bupropion Pearls

1. The earliest effects of bupropion can take some time to accumulate. Four weeks of pretreatment is not an unusual requirement and can sometimes extend to several months before the patient feels control over the compulsion to smoke.

2. Bupropion works best when combined with nicotine replacement, leveraging the dual biological activities inherent to the two different classes of controller.

3. Patients treated with bupropion are less likely to gain weight during their abstinence attempt.

4. There are good data supporting the use of bupropion for the prevention of relapse in patients who feel vulnerable to nicotine after a period of prolonged abstinence.

Telephone Encounter Record: Bupropion Side-Effect Report

Patient Lawrence B. (DOB: 05/05/55) called this morning to inform you that he had to stop taking bupropion due to hallucinations. Patient states that his dog started barking very loudly at the front door last night. When he looked outside, he saw what appeared to be a shopping cart filled with clothes parked on the sidewalk. Mr. B went upstairs to get a flashlight and call the police. When he returned, the cart was gone. Wife suggested he stop the bupropion for fear it was causing visual hallucinations.

I was able to confirm that Mrs. B also heard the dog barking so I tried to reassure the patient that this was an indication of an alternative explanation for the cart's disappearance and not a hallucination.

The patient and his wife remain concerned and would like a callback from the doctor. Please advise.

VARENICLINE

Varenicline is thought to primarily be an agonist-antagonist of the α4β2 nicotinic receptor. Despite rumors to the contrary, varenicline has proven itself to be very safe and well tolerated. Increasingly, varenicline has become an acceptable option to patients because of its ease of use and its effectiveness as a controller medication. The clinical effect of varenicline is to reduce the survival salience of environmental cues associated with smoking. By undermining the salience effects of nicotine, patients experience a progressive distancing of their relationship to the cigarette. In effect, varenicline helps the breakup happen on the inside before the breakup happens on the outside. The typical course for varenicline is 1 milligram twice daily for three months, though there is increasing evidence that treatment courses longer than six months provide long-term abstinence advantage.

The manufacturer's package insert recommends a one-week up-titration period, beginning with 0.5 milligrams once daily and progressing quickly to the target dose of 1 milligram twice daily. The objective of the up-titration strategy is to minimize the occurrence of nausea. About 10% of patients starting varenicline will experience the same kind of queasy nausea that novice smokers sometimes experience during the early days of initiation. In our experience, the titration schedule can be confusing for some patients, particularly those who have been subjected to a temporary pause in treatment followed by restart of the medication. We typically instruct our patients to take a 1-milligram pill twice daily with food (one pill with breakfast, one with dinner), which achieves the same protection against this aversive, sometimes treatment-limiting symptom.

The nausea is easy to manage with a few simple maneuvers. First, ensure the patient is taking the medication directly after a meal. A full stomach can substantially reduce the incidence of gastrointestinal distress. If a meal is impractical, a large glass of milk or water will sometimes be sufficient. Second, consider reducing the dose to 0.5 milligrams twice daily unless the nausea only occurs around one or the other administration, in which case it is appropriate to reduce only the dose that causes the problem. When this situation does occur, it is most commonly seen with the morning dose. Third, it is possible to abate the nausea by instructing the patient to take a chewable bismuth tablet just before varenicline administration. This may affect absorption of the medication, so it is advisable to discontinue the bismuth after a few days, once the brain has accommodated to the varenicline and the nausea has resolved.

Another main side effect of varenicline is sleep disturbance. This may be experienced as insomnia or vivid dreams and happens in about 10% of patients. By instructing the patient to take the second daily dose of varenicline with dinner instead of at bedtime, the additional few hours before sleep are often enough to mitigate this symptom. If vivid dreams persist, consider administering the second dose even earlier in the afternoon, changing the dosage to 1 milligram in the morning and 0.5 milligrams in the afternoon, or in extreme cases discontinuing the evening pill altogether. Some patients will experience a vaguely uncomfortable, dysphoric feeling early in the initiation of varenicline. This has been described variously as a "foreboding," an "out-of-body feeling," or sometimes a "just not right" uneasiness. This is distinct from a depressed mood and generally reflects an overrepresentation of the antagonist activity of varenicline. In effect, over-antagonism leads to an abrupt withdrawal sensation and can sometimes be resolved easily by reassuring the patient and adjusting the dosage downward to 0.5 milligrams twice daily.

Concerns over severe neuropsychiatric side effects, including clinical depression and suicidal ideation, have been overstated and should not represent a barrier to using varenicline in people who have mental illness. A meta-analysis performed by the American Thoracic Society during production of the Initiating Pharmacologic Treatment of Tobacco Dependence in Adults clinical practice guideline calculated that the relative effect of varenicline was 30% greater than that of nicotine replacement. Despite the apparent vulnerability of patients with mental illness, the harms were found to be equivalent, with undesirable effects of treatment judged as trivial. The 2016 Evaluating Adverse Events in a Global Smoking Cessation Study (EAGLES) trial compared four thousand patients who smoke and have serious mental illness to matched patients without mental illness. The study documented parity in side-effect rates comparable to placebo, regardless of which controller medications were used. Some clinicians have avoided the use of varenicline in patients with a history of depression or another behavioral disorder for fear of exacerbating their mental health condition or destabilizing control over symptoms. Varenicline has an equivalent relative effect size in patients with preexisting behavioral health diagnoses as it does in the non–mental illness population. There is no reason to withhold this important therapeutic intervention over concerns for neuropsychiatric stability.

No absolute contraindications to varenicline use exist. The manufacturer cautions clinicians to use judgment when prescribing varenicline to patients with heavy alcohol use or a seizure history. In general, it makes sense to avoid starting a new central nervous system drug if the patient is experiencing poorly controlled seizures, but a remote or well-controlled seizure history should not be an absolute contraindication to use. Patients with renal insufficiency require dose adjustment based on creatinine clearance rates. Start with 0.5 milligrams once daily in patients with a creatinine clearance rate less than 30 milliliters per minute and move up to 0.5 milligrams twice daily if well tolerated. Patients on dialysis should be prescribed a maximum dose of 0.5 milligrams once daily.

Varenicline Pearls

1. Start it early—and do not stop it too soon. The effects of varenicline accumulate over months. In fact, there are some data suggesting that quit rates continue to rise even after three months of "pretreatment." Starting the varenicline five weeks before the anticipated quit date rather than the recommended one week has been shown to double the long-term abstinence likelihood.

2. Even in patients who are resistant to change (Chapter 8), the idea of starting varenicline to simply evaluate its effects can be palatable and often represents a useful "toehold" in clinical conversation. Patients who are unwilling to quit may be more willing to explore the possible effects of varenicline if the clinician doesn't press for abstinence. The data suggest that varenicline treatment will lead 30% of patients currently unwilling to quit to go on to abstinence within three months of starting therapy. The American Thoracic Society meta-analysis calculated that clinicians can help more than three hundred additional patients stop smoking per thousand treated just by starting varenicline well before the patient expresses a readiness to quit.

3. Patients and their families will frequently express reluctance to use vareni-cline because of popular myths and misunderstandings. Clinicians should not interpret this as a refusal per se but rather as an opportunity to understand the source of misgivings while providing reliable information. "Varenicline is definitely not our only option, but I want us to both have the same information before we make this decision together."

4. Despite its presumed biologic activity as an agonist-antagonist, varenicline's effectiveness is augmented by combining it with nicotine replacement therapy. To date, it remains unclear why this is the case, but clinicians can expect to help over a hundred additional patients stop smoking per thousand treated by employing this simple maneuver alone.

Chart Note: March 3, 2020; 1530 hrs

Chief Complaint: "I'm here because my doctor made me come."

Present History: Steven K. is a 59-year-old pipe fitter who works at the Philadelphia shipyard. Has a history of severe peripheral vascular disease, with multiple hospitalizations for intractable right lower extremity pain. Recently underwent right lower extremity amputation below the knee. Pain better but not resolved. Following amputation, surgeon arranged for visit to tobacco clinic. Presents today with somber affect, courteous but direct: "I'm here because I have to be, not because I want to be. I cut down a lot, but I really like smoking and I have no intention of stopping."

Pertinent tobacco history includes terrible experience with varenicline in past. Vivid dreams/nightmares quickly became intolerable. Physical exam significant for thin, asthenic build—now status post amputation.

Impression: Severe dependence, strong ambivalence. Anger and loss of agency complicate intervention. Current substage = resistance. Low body weight and apparent small volume of distribution suggest dose of varenicline may have been too high on earlier trial.

Plan: Focus on restoring autonomous control, including potential for control over identification of "right dose" of varenicline. Discussed nature of nicotine addiction and instructions for managing medication titration. Suggest varenicline 0.5 milligrams once daily with food in AM, then followed by increase to 0.5 milligrams twice daily with food if well tolerated. Patient to continue smoking but will track daily routines to observe for indications that relationship to cigarettes may be loosening. Return to clinic in four weeks to report on progress. Given phone number to call with questions/concerns.

NICOTINE GUM

Nicotine gum is a classic example of a reliever medication. Its greatest utility is in giving the patient an active means of turning off negative prediction error signaling in the face of environmental smoking cues. Rather than having patients passively wait for the cravings to subside or hoping they can distract themselves from the desire to smoke long enough for it to pass, patients can be counseled to play an active role in ameliorating the impulse to smoke by anticipating the daily circumstances where smoking would otherwise be routine and using a piece of gum to "smooth over" the triggered desire for a cigarette. The combination of cognitive focus on the gum as an alternative reinforcer, the motor activation necessary to deploy the gum, and the acute elevation in blood nicotine levels accomplished shortly after its appropriate use can give patients a short-term means of rebalancing the signals produced by the mesolimbic system in favor of volitional control.

It is not uncommon for patients to initially frame nicotine gum use in reactionary, "for-emergency-use-only" terms. Though some cues will naturally happen unexpectedly, in our experience the majority of cue-induced cravings happen during anticipatable circumstances. In our practice, we encourage patients not to rely on a reactive strategy for gum dosing but instead to use a two-week learning period to identify ways of inserting nicotine gum into what would otherwise be their smoking routines. It is often useful to use the metaphor of "grease for the gears" that makes it easier to function—as opposed to the metaphor of a "fire extinguisher" putting out a fire—to make this point. Patients should be encouraged to use the gum liberally in the early stages until they develop a more precise understanding of their own optimal pattern of use.

Nicotine gum is available in both 2- and 4-milligram strengths. The typical dosage recommendation when using the gum alone is one piece every hour or so as needed, up to a maximum of sixteen pieces daily. The manufacturer uses the time to first cigarette as an indication of dose requirement, recommending 2-milligram gum for patients whose first cigarette is more than thirty minutes after waking and 4-milligram gum for patients who smoke within the thirty-minute cutoff. In our experience, it is more straightforward to simply recommend the 4-milligram strength for all patients, reducing it to 2 milligrams only in patients who find the higher strength aversive. The duration of therapy varies along with duration of compulsion to smoke, as described in the paragraphs above. However, it is not uncommon for patients to continue reliever use for a short time following discontinuation of their controller, until they gain confidence in their ability to abstain without pharmacologic support.

Patients should be instructed to chew the gum just long enough to soften the polacrilex vehicle and then park the gum in direct contact with the inner cheek. Absorption is a function of contact area as well as duration of contact, so our instructions always include a suggestion to use the tongue to spread the gum into a wide, flat disk, placing it against the inside cheek or under the tongue, and leaving it in place as long as tolerated. There are no contraindications to nicotine gum use, and side effects are limited. Local irritation is not uncommon after a prolonged therapeutic course, and gum that is used incorrectly (that is, chewed without parking) can frequently cause nausea or hiccups. These side effects can typically be managed by reviewing the proper technique with the patient or decreasing the recommended strength.

Nicotine Gum Pearls

1. Using one form of nicotine replacement (for example, a patch) will double the patient's likelihood of abstinence; supplementing that with a second form for more acute delivery (for example, gum) will triple the likelihood from there.

2. Patients without teeth and those with poor dentition can find it difficult to chew through the candied shell to kick-start the application. It is acceptable for these

patients first to park the gum whole, allowing saliva to dissolve the coating before kneading it into place. Patients for whom this remains uncomfortable can be switched to the nicotine lozenge.

3. For patients who experience local irritation from nicotine gum use, before discontinuing the gum outright, try recommending a mentholated cough drop to provide immediate relief and a cooling sensation in the throat. In severe cases, a daily antihistamine can be used to minimize the discomfort produced by histamine release in the posterior pharynx.

4. Patients may find buccal placement to be uncomfortable and to interfere with normal speech. Placement under the tongue may be more comfortable and has excellent absorption characteristics.

NICOTINE LOZENGE

Functionally, the nicotine lozenge acts the same way as the gum. It is another familiar example of a reliever medication, an active means of turning off cue-induced cravings rather than passively waiting for the impulse to subside. Like the gum, delivery depends on mucosal absorption, so placement instructions are important. Patients should be encouraged to place it between the cheek and gums and leave it in place as long as tolerated. Both the 2-milligram and 4-milligram lozenges are available in two sizes; the full-size lozenge is about the size of a nickel (about 15 millimeters) and can take a little longer to dissolve than the mini-lozenge (5 millimeters) counterpart. Pharmacologically, the two forms are essentially equivalent. However, each has strengths that may favor one over the other in a particular patient. For example, the larger lozenge is reminiscent of a hard candy in size and shape and may resonate with patients who have found candy mints to be helpful in the past. Conversely, it also has the potential to leave a chalky residue behind and can be off-putting to some as a result. The mini lozenge has the advantage of small size and relatively quicker dissolution. It is well tolerated and can deliver nicotine well when placed under the tongue. The option makes it possible to use the mini lozenge in situations where the larger lozenge is impractical. Conversely, the similarity between mini lozenges and shaker mints can sometimes lead patients to chew or swallow the mini lozenge once the effect has been achieved. Patients prescribed the mini lozenge should be educated to expel any residual matter rather than ingesting it; swallowed nicotine in the stomach will frequently make patients feel nauseated and cause hiccups or gastric distress and won't do anything to help with the urge to smoke.

Nicotine Lozenge Pearls

1. The nicotine lozenge's indications, contraindications, side effects, and duration of therapy are the same as for the gum. The decision on which form to use should be based on patient preference and availability.

2. Some patients prefer to alternate use of several forms of reliever nicotine, based primarily on the circumstances operant at the time of the craving. The forms are essentially pharmacologically equivalent and can be mixed and matched to the patient's needs.

3. Nicotine lozenges are available in several flavors. Sometimes trouble with palatability of the product can be managed by trying a different flavor rather than discontinuing the medication. A variety of natural and artificial sweeteners are used to flavor both the lozenge and gum. However, the amount of sweetener is quite small and does not interfere with blood glucose control in patients with diabetes.

4. Like the gum, the lozenge is available over the counter. Remember that prescribers should still write a prescription when recommending these products in case the product is covered within the patient's insurance plan formulary.

NICOTINE INHALER

Unlike the more recognizable asthma inhaler, the nicotine inhaler does not require activation, uses no propellants, and does not deliver a set dose with each use. The nicotine inhaler is a hollow plastic tube, or holder, that splits apart in the middle, into which a small (2.5-centimeter) cartridge containing nicotine is loaded. The cartridge has a small sponge in the middle that is impregnated with liquid nicotine. Once loaded, the patient simply puffs gently on the holder mouthpiece, delivering a fine mist of atomized nicotine droplets to the posterior pharynx. Absorption of nicotine is almost completely mucosal, with only a small portion of the nicotine making it past the larynx into the lungs.

The nicotine delivered via the inhaler is not released in the free-base form and consequently is an airway irritant. Patients, conditioned over a lifetime to inhale their cigarette smoke deeply into the lungs, will frequently inhale too deeply on initiation and should be educated to puff gently, aiming to produce a "peppery" sensation in the back of the throat. Multiple small puffs are tolerated better than fewer large puffs, at least at the beginning of treatment. Consequently, while the upper airway begins the process of accommodating to the nicotine droplets, patients should be encouraged to experiment with their inhaler technique until they find the right combination of puff volume, flow rate, and frequency to produce the desired effect. Nicotine droplets that do make it to the lung will stimulate cough; patients will sometimes interpret this as harmful to the lungs. Clinicians should be prepared to allay these fears, and remind patients that technique is important to minimizing the benign, but annoying airway irritation. Remember that the inhaler, despite its vague similarity in size, shape, and color to a cigarette, is not intended to re-create the experience of smoking; instead it gives the patient an active means by which to reduce the intensity of negative prediction error signaling in response to environmental cues.

Once the cartridge seal is broken by the holder, the nicotine begins evaporating. Even unused cartridges will become ineffective within about two to three days once the seal is broken. The inhaler is functionally similar to the gum and the lozenge but has the added advantage of being exquisitely titratable by the patient. We instruct patients to begin by using a cluster of five to ten puffs every hour or so to begin getting a sense of how much is enough and, just as important, how much is too little. Giving patients license to vary the number of puffs and puff frequency based on the day's circumstances often gives them an important sense of control over their craving impulses.

The inhaler is nothing fancy; there are no lights, no electronics, and, crucially, no imitation smoke or artificial flavorants. It's just pure nicotine. Puff on it, and get nicotine absorbed from the oral mucosa. Despite the manufacturer's marketing claim to the contrary, in our experience the main advantage of the inhaler is not in its ability to reproduce the fabled hand-to-mouth motion of smoking but rather in its dosing flexibility. While some patients will initially emulate the smoking motions with the inhaler, few maintain that pattern very long. Still others see the reminiscent patterns as too close to smoking and worry that it will trigger relapse to cigarettes. Either way, it is advisable for clinicians to frame the device as a titratable nicotine delivery system rather than a substitute for the cigarette since it can't reproduce the experience of smoking.

There is ample evidence in favor of the inhaler's safety and efficacy, including multiple randomized clinical trials with results pointing in the same direction. For this reason, the inhaler is an excellent reliever choice for patients who have expressed interest in using the electronic cigarette to help them stop smoking. Because there are no additional organic aerosol constituents, there are fewer toxicity concerns. And because it is available by prescription, the inhaler is often covered by insurance plans. While the efficacy of electronic cigarettes in clinical situations remains an unresolved question, the efficacy of the inhaler does not; the nicotine inhaler doubles the odds of quitting.

Nicotine Inhaler Pearls

1. To describe the proper inhaler technique, it can be helpful to use the cigar as an analogy. Patients are familiar with the idea that cigar smoke is often not inhaled but instead puffed in short, shallow, repetitive bursts. Acting out the differences between the deep inhalation of the cigarette and the shallow puff of the cigar, including the differences in how the hand holds each device, can sometimes give the patient sufficient initial guidance to minimize the potentially off-putting experience of inhaler initiation.

2. Because the inhaler can take some practice, it may pay to recommend a two-week period of experimentation, during which the patient is instructed to concentrate only on perfecting their technique rather than focusing on the device's ability to forestall smoking. The metaphor that seems to help relates the patient's experience to learning to ride a bicycle. It takes multiple attempts, with dozens of small adjustments, before the rider begins to feel like riding is second nature.

3. Sometimes, particularly when patients have a heavy smoking history, the inhaler cannot deliver enough nicotine to create a sensed experience in the throat. In those instances, it is possible to have the patient tape two cartridges together—ensuring the foil barrier between them is punctured—to produce an aggressive "hit" on inhalation. Of course, the holder can't be snapped closed in this situation, but the resourceful patient can often find a way to make this work long enough to help them discover the correct technique and frequency needed to make the inhaler work.

4. Because of the external similarities, patients will often adopt a strategy of employing the inhaler only when they feel they need a cigarette. Clinicians should counsel patients to avoid restricting use of the inhaler as a metaphorical "fire extinguisher" and to remember instead that its greatest utility is as metaphorical "grease for the wheels."

No Need to Write That Letter

Electronic cigarettes and their potential to help people suffering from tobacco dependence is a topic that has generated a lot of heated discussions. People from across the medical-scientific spectrum, with only the best of intentions, have been struggling to resolve a whirlwind of partial information in search of answers to the fundamental question: do e-cigarettes represent a public health blessing, or are they a social affliction destined to undermine fifty years of progress in controlling the tobacco epidemic? The search for answers is confounded by the sense of desperation produced when the intransigence of smoking comes face-to-face with the mortal damage it produces—and, of course, by the motivated reasoning sometimes fed by manufacturers and others with a financial interest in a particular conclusion. It is reasonable to agree on a few things:

1. E-cigarettes are not just one thing. There is enormous variation in design characteristics of the device types currently available for purchase on the market, even though the world has lumped them all together colloquially as "vapes" or "e-cigarettes." Even within a single category of device, there is enormous variation in the aerosol characteristics they produce. Things like particle size, aerosol density, viscosity, and heating element temperature are all important variables to consider when delivering a pharmacologic agent to the lung. Finally, even in a situation where you might imagine only a single available device, there is still enormous variation in the chemical constituents of the "vape juice" employed to produce their effect. Now that you know what William Dunn knew in St. Martin fifty years ago, you can never again make the mistake of imagining that the chemistry and physics of nicotine delivery can be conveniently ignored.

Enormous variation × enormous variation × enormous variation = a far greater degree of variability than clinicians traditionally accept when thinking about reliability in patient care. Imagining these devices to be functionally similar to each other in their pharmacologic effect is like imagining all vehicles behave like bicycles. They may someday prove to be a useful tool for the right application, but for now their variability makes them unreliable and therefore not recommended for clinical applications.

2. Wishful thinking is not the same as science. The collective desperation that leads clinicians to feel like we need to capitulate to something! anything! that might help us solve this problem is the by-product of the cessation model of tobacco intervention. Impotence is not a function of the efficacy of the currently available tools, neither behavioral nor pharmacologic. Rather, perceived ineffectiveness is an offshoot of the many misunderstandings surrounding the proper approach to tobacco dependence. As clinicians get better at longitudinal management of dependence, the need to rely on hope alone disappears. When making clinical decisions, stick with the stuff that is based on science and focus on getting better at it rather than leaving patients to the whims of hopes and prayers.

3. If it sounds too good to be true, it probably is. In 2016 the Royal College of Physicians published a seminal monograph entitled *Nicotine Without Smoke: Tobacco Harm Reduction.* The monograph made hay out of a claim that using e-cigarettes would lead to a 95% reduction in harmful health effects compared to conventional smoking. "Although it is not possible to precisely quantify the long-term health risks associated with e-cigarettes, the available data suggest that they are unlikely to exceed 5% of those associated with smoked tobacco products, and may well be substantially lower than this figure." In a single sentence, the statement cited (1) the impossibility of knowing, (2) what was assumed to be known, and (3) that the assumptions probably underestimated the truth. That figure would prove to be too hard to ignore.

However, a careful look back at the research that led to this claim revealed that the "available data" cited was in fact a single report of the average opinion of twelve people on an expert panel. Those twelve participants, including public health advocates, lawyers, and tobacco company representatives, may have had the best intentions, but their words would go on to be misused. The opinion of twelve people, derived in an open forum, would go on to form the basis of national public health policy. That is wishful thinking on an enormous scale. A number of reputable professional societies have gone on to warn that the harmful effects of e-cigarettes should be considered unknown until they are known.

4. Common sense is not necessarily logical. It's appealing to rely on common sense when judging the value of a particular intervention for an individual patient. If smoking equals death, then not smoking equals not death. Unfortunately, common sense sometimes leads us down a path toward just-plain-wrong conclusions by virtue of several common logical fallacies. Watch out for these as best you can, and avoid them when applying your judgment in the clinic. Here are a few examples:

A *synecdochical fallacy* is when we assume that what's true for a part must be true for the whole. We fall prey to this fallacy when we assume that (1) because some patients can switch from traditional to electronic cigarettes, all patients could; (2) because e-cigarette use reduces the risk of a given disease, it reduces overall harm; or (3) because a particular device has been found to deliver fewer carcinogens, all similar devices do the same.

An *ecologic fallacy* is when we assume that what is true for the average must be true for the whole. We fall prey to this fallacy when we assume that (1) because the average toxicant concentration produced by a given device is low, that total toxicant delivery is similarly low; (2) because the average risk of a given disease within the overall population is reduced, an individual's risk of the same disease is also reduced; or (3) a general population's experience with e-cigarette toxicity accurately represents the experience of the various subgroups within that population.

Overstatement bias is the tendency to anchor our judgments to pre-vious experience, particularly when that experience has a high emotional valence or is otherwise "available." Common expressions of overstate-ment bias include (1) "It just *has to be* better than smoking"; (2) "It's just water vapor"; (3) "Being addicted to nicotine is just like being addicted to caffeine"; and (4) "Although it is not possible to precisely quantify the long-term health risks associated with e-cigarettes, the available data suggest that they are unlikely to exceed 5% of those associated with smoked tobacco products, and may well be substantially lower than this figure."

To help clinicians, researchers, and policy makers avoid these com-mon rhetorical pitfalls in the future, the American Thoracic Society pro-duced comprehensive guidance on the appropriate construction of harm reduction claims. Two key points: Talk to your patients about harm, using lay language and being careful not to exaggerate effects, and be explicit about the range of possible outcomes expected.

Nicotine Nasal Spray

Nicotine nasal spray is similar in style to pump-action cold sprays but is only available by prescription. The device delivers a huge hit of nicotine di-rectly to the highly vascular nasal mucosa, which is both a blessing and a curse. On one hand, the spray device is very effective in relieving cue-induced crav-ings by producing a reliable increase in blood nicotine levels rather quickly. On the other hand, it can be difficult for patients to tolerate the side effect produced when applying that much nicotine to the nose. Patients often experi-ence the "pepper-in-the-nose" effect, with nasal irritation, persistent sneezing, watery eyes, and runny nose. Patients should be counseled to begin using the spray device gently—with a single, gentle squeeze on first application. Patients will usually acclimate to the effect of nasal nicotine within a few days, but the symptoms can limit the utility of the medication if patients are not sufficiently prepared for the initial experience. Once the patient is fully accustomed to the sensation, they can be instructed to titrate up to the target dose of one spray in each nostril every hour as needed to control the compulsion to smoke.

There are no absolute contraindications to nasal spray use. However, one of the distinct features of nasal spray nicotine is its ability to result in the depen-dence phenomenon. The nicotine preparations discussed so far all have a very limited addictive potential; nicotine delivery is just too low and too slow to create the necessary changes in mesolimbic function. However, the delivery of nicotine in the spray is much closer to the delivery of nicotine in a cigarette. As a result, 10% of patients using the nasal spray will report the same anticipatory anxiety, feeling of connection, and automatic behaviors produced by cigarettes. Whereas some patients using gum, lozenge, or patch will feel like they are still vulnerable to cigarette relapse if they discontinue, the difference is about which nicotine delivery device they are beholden to. No one goes outside for a nicotine gum break, but some folks actually do go out for a nasal spray break. Clinicians should not let the addictive potential of nicotine nasal spray dissuade them from using it, but it is important to discuss this possibility with patients before starting the medication.

Nasal Spray Pearls

1. Clinicians can sometimes help patients overcome the initial nasal irritation in those who find nasal spray difficult to tolerate. For example, in our practice, we will sometimes advise patients to apply a drop of nasal spray to a cotton swab and use the applicator tip to deliver nicotine to the nasal vestibule. By slowly advancing the swab, the nasal septum can be lightly exposed to nicotine for a few days before advancing to a gentle spray. Patients for whom this technique is ill advised can alternatively be counseled to take an over-the-counter anti-histamine in the morning and wait two hours before introducing the spray. In either case, once acclimation is complete, patients should resume the normal recommended method of administration.

2. On rare occasions, patients will not be able to tolerate any method of nasal administration. For those who absolutely require the high-dose delivery of nasal spray, we sometimes recommend they try application under the tongue. The acrid taste can be masked by a mint or menthol cough drop.

3. Patients who develop an apparent dependence on the nasal spray can be managed by treatment with any of the pharmacotherapies listed above. The nicotine patch can be effective at reducing the impulse to spray, and instructions to intersperse occasional doses of 4-milligram nicotine gum or lozenge can help reduce the frequency of spray dosing.

4. Patients prescribed nicotine nasal spray should be counseled to store their medication in a secure location, away from children or pets that could suffer overdose if accidentally ingested. The amount of nicotine in one bottle of nasal spray is approximately equivalent to twenty-five pieces of 4-milligram gum. This last pearl is really good general advice for any medication, regardless of whether it is available over the counter or by prescription.

Chapter 9 Learning Points

- Medications do not replace smoking. They merely help create the conditions for change. In that sense, they do not replace the work of quitting; they are only one tool that makes it possible.
- Tobacco-dependence pharmacotherapy has several useful clinical effects. However, none of those effects are universally experienced by all patients who use them. A mechanistic perspective on the role of medication is useful in explaining the wide variety of effects and in individualizing patient expectations.
- Understanding the impact of pharmacotherapy on conditions for change requires thinking probabilistically, not linearly. Even small changes in the probability of moving between states can have a profound impact on the likelihood of abstinence within large groups of dependent patients.
- As with other chronic disease conditions, medications may not necessarily represent cure, only control. In a chronic disease model of care, clinicians expect to use medications to exert control over the compulsion to smoke—as needed over a lifetime.
- Both pharmacodynamics and pharmacokinetics are important when choosing a medication approach. Do not think about tobacco-dependence pharmacotherapies as interchangeable; think about the important differences in both biologic activity and rate of delivery when tailoring recommendations.
- Medication basics include an understanding of dose, contraindications, and anticipated effects. It also includes thoughtful, creative solutions to predictable obstacles to adherence.
- Though a source of contention within the public policy and public opinion domains, thinking about the electronic cigarette in the clinical context is very straightforward: they are neither approved nor recommended for use as cessation pharmacotherapy. Keep scientific and wishful thinking separate in your head.
- Do not be afraid to use pharmacotherapy to help patients control their smoking. All guidelines written since 1998 have recommended the use of pharmacotherapy for all smokers, regardless of their level of dependence. Doses, durations, and desired effects vary on an individual basis.

Chapter 10
Management

My whole family hates my smoking, but not as much as I hate myself for smoking.

—Homer G., 74 years old

"Everyone is different, and this is not a contest," Kathy tries to remind Helen. Kathy started the nicotine patch two months ago and was no longer interested in smoking. Helen, on the other hand, was on her sixth month of this quit attempt and still struggling. She would do well for a week or so and then suddenly feel compelled to go to the corner store and buy a few loosies. She was happy for Kathy but couldn't really understand how this was possible. It didn't seem fair. "I am the one who went to the doctor and tried multiple medications. Why is this so much harder for me than it is for her?" she asked herself. "I wish I had her strength, but I am just too weak."

Patients do not always follow the prescribed directions when taking their medications. Even when they do, the medications do not always work as expected. This should not come as a surprise. It is the same observation every clinician has made about every other illness in every other aspect of practice. But we sometimes lose track of the universal importance of mediators and moderators of a drug's effect when we focus our attention exclusively on "quit rates" as a means of describing anticipated results. Focusing on quit rates as a measure of pharmacologic success puts us in a position to imagine outcomes as a function of the drug alone, when the truth is so much more complex. Quit rates might be a useful way to measure a drug's comparative efficacy in a research trial, but they do not translate well into measures of effectiveness in the clinic. At the risk of being repetitive, remember that to the clinician, the therapeutic goal is always to help patients achieve abstinence, but the therapeutic effect we seek from our interventions is to help patients achieve control over the compulsion to smoke. Our effectiveness is a function of the complex interactions between medication effects, patient-level variables, and the intervention characteristics under providers' control.

A number of predictable issues influence day-to-day effectiveness in the clinic. Just like in other aspects of clinic life, providers do their very best to manage as many of these determinants as possible in an effort to maximize impact. In short, never underestimate the inevitability of adjustments to the plan. Clinical decision-making is always iterative; specialized cognitive processes are applied in an effort to determine the patient's status, their response to recent interventions, any required modifications to the initial approach, and the need to employ additional tools to accomplish a prespecified end.

Generally, one of the most important patient-level mediators of pharmacotherapeutic effect is the degree to which a patient adheres to the medication regimen. One of the oldest clichés in medicine is that medications work best when the patient uses them. Incidentally, it is equally true that medications work best when providers prescribe them, but that is a matter for discussion in Chapter 12. Patient adherence to any medication regimen, for any problem, is always a fragile issue, constantly under threat of incremental deformation because of a variety of pressures. For instance, a preexisting sense of ineffectiveness may conspire with a difficult administration schedule to tip the balance in favor of inaction. Patients with limited cognitive abilities may have trouble interpreting, then reinterpreting or remembering instructions for use. Those taking multiple medications may find themselves merging dosing regimens either intentionally or not. Certainly, side effects may lead to a self-directed change in dose or timing of administration. These pressures are natural and make imperfect adherence a near-certainty for most conditions.

Intentional Nonadherence: The Rational Mind

Mark T. is a 35-year-old local businessman. On the recent birth of his daughter, he resolved to take the necessary steps to stop smoking. He was particularly energized by his newfound understanding of the neuronal distortions that help explain his dependence behaviors. Feeling empowered, he agreed to a plan that included pharmacologic support with varenicline. Unfortunately, by the second day of his pretreatment period, Mr. T. began experiencing nausea throughout the day, limiting his ability to perform his work duties. He experimented with a few ways to manage this side effect, including waiting until later in the day for the first dose, drinking milkshakes before dosing, and discontinuing his morning pill altogether. When the nausea persisted despite these maneuvers, he decided to stop the medication. On the follow-up visit, he reported, "Sorry doctor, I really tried to push through, but it was keeping me from doing my job. I had to stop."

Preexisting health beliefs influence adherence in any condition. Tobacco-dependence treatment plans may be especially at risk of intentional nonadherence because of the ubiquity of myths unique to smoking, including the notion that unassisted abstinence attempts are "better" (Table 10.1).

Table 10.1. Commonly Expressed Tobacco Health Beliefs Affecting Adherence.

"It's just a matter of willpower." (prioritizing lay knowledge)
"I tried that stuff in the past, and it didn't work." (prioritizing past personal experience)
"I have a friend who tried that and nearly went crazy." (prioritizing indirect experience)
"I just have to do it—today." (prioritizing instant status change)
"I'm not going to remember to take my pill while I'm at work." (avoiding inconvenience)
"That stuff is expensive. At least cigarettes make me happy." (emphasizing relative utility)
"I started this. I'll end it." (prioritizing self-reliance)

Another issue shows up all the time in the clinic but does not fit easily on a list of reasons for intentional nonadherence. Ambivalence is a powerful distorting pressure, affecting adherence in ways that sometimes defy words but is often evident in the patient's body language and behaviors.

Ambivalence Impersonating Nonadherence: The Duality of Mind

Ruth G. is a 54-year-old mother of two and a resident of West Philadelphia. She presents on the advice of her pulmonologist after recently being diagnosed with moderate chronic obstructive pulmonary disease (COPD). She was told that her COPD would inexorably worsen unless she stopped smoking. On discussion with her adult sons, their obvious concern for her well-being and her own sense of responsibility for the problem prompted a visit to the tobacco clinic. During her initial interview, her distress was palpable, with pressured speech, intermittent tearfulness, and expressions of hopelessness. "Doctor, you just have to help me stop smoking, you just *have* to." After a careful history and discussion of the options, the nicotine inhaler was recommended: "five to ten puffs every hour or so as needed to keep the impulse to smoke at bay." Ruth was visibly excited by the possibilities. "This is *great*! I think it is just what I need. Oh, thank you, doctor!"

When she returned for her follow-up visit, Ms. G. again seemed distressed. "Doctor, *please* help me stop smoking. I just have to. I do not want to die." "Well, tell me about your experience with the inhaler," the doctor asked. "Oh, I didn't use them," Ruth replied. Assuming systematic obstacles to the plan, the doctor inquired about how much the pharmacy was going to charge her for the medication. Ms. G., in a raw display of self-awareness, became tearful as she explained, "No, they were free. I picked them up, took them home, and put them in a kitchen drawer. They are still there, in the wrapper, waiting. I know it sounds ridiculous— doctor, please help me—but I didn't use them because *I was afraid they might work.*"

When ambivalence is resolved through escape, it can sometimes be camouflaged as intentional nonadherence. Seemingly a reasonable act at first glance, escape nonadherence is characterized by motivations that break down on examination. If accepted on its face as intentional nonadherence, escape can be a source of significant frustration from the clinician's perspective, given that the rationale can seem trivial or even illogical.

Escape as Nonadherence: Resolving Ambivalence

Gordon W. is a 76-year-old retiree, currently living alone in a New Jersey seaside community. On his last visit to his cardiologist, Mr. W. was surprised to hear his echocardiogram showed progression of his heart failure. He presents to the tobacco clinic on the advice of his doctor. After a careful history and discussion of the options, varenicline was recommended at the standard dose. Mr. W. articulated his understanding of the plan and expressed enthusiasm for getting started, stating "maybe I can help myself live a little longer." When he returned for his follow-up visit, the patient reported being unable to take the medication as prescribed.

Clinician. What happened?

Mr. W. It just didn't feel right.

Clinician. Can you describe your experience?

Mr. W. It just wasn't good. It felt weird.

Clinician. What part of your body felt weird?

Mr. W. I don't know. All of it.

Clinician. OK, maybe we can change the dose or . . .

Mr. W. It wasn't working anyway.

Clinician. How many days did you take it?

Mr. W. I just took it once.

Clinician. Shall we try again? Maybe we can change the dose.

Mr. W. My wife doesn't want me to take it. How about the patch?

The artful practitioner probes and questions to discern the difference between intentional and escape nonadherence. The tangential nature of Mr. W.'s rationale is in marked contrast to the congruent narrative in the first example despite the superficial similarities. It is conceivable that Mr. W.'s decision to stop the medication after one dose was a response to an unanticipated biologic effect of the drug, but it is much more likely that his nonspecific side-effect experience was the result of mesolimbic threat detection. Stopping the medication offered a means of resolving ambivalence through escape. Keep in mind that resolving ambivalence through escape is not an indication of perfidy; threat detection in the instinctive mind powerfully frames the patient's cognitive experience of the world.

Clinical Patterns

At the risk of sounding obvious, quitting is not the same thing for everybody. Neither the clinical presentation of tobacco dependence nor the course of its treatment are monolithic. But is it random? Chaotic? Infinite? Or are there discernible patterns that can help us predict important treatment-related variation? Recognizing clinical patterns can help clinicians better understand what to expect, can improve tailoring of approach, and can reduce the corrosive effects of unmet expectations.

There are a few patterns that help to understand what to expect in the clinic. The most recognizable is the archetypal pattern. Approximately a third of patients will follow the expected clinical trajectory, wherein appropriately placed patient education and counseling, supplemented by some medication, is followed by pretty good patient adherence to the plan and eventual smoking cessation. This is the ideal situation: talk to patients about triggers, help them modify some of their routines, teach them how to wear a patch, and watch change happen. Patients displaying the archetypal pattern are characterized by their ability to use the general, abstract concepts discussed in the clinic to identify concrete action steps specific to their personal needs. Archetypal patients are sometimes surprising in their creativity and will frequently engender a feeling of intense gratification among clinical staff.

The second, somewhat stereotypical clinical pattern is referred to as the dependent pattern. When working to control their compulsion to smoke, another third of patients follow a pattern more akin to substance-use recovery. These patients toil to reach a new understanding of tobacco use and achieve behavior change. Despite following the clinicians' advice, they seem to initially have trouble getting their compulsion under control. Patients displaying dependent patterns experience incomplete medication effects, early lapses, and multiple relapses before finding their new pattern of patterns. Dependent patients often require multiple and prolonged interventions before achieving control.

The third clinical pattern is often the one most difficult to understand. About a third of patients will experience a clinical course notable for a pattern of recurring escape nonadherence, referred to as the compulsive pattern. Patients demonstrating the compulsive pattern may superficially appear to be intentionally ignoring clinical advice, seemingly operating on two levels, assenting to a prespecified plan while in the clinic but quickly moving off that plan once left to their own devices at home. Because escape nonadherence can be easily misidentified as intentional nonadherence, patients displaying compulsive patterns can engender a sense of frustration and hopelessness among clinicians. Interestingly, these patients often display significant subjective distress at not being able to move treatment forward or attain their abstinence goals. Individual interactions are often marked by a sense of urgency that accompanies a clearly articulated rationale for abstaining (for example, "This is killing me; I just have to stop!"). Commonly, the patient's sense of desperation leads to alternative suggestions for treatment (for example, "How about the patch?"). From the clinician's perspective, this is often experienced as consistently trailing one step behind the best patient-centered approach, an experience not unlike that produced by the carnival game Whac-A-Mole.

Compulsive patients require a great deal of intensive, individualized attention. They often find it difficult to modify their daily smoking rituals and equally difficult to explain why. This clinical pattern is marked by frequent false starts and a chaotic quality to the treatment trajectory. Patients may report invasive thoughts of smoking and high impulsivity in response to short periods of attempted abstinence. Relapse is impulsive. The approach to these patients is intensive and requires a focus on creating awareness of emotional responses to threats of abstinence and the influence these emotions have on decision-making. Small process steps and a commitment to longitudinal monitoring are the norm, and they often require years of intervention and reintervention before confidence in control is established.

At this juncture, it remains unclear whether these clinical patterns represent distinct subgroups of disease, with distinct biological and/or social antecedents, or simply touchpoints on a continuum of disease severity. However, this is beside the point. At minimum, it is worth noting the range of clinical diversity if only to make plain the need for treatment strategies that extend beyond the current one-size-fits-all model. More significantly, by acknowledging the diversity in clinical presentations, we can begin to visualize care models that seek to match patient needs with the required intensity of treatment. For example, the various available modalities of counseling (individual, group, internet, telephone) may no longer be viewed as interchangeable vehicles of similar information but rather as tools to be matched to the details of clinical phenotype as needed. Medication choices may no longer be based on pharmacology alone but rather in response to the specific functional distortions identified in phenotypic groups. Finally, health system policies, including prescription formulary coverage, training priorities, and availability of advanced resources, might be retooled to match the range of phenotypic variation and avoid one-size-fits-all solutions.

> *Does a 30% quit rate imply the medication was effective in 30% of patients, or that it worked in nearly all the 30% of patients for whom it was the right choice?*

Clinic Insight: Loss to Follow-up

In tobacco-dependence research, when a subject fails to return for a scheduled follow-up visit, the most stringent way to evaluate the intervention being studied is to consider the loss to follow-up to be a sign that the subject continues to smoke. When a subject is lost to follow-up, information about their status remains unavailable at a predetermined measurement timepoint in the study protocol. In a statistical process called point censoring, the researcher imputes a value for that subject's status based on common assumptions about the condition being studied. It is estimated that as many as 30% of subjects who enroll in clinical studies of all types will be lost to follow-up at some point in the study. Because relapse is common in tobacco-dependence treatment, missing values in study protocols are often censored as "currently smoking." If the researcher can still prove the intervention is effective despite the most conservative assumption, she can be more confident that the intervention will work in "real-world" situations.

In the clinic, as many as 20% of patients who present for care will be lost to follow-up after only a few visits. This is true for all conditions in medical practice, but it is particularly important in tobacco dependence. Often, clinicians will implicitly apply the same conservative point censoring assumptions to lost patients and assume that failure to return implies a de facto "currently smoking" status. Given what we know about adherence and the myriad ways in which patient behaviors may be affected, the same conservative assumptions that make sense in the research context become counterproductive in the clinic. It may be that the patient needs transportation, cannot afford the co-pay, or mistook the date. It certainly could be a means of sabotage (Chapter 8), but it could also be that the last visit resulted in abstinence. Keep in mind that no one really loves a trip to the clinic if they have already achieved their goals. Find a way to get in touch with patients who fail to show up as appointed. Find out what is going on. Expect nonadherence and manage it. The last thing that belongs in a tobacco-dependence clinic is a prevailing assumption of failure.

Biological Phenotypes

One of the earliest indications that there may be a biological basis for variation in smoking patterns came from a cohort study of Danish twins, born between 1870 and 1910. The study plotted the rate of behavioral concordance (whether both twins smoked or didn't) against the prevalence of smoking in the regions of Denmark in which they lived. The reasoning was simple: if the propensity to smoke was a simple matter of social influence alone, concordance rates in twins should mirror the prevalence of smoking in their immediate environment. The more smoking there was in the community, the more likely both twins would be smokers. If, however, there was a biological basis for smoking, people who share genes should share behaviors more frequently than the community rates would predict. The study confirmed that environmental factors do influence smoking rate but showed a significant increase in concordance among twin sets. Further, monozygotic (identical) twins, who share exact copies of their genes, had higher concordance rates than their dizygotic (fraternal) twin counterparts, who share genetic material to the same degree as nontwin siblings, regardless of the surrounding prevalence of smoking. Shared genes means shared probability of smoking. The effort to identify the genetics of tobacco dependence was in full swing after that.

It is now generally accepted that a significant portion of the variability in smoking initiation is attributable to genetic factors, approximately equivalent to the influence of environmental factors like cultural acceptance and availability. Even siblings who are adopted and raised in separate environments show concurrence and have a greater likelihood of becoming heavy smokers together. As much as two-thirds of the variability in the ability to control the compulsion to smoke has been attributed to genetic factors, including the severity of withdrawal symptoms and the response to pharmacotherapy. With a better understanding of nicotine's effect on the brain comes a growing understanding of the numerous ways genetics might explain the clinical variation experienced in the clinic.

One of the targets that shows great potential to have direct clinical relevance involves measurements of how quickly the patient metabolizes nicotine. It is unclear in exactly what manner the rate at which the body removes nicotine from circulation impacts the neurobiologic effects of nicotine exposure, but it is pretty clear that it is an important marker for some effect that has direct clinical relevance. Most of the nicotine is metabolized by the liver enzyme CYP2A6. Several genetic variants of the CYP2A6 gene have been identified, each coding for slightly different versions of the enzyme with resulting differences in enzyme activity. The problem is that it is hard to discern differences in CYP2A6 activity between individuals because the rate of nicotine metabolism is also influenced by other factors, like concurrent medications and use of oral contraceptives. Adding to the problem is the fact that there is substantial day-to-day variation in nicotine metabolism, even among individuals with the same genotype. Thankfully, a biomarker for CYP2A6 activity was identified that correlates well with CYP2A6 genotypes. The nicotine metabolite ratio is a measure of the relative concentration of two important metabolites of nicotine and is sometimes referred to as the 3-hydroxycotinine–to–cotinine ratio. This metric is insensitive to things like gender, race, medications, and hormone status; is independent of time since last cigarette; and is reliably measured in both saliva and plasma.

The first study to examine the effect of the nicotine metabolite ratio on response to treatment suggested that subjects with a low ratio (slower metabolizers of nicotine) responded significantly better to nicotine patch therapy than did subjects with a higher ratio (faster metabolizers). At the end of six months of follow-up, nearly three times as many slow metabolizers were still not smoking compared with their fast metabolizer counterparts. Interestingly, fast metabolizer subjects treated with a self-titratable form of nicotine (nasal spray) were able to overcome this handicap and achieve abstinence rates similar to the slow metabolizer group. Besides better abstinence probabilities, lower nicotine metabolite ratios have also been associated with consumption of fewer daily cigarettes, smaller puff volumes, and fewer puffs per cigarette. These observations culminated in a large, prospective, double-blind study of the effect of nicotine metabolic ratio on pharmacologic outcomes. More than 1,200 subjects were grouped by nicotine metabolite ratio, then randomly assigned to receive the nicotine patch, varenicline, or placebo. All subjects received counseling on ways to stop smoking. Slow metabolizers of nicotine again did much better when treated with the patch than did their fast-metabolizing colleagues. Treatment outcomes with varenicline were not affected by nicotine metabolism, but there was an interesting increase in rate of side effects experienced by slow metabolizers (Table 10.2). Always consider biological differences when evaluating the impact of your intervention.

Table 10.2. Potential clinical impact of personalized approach to treatment selection based on biologic phenotyping.

Nicotine Metabolite Ratio	Metabolic Rate	Treatment Response (Patch Controller)	Treatment Response (Nasal Spray Reliever)	Side-Effect Probability (Varenicline Controller)
Low	Slow	↑↑	No difference	Increased
High	Fast	↓	No difference	Low

Concurrent Conditions

A few important and prevalent conditions have profoundly affected clinical decision-making in the past. The good news is that more data have become available over the past decade suggesting that the treatment of nicotine dependence is safer than we thought, even in groups previously felt to be "high risk" or otherwise especially vulnerable. For example, while treating tobacco dependence is a key component of reducing the disparity in morbidity and mortality suffered by people with serious mental illness, long-standing worries about the possibility of destabilizing psychiatric control and misapplied concern for patient autonomy have conspired to keep rates of integrated tobacco treatment low. Early laboratory observations about the vasoactive properties of nicotine have kept effective treatments out of the hands of patients at high risk of cardiovascular events, despite the proven impact of abstinence on morbidity. Finally, outdated notions regarding the nature of willpower and nicotine addiction have limited our willingness to offer pregnant women pharmacotherapy, leaving them alone and to the considerable detriment of the fetus.

BEHAVIORAL HEALTH

A significant mortality gap is experienced by people with serious mental illness (SMI) compared with their non-SMI counterparts. Essentially, their illness condemns them to living only two-thirds of a full life. The premature mortality experienced by this group of people is the result of a complicated mix of factors, including poorer physical health, limited financial and housing resources, and obstacles to high-quality healthcare. However, one of the major contributors to this gap is the prevalence of smoking in this group. On average, people with SMI smoke more aggressively than people without SMI and suffer smoking-related illness at about three times the rate of the general population. That is a travesty. This disparity persists in part because of several pervasive myths concerning tobacco treatment in the mentally ill (Table 10.3).

Table 10.3. Misconceptions regarding treatment of tobacco dependence in behavioral health.

Behavioral Health Myths	Tobacco Dependence Facts
People with mental illness will not quit smoking.	Patients with serious mental illness (SMI) report interest in quitting at the same rates as the general population.
People with mental illness cannot quit smoking.	Patients with SMI experience the same relative effects of pharmacotherapy when treated.
Smoking makes it easier to treat SMI.	Patients with SMI who smoke are several-fold more likely to leave treatment against medical advice.
Continued smoking is important to maintaining stable blood levels of SMI medication.	Smoking can increase clearance of common medications, making them much less effective.

People with mental illness cannot quit without experiencing negative consequences.	Both positive and negative affect scores remain stable after quitting with treatment.
People with substance use disorders cannot effectively pursue recovery if abstaining.	Tobacco dependence treatment supports recovery from other addictions.
Staff at mental health facilities sometimes use access to smoking privileges as a reward for good behaviors.	OK, that one is true.

Over the past decade, a number of sophisticated studies have been performed evaluating the safety and efficacy of tobacco-dependence treatment in people with SMI and substance-use disorders. Large-scale observational studies, involving progressively larger cohorts of patients with sample sizes reaching the tens of thousands, consistently demonstrated that initial concerns may have been unwarranted. Analyses of prospective trial data that included subjects with preexisting SMI proved too insufficient to overcome long-standing reluctance to use pharmacotherapy in this group, that is, until a seminal study was published in 2016 laying the question to rest. Designed specifically to evaluate the impact of pharmacologic treatment on the rate of adverse events in patients with SMI, the EAGLES trial enrolled a massive 8,144 participants across 16 countries, about half of whom had SMI. Each subject was randomly assigned to receive one of four possible pharmacologic treatments—varenicline, bupropion, patch, or placebo—in addition to counseling. The subjects were matched so that the only significant difference between the groups was the presence or absence of SMI. To reduce any potential bias when evaluating the results, all subjects and investigators were blinded to the assigned treatment being used.

In terms of efficacy, the medications performed about as expected. The subjects treated with varenicline experienced the highest proportion of abstinence, followed by those treated with bupropion or patch, while counseling alone (placebo medication) performed least well of all the options. What was notable was that this pattern was the same for both the SMI and the non-SMI control group; while the absolute numbers of patients with SMI who quit were a bit lower, the relative impact of adding the medication to counseling was the same. This finding highlighted two important points. First, while one might expect people with SMI to face more complicated obstacles to quitting than their non-SMI counterparts, the ability of medications to change the probabilities of the target outcome were the same for both groups, regardless of preexisting mental illness. Thinking probabilistically instead of linearly, this effect cannot be ignored. Second, denying people with SMI access to these medications, particularly in light of the disproportionate toll tobacco takes on their lives, is inconsistent with a philosophy of nondiscrimination based on mental illness and contravenes the long-standing International Covenant on Economic, Social, and Cultural Rights in mental illness.

The study was specifically powered to be able to detect the impact of tobacco-dependence pharmacotherapy on the rate of adverse events in the setting of mental illness. If treating tobacco dependence makes it more likely that SMI symptoms worsen—or that likelihood of suicide increases—one would expect to see this effect overly represented in the cohort of subjects with preexisting SMI. This was not the case. Not only were rates of adverse events low in both groups; they approximated the event rates observed in the placebo treatment group, regardless of which active pharmacologic treatment they received. Unfortunately, there was one suicide that occurred, in a non-SMI subject receiving placebo—an overall suicide rate approximately equivalent to the observed global suicide rate.

CARDIOVASCULAR DISEASE

In the late twentieth century, laboratory studies confirmed that nicotine can lead to increases in heart rate and blood pressure in patients with poor baseline control. Additionally, there was concern that the vasoactive properties of nicotine would cause coronary vasoconstriction and potentially worsen critical blood flow in patients with preexisting vasculopathies. For a long time, clinicians were cautious about prescribing nicotine-based therapies to their tobacco-dependent patients with cardiovascular disease. Unfortunately, excessive caution became the norm. The situation is better now that there are non-nicotine treatments available, but concern over cardiovascular side effects remains a major contributor to persistent fears of nicotine overdose, among clinicians and patients alike. Keep in mind that no matter which form of nicotine treatment is prescribed, smoking leads to arterial blood nicotine levels as much as ten times higher than those produced by pharmacotherapy (Chapter 6), even if the patient continues to smoke during treatment.

The vasculopathic effects of smoking, including the impact on microvascular blood flow during wound healing, are the product of several complicated distortions in vascular biology produced by smoke, not nicotine. The non-nicotine components of cigarette smoke promote cardiovascular injury by delivering significant concentrations of carbon dioxide to the arterial blood, lowering circulating oxygen content, and causing a reciprocal increase in compensatory cardiac work. Platelets and fibrinogen, the blood's circulating sealants, begin to clump and form microclots in the tiniest of blood vessels, reducing local oxygen supply. Neutrophils, the immune system's front line of defense against environmental injury, get activated and release powerful oxidizing enzymes into the system, promoting ongoing oxidant injury long after the smoke has cleared. For these reasons and others, the impact of helping people stop smoking on cardiovascular future morbidity is significant and immediate.

The first seminal study to evaluate this prospectively was published in 1996 and included 584 veterans with documented cardiovascular disease who were cared for across 10 Veterans Affairs health centers. They received either a ten-week patch taper or placebo. Those receiving the patch were more likely to quit and showed no additional risk of death, cardiovascular events, or hospitalization for any reason. Since then, several studies have been performed in various settings, with subjects suffering varying degrees of cardiovascular acuity. The results all seem to point in the same direction. In one study, researchers found that intensive tobacco-dependence treatment reduced all-cause mortality among high-risk smokers hospitalized with acute cardiovascular events from 12% in the usual-care group to only 2.8% in the intensive-treatment group. That is a huge absolute risk reduction of over 9% during the two-year follow-up period. That means treating tobacco dependence in eleven high-risk smokers will save one extra life.

PREGNANCY

Though pregnancy is not exactly a medical "condition" in the classical sense, treating tobacco dependence during pregnancy is encumbered by deep-seated societal notions of maternal obligation. Clinicians are commonly confronted with two contradictory ideas. On one hand, if a woman needs pharmacotherapy to help her stop smoking while she is pregnant, she may be seen as not having sufficient willpower to match her newfound responsibilities. On the other, if she admits she does not have enough willpower to quit despite being pregnant, cultural expectations may compel her to work to find more willpower, not pharmacotherapeutic help. Somehow, it is easier to ignore the variability in tobacco dependence when a woman is pregnant, as though a baby makes decades of complicated neurophysiology suddenly trivial. Some women stop smoking without assistance, but that is not a rebuttal to variability; it is proof of the point. By expecting all pregnant women to be of the archetypal phenotype, clinicians are exacting a kind of redistributive injustice, accepting the chance that the baby will pay the toll of continued smoking in exchange for the convenience of not recommending tobacco-dependence pharmacotherapy under complicated circumstances.

Both the U.S. Public Health Service and the American College of Obstetrics and Gynecology have produced recommendations which deal directly with treating tobacco dependence during pregnancy. Neither organization makes a direct recommendation to use pharmacotherapy in pregnant women, favoring instead intensive individual counseling, cognitive behavioral therapy, and telephone quit-line support. This probably goes without saying, but clinicians should not use pharmacotherapy to treat any problem when it is not required. When nonpharmacologic interventions prove insufficient, however, clinicians are forced to face the reality they have rather than the one they want. In that case, the decision to use pharmacotherapy can only be made after carefully weighing the totality of risks and benefits and estimating how they line up with the patient's understanding and needs. It is a personalized decision that requires careful discussion with the patient and careful monitoring for any indication that the plan needs to change. To be fair, neither organization recommends against using pharmacotherapy; they just could not find a way to recommend its use given the poor quality of data available at the time the guidelines were produced.

In a 2012 fixed-effects meta-analysis of five randomized controlled trials, one quasi–randomized controlled trial, and one prospective study (1,386 pregnant women who smoke), pharmacotherapy (nicotine replacement or bupropion) had a significant effect on the mother's ability to achieve abstinence (risk ratio, 1.8), and no discernible negative impact on fetal development or obstetric complications. The gestational safety of pharmacotherapy during pregnancy was again confirmed in a 2016 analysis of data derived from 900 pregnant women who smoke who were enrolled in the Quebec Pregnancy Cohort, in which both nicotine and bupropion reduced the risk for premature delivery by about 80%. The 2020 Cochrane meta-analysis of eleven trials (2,412 pregnant smokers) again confirmed the safety of treatment and found nicotine replacement produces a significant difference in abstinence rates in later pregnancy (risk ratio, 1.37), but this effect size decreases when the analysis is limited to only studies with placebo controls (risk ratio, 1.21).

Here is the problem: a paucity of high-quality evidence regarding use of tobacco pharmacotherapy during pregnancy may not be sufficient justification for avoiding more aggressive interventions given the potentially catastrophic impact of continued maternal smoking (Table 10.4).

Imagine Miracle Drug X were being evaluated for its potential to reduce placenta previa, premature birth, and perinatal deaths. Given the dramatic, life-altering nature of these events, how strong would the evidence in favor of Miracle Drug X need to be—in how many trials, over how many years—before clinical opinion shifted toward universal acceptance? Would we tolerate study designs plagued by nonadherence with Miracle Drug X as evidence of ineffectiveness? Would we accept study designs that require proof that the patient had sufficient resolution to achieve the effect of Miracle Drug X before offering the intervention? Imagine how different the clinical conversation would be if tobacco-dependence pharmacotherapy were framed as an intervention to reduce fetal morbidity and mortality rather than as an intervention aimed at modifying maternal behavior.

Table 10.4. Effects of smoking and pharmacotherapy on pregnancy. A paucity of high-quality evidence regarding use of tobacco pharmacotherapy during pregnancy may not be sufficient justification for avoiding more aggressive interventions given the potentially catastrophic impact of continued maternal smoking.

Continued Smoking		Pharmacotherapy
Social stigma Placenta previa/abruptio Reduced fetal measurement Low birth weight Premature birth Infant wheezing Perinatal death	vs.	The quality of data on effectiveness is mixed.

Chapter 10 Learning Points

- Adherence is an important mediator of pharmacotherapeutic effect. Managing adherence is an important responsibility of clinicians seeking to achieve that effect.
- As in all other medical interventions, nonadherence with tobacco-dependence pharmacotherapy may be intentional or nonintentional. However, unlike other medical conditions, the ambivalence of dependence may also manifest as escape nonadherence. To the untrained eye, this can appear to be intentional.
- Escape is not deceit. It is threat response. Gentle probing reveals a subtle incongruence in the patient's narrative details—the hallmark of escape nonadherence.
- Not all quitting is the same. Three distinct clinical phenotypes represent three different clinical trajectories and require three different clinical approaches to care.

- In contradistinction to research, loss to follow-up in the clinic does not necessarily indicate continued smoking. Clinicians should follow up with patients to find pragmatic solutions to longitudinal care impediments.
- The nicotine metabolite ratio is a useful biological marker that appears to have important clinical implications. In the future, medication choices may be driven by biology rather than incorrect notions of therapeutic equivalence.
- Patients with psychiatric comorbidities should be treated. Patients with known elevated risk for cardiac events benefit significantly from the treatment of their tobacco dependence.
- Pregnant women who smoke sometimes need clinical help to stop. When evaluating the evidence in favor of treatment, frame the intervention in terms of reducing gestational and perinatal morbidity.

Chapter 11
Routines

Coffee and cigarettes just go together perfectly. Neither one tastes right without the other.

—Eileen B., 45 years old

"What is that CPT code for smoking?" David mutters as he searches the long list of billing codes on his computer, trying to finish his notes and leave the office. "That was definitely more than ten minutes of counseling with Helen." She had met with the surgeon, and as expected, she needs to quit smoking before her hip surgery. She was clearly struggling, but it was difficult to develop a plan that she would follow and that would have an effect. Helen complained, "My morning coffee is not the same without a cigarette, and it is impossible not to smoke a cigarette after dinner." David remembered having dinners with his brother John, who also smokes, and watching his brother jump up from the table after dinner—always making some excuse to go outside. John's wife often cornered David at family gatherings, desperate to see if there was anything that could help her husband stop smoking. He recommended buying the patch or gum, but now he wondered if his brother was struggling in the same ways as Helen. David tried suggesting to Helen that she change her routines around a little, but she was stubborn. "I've sat in the same chair every morning enjoying my coffee and cigarette for over thirty years. There's nowhere else for me to sit." When he suggested different ways of talking to Kathy that didn't require sitting on the porch chairs, she dismissed this as well. Helen mentioned that Kathy was no longer smoking, so David thought they could sit inside or talk on the phone. Both of those ideas were emphatically rejected as "not possible," although it was unclear why. David's brother was infamous for putting up roadblocks to any suggestions regarding quitting, and his family blamed his inherent stubborn nature. As David finishes his note about Helen's visit, he thinks, "I doubt that Helen will take any of my advice. My own brother doesn't take my advice. This must be more than stubbornness."

———

David counseled Helen to stop smoking. As a transitive verb, "counseling" implies the act of giving advice, urging a course of action, or recommending the adoption of a specific plan. So when Helen doesn't follow David's advice, engage in his preferred course of action, or adopt his specific plan, "counseling" acquires a strange duplexity. It is simultaneously trivial and easy to accomplish, yet complicated and requires years of training. Counseling conjures both the summer camp and the Freudian couch. It is no wonder the practice remains just short of satisfying so often and for so many clinicians.

Chapters 9 and 10 dealt with rebalancing the chemical milieu of the meso-limbic system so that positive change becomes possible. Though medications help to improve the probability of recovery, medications do not make change a certainty. If David expects Helen to stop smoking just because she wears a patch, he has missed the point of using medications. No amount of medication can take the place of the inner work that is necessary to achieve abstinence, yet Helen's inner work cannot be left to chance alone. If nicotine has changed the pattern of patterns in Helen's brain, affecting how she thinks about smoking, what David needs in response is an active way of helping Helen reset the patterns back to the time before she began to smoke. As a noun, "counseling" can be conceived of as a set of tactics that David can use to guide Helen toward a new mode of thinking about smoking—not a way of convincing her to think differently but a way of facilitating Helen's thoughtful movement toward a new way of thinking. In the tobacco clinic, "counseling" (the noun) refers to a set of meta-cognitive skills that help new patterns, emotions, and reactions emerge from within the patient herself (Table 11.1).

———

Table 11.1. The functional difference between framing "counsel" as a transitive verb rather than as a particular set of clinically effective skills.

Helen: "What should I do to stop smoking?"	
David counseled (verb): "Try reading a book or taking a walk."	David applied counseling skills: "What do you think might work?"

In a way, clinical counseling in tobacco dependence is about using cognition to manage cognition. As medications affect the brain in hopes of changing the mind, cognitive management seeks to change the mind in hopes of reordering the disordered patterns within the brain. David can get to Helen's mesolimbic system through the bloodstream, but he can also get there through her ears. By guiding Helen toward a change in her thinking about smoking—and her visceral response to the threat of abstinence—David is actively promoting change in the physical function of her threat detection system just as the cardiologist changes the strength of a heartbeat through advice to exercise.

Think of cognitive management as a subset of cognitive behavioral therapy (CBT), a well-validated form of therapeutic counseling that has shown excellent effectiveness in a variety of disorders in which destructive behaviors exist at the intersection of abnormally amplified emotional motivators and the maladaptive thought patterns that result. CBT proper rests on the idea that behavioral problems are often based on a foundation of faulty or unhelpful ways of thinking and that those learned thinking patterns need to be actively unlearned and replaced with better ways of coping. The professional practice of CBT usually involves helping patients recognize the distortions in thinking that are creating the problem, reevaluate them in light of reality, and gain problem-solving skills to help manage anticipatable difficulties. Therapists help patients develop a greater sense of confidence and a willingness to face fears instead of avoiding them. Professional CBT practice requires specific in-depth training and resources that are beyond the scope of the typical tobacco-dependence clinical practice. However, that does not mean clinicians cannot adopt the pertinent aspects of CBT theory, learn from the tactics employed by CBT professionals, and integrate the lessons learned into a set of cognitive management skills that will help them become even more effective.

Defining the Problem

Imagine a therapist concerned with helping clients manage their depression. Both the therapist and client would have a similar overall goal for therapy—to resolve the depression. When describing the impact of depression on their life, new clients might define their problem in a number of possible ways. For example, a problem statement might be something like, "I just do not have the energy to participate in daily tasks anymore," or "I feel sad inside and I do not really know why." It is less likely that the new client would state their problem as "Tell me what to do to resolve my depression." Problems are experienced while goals are tangible outcomes.

In tobacco dependence, the problem statement is often conflated with the goal. It is not unusual to hear patients state their problem as "I just have to stop smoking." That is an outcome. Their experience of ambivalence can be so deeply embedded in their thinking that it becomes difficult to notice the problematic connections that have kept them from achieving their goal. A good place to start the process of cognitive management is by helping patients to discern the two ideas, focusing their attention on the experience of ambivalence rather than their desired outcome. Doing so allows the patient to shift the emphasis away from "quitting" and concentrate more fully on the obstacles that keep them from achieving their goal. Helping the patient recognize the experience of ambivalence helps them remove "I can't" from the problem and replace it with awareness of distortions in threat detection (Table 11.2).

Table 11.2. Common expressions of ambivalence in the clinic.

It's not really a craving, it is more like a wake-up call. When it happens, you just smoke. That's it. I can't really explain it. It's weird.
I really hate the way it smells, the way it tastes—everything about it. But sometimes I just need a little taste—a few puffs—and then I'm back in business.
I know I have to stop, but I do not want to. I love smoking. I'm afraid I'll never quit.
I can quit if I want to; I've quit lots of times before. I just can't seem to stay away from the cigarettes for very long afterward.
I can't imagine my life without smoking. What am I supposed to do without my best friend, my security blanket?
I quit about a month ago. But my husband still smokes in the house, so I spend my days desperate for a cigarette.
My mother died from lung cancer last month. She made me promise I would stop smoking. I promised her I would, but then I smoked at her funeral. What kind of person does that?

As ambivalence problem statements emerge, they provide a good starting point for exploring ways to talk about the neurophysiology of nicotine in ways that are accessible to patients and relevant to their experience. The provider's distillation should be complete enough to be factual, individualized enough to meet the patient's specific needs, and direct enough to be appropriate to the context of a clinical visit. Do not expect to have this distillation perfected on the first try; be willing to first break down complex ideas into rudimentary teaching points, then practice and refine each rudiment until the delivery is comfortable and efficient. At this stage of cognitive management, do not be afraid to gently educate rather than listen, always taking care not to be overly pedagogical. A small investment in education initially will help define the contours of the problem and give the patient a touchstone against which to explore the problem of ambivalence. This is the time to take a moment to talk about the process, discuss intermediate clinical objectives, or undo the burden of artificial timelines. Remember to avoid unwarranted emphasis on the overall therapeutic goal at this stage. A spontaneous doodle or prepared handout can really help here (Figure 11.1).

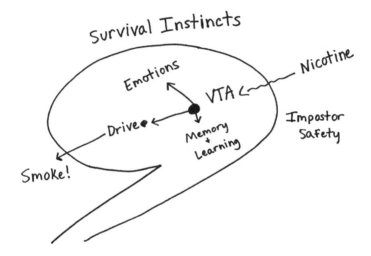

Figure 11.1. Making complex ideas accessible to the patient: a rough sketch of mesolimbic functions and the distorting effects of nicotine.

Make It Cognitive

A sensory input triggers the signal to smoke, which Helen responds to immediately by smoking. The nature of the actual signal to smoke, the type of emotional response it engenders, and the connections that activate the motor sequence capped off by the cigarette to the lips are not easily recognized. In order for Helen to recognize the distortions that drive her smoking, she must understand the influence the mesolimbic system has on her decision-making. For that to happen, her reactions need to be "slowed down," reviewable moment by moment. She needs to notice the triggers, the instinctive reaction, the irrational drive, the anticipatory anxiety, the automaticity of thought, and the behavioral sequence that gets activated as a result.

How does a clinician help the patient deconstruct that experience? The best way is asking questions instead of giving answers. Questions force a search for the proper word to express a feeling or idea, which in turn forces feelings and ideas to transform from gut-level ambiguities to conscious specificities. By asking questions about the nature of triggers, the emotional response to the signal to smoke, and the automatic assumptions that constrain the resulting thoughts, the clinician effectively guides patients to a place where they begin to recognize holding two dissonant ideas simultaneously.

CLINICIAN. Tell me about your smoking routines.

PATIENT. I do not have any routines. I smoke all the time.

CLINICIAN. Do you smoke after dinner?

PATIENT. Yes.

CLINICIAN. Every night?

PATIENT. Yes. (hmmm . . .)

CLINICIAN. Before or after washing the dishes?

PATIENT. After. Always after. I like to get them done before my girlfriend calls at 7:00 o'clock.

CLINICIAN. What do you do when she calls?

PATIENT. I grab my cigarettes. I go up to my room. We talk. And I smoke. I guess I do have routines.

CLINICIAN. What would happen if she called but someone had moved your cigarettes, so you couldn't find them?

PATIENT. I would look for them first, then call her back once I found them.

CLINICIAN. What if you couldn't find them?

PATIENT. Oh, God. I don't know. [agitated] Go to the store maybe? That would suck.

Guiding patients toward a dissonant position is an important part of cognitive management for two reasons: (1) it provides an opportunity to relate the source of dissonance back to the conflict between the instinctive and cognitive brains, and (2) a first-person experience of incongruence can be more effective at facilitating change than the more typical bystander experience of having the clinician point out narrative inconsistencies.

The Principal's Principles?

Ms. Lewis was a 63-year-old principal of a West Philadelphia middle school. She first presented to the tobacco clinic on the advice of her primary care provider in March 2006, seeking assistance with her tobacco dependence. She had smoked for nearly fifty years at that point, having attempted abstinence on many occasions over the years. Ms. Lewis was always impeccably dressed, professional, easygoing, and quick with a smile. By April of that year, she had successfully controlled her compulsion to smoke, using a combination of bupropion and nicotine inhaler. She had excellent insight into her triggers and was always adherent with both her pharmacologic regimen and the behavioral work prescribed during her clinic visits. On her July visit, Ms. Lewis appeared noticeably agitated. Though she was never overtly unkind or angry, her answers had become uncharacteristically short and directed. She reported remaining continuously abstinent since April, but she was becoming increasingly frustrated that her connection to cigarettes had not yet "gone away." She was tired of quitting and wanted to simply be done with the process.

Ms. Lewis reported that in an effort to accelerate her recovery, she had recently bought a pack of her favorite brand of cigarettes and placed them on top of her china cabinet, where they remained out of sight. When asked whether she thought this was a risky strategy, potentially a significant step toward relapse, Ms. Lewis explained that "this is the way to handle problems in life." Pressed for more details, she went on to state, "This is the way my family has always handled our problems. You have to stare your problems straight in the face and just plain beat them on principle. My father handled all of his problems that way." "Can you describe another life problem that you or your family have dealt with this way?" the clinician asked. After a long pause without an obvious answer, the clinician rephrased: "OK, maybe that's too hard to recall on the spot. How about in school? Are there problems that your students experience where you might advise them to use a similar coping principle?"

At that point, Ms. Lewis became tearful, her confusion and exhaustion evident in her body language. "No," she said, "that's bad advice. I don't know. We don't really handle problems that way. It just seemed like maybe it was a good idea, even though I knew it was a bad idea. I'm just so tired."

Remember that triggers can be internal, too. Emotions, particularly negative emotions like fear, anger, loss, sadness, frustration, or boredom, can be powerful triggers to smoke. The problem is that unlike the 7:00 p.m. phone call each night, negative emotions are more like rolling waves that ebb and flow and less like discrete events that can be easily anticipated. While the emotion itself may be a reliable stimulus to smoke, the events that produce the emotion are varied and often occur unexpectedly. It pays to spend some time helping patients identify the warning signs that indicate negative emotions are on the horizon. For example, a patient might expect an increased level of anxiety on the night before weekly staff meetings. Another might identify the end-of-month billing period as a stressful time. Many patients identify their evening television routines as a source of boredom, responsible for a significant increase in smoking. Clinicians shouldn't feel powerless if the underlying problems can't be resolved per se (that is, anticipatory anxiety in preparation for a staff meeting may actually be adaptive, the patient's financial pressures cannot be made to disappear, and so on). The objective is to help patients distinguish the influence of the context (for example, evening television) from the influence of the emotion (for example, boredom).

> *Emotional responses to external circumstances*
> *should be accepted as natural fact.*
> *Smoking in response to internal emotions*
> *is an unnatural, learned fiction.*
> *It is OK to be [insert emotion] without smoking.*

Guiding patients toward an awareness of their automatic responses to emotional triggers is another important part of cognitive management for two reasons: (1) it provides an opportunity for patients to reflect on the ordinariness of those emotions and the role of emotion in the genesis of automatic smoking, and (2) it provides an opportunity for the patient to identify instances in their life wherein the same emotion isn't inevitably followed by smoking. These ideas provide observable "proof" that patients have the nascent skills to cope without nicotine.

Managing negative emotional states can cost the patient a significant investment of energy. Depletion, a state of emotional and cognitive fatigue, increases impulsivity and is a significant risk factor for relapse. Clinicians should make patients aware of the possibility of depletion and the potential consequences thereof. Proper rest, attention to nutrition, alcohol avoidance, and the pursuit of alternative reinforcers like social gatherings, exercise, and other forms of entertainment can be effective at preventing depletion and can restore energy reserves necessary for resilience.

Anticipate Forecasting Errors

Anticipatory anxiety in the face of impending abstinence is a hallmark of dependence. But anxiety forecasting (being anxious about the possibility of being anxious in the future) is a form of affective prediction error that can keep some patients frozen in place, despite a desire to change. Statements like "I'm worried about how I'll be able to manage" or "What will I use to help me calm down after I quit?" can be clues that this form of emotional prediction error is in play. Left unchecked, anxiety forecasting tends to result in a significant overestimation of the intensity and duration of negative emotions experienced as a result of abstinence. In other words, molehills become mountains, and challenges become catastrophes. "My doctor said I'm anxious, but I'm really worried it is something worse."

Part of the clinician's role in cognitive management is to minimize the influence of unworkable affective predictions. Decatastrophizing is a strategy for reducing catastrophic thinking by acknowledging, not denying, the emotion and promoting a more balanced response. Careful always to ask questions instead of giving answers, decatastrophizing guides patients toward more realistic predictions through use of "So . . . what if?" questions. Here are some examples:

- So . . . what if you feel like you need a cigarette but do not have one? What would realistically happen if you had to go without?
- So . . . what if you feel stressed at work at a time when smoking is not appropriate? How do you usually manage? If smoking in the house becomes inappropriate, what would realistically be different from the way things are at work?
- So . . . what if you feel anxious for a little while? Could you accept that? Other than being uncomfortable, is being anxious harmful? Is there another way to think about discomfort that does not mean it is "bad"?
- So . . . how do athletes deal with the stress of a close game? Are there any lessons in there for the rest of us? Can the stress resulting from the need to perform be a good thing?
- So . . . imagine being forced to go a whole day without smoking for some reason. How would you cope if that happened? What would realistically be different about your life on that day? Can you list the parts of your day that would be the same regardless?

Lock in the Future You Want, Not the One You Get

Many tobacco-dependent patients mistakenly place their faith in their strength of will and resilience. Encouraging patients to prethink ways to avoid temptations before they arise is a way of making the problem cognitive and will empower patients to find ways to avoid the salient temptations. Here is an example:

CLINICIAN. Tell me about the one thing you think will keep you from achieving your goal.

PATIENT. I can go all day without a cigarette, but when I pass the bodega on the corner, I always seem to just go in there and get two loosies. Every time.

CLINICIAN. When do you pass the bodega?

PATIENT. Every time I come out of my house.

CLINICIAN. When you walk out your front door, which way do you have to turn to walk past the bodega?

PATIENT. Right. I always turn right.

CLINICIAN. Could you turn left?

PATIENT. Not really. My street is one-way, and I park my car to the right. I have to go that way.

CLINICIAN. Is there anywhere else you could park your car?

PATIENT. I guess I could park around the corner on 21st Street. That should be OK.

CLINICIAN. Let's make that our new rule. Always park on 21st Street so you can turn left coming out of the house.

PATIENT. OK. Sounds good.

Prethinking a plan for avoidance is clearly important, but prethinking a legitimate response to unavoidable encounters is also essential. Preplanned behaviors, in the form of "if this problem, then that solution," makes those behavioral solutions more readily available to the patient and more likely to be implemented with less effort when the obstacle does arise. Preferred behavioral responses become more automatic, requiring fewer cognitive resources if they are prospectively planned.

However, prethinking solutions can sometimes be challenging. For most of us, our brains are oriented toward goal-intention thought. "I want to stop smoking." Sometimes, it is difficult for patients to move away from goal-intentioned thinking to implementation-intention thinking without a little coaching. "In order to stop smoking, I will first X, then I will Y, and if Z happens, I will A, B, and then C." It is easy to see how much more complicated this form of prospective planning might be. Despite the extra effort it may take, it is important for clinicians to help patients accomplish this because implementation-intention thinking significantly increases the likelihood of reaching a behavioral goal (Table 11.3).

Table 11.3. Clinical conversations reflecting goal intention versus implementation intention.

Goal-Intention Speech	Implementation-Intention Speech
CLINICIAN. What will you do when the urge to smoke hits? PATIENT. I won't smoke. No way. I just have to remind myself that I really don't want to smoke. CLINICIAN. How will you avoid it? PATIENT. I just won't pick up a cigarette. CLINICIAN. What can you do to help yourself not pick it up? PATIENT. Trust me. I won't.	CLINICIAN. What will you do when the urge to smoke hits? PATIENT. Use my nicotine inhaler. CLINICIAN. How will you know you're using enough? PATIENT. I will use five to ten puffs at a time, and keep using it every few minutes until the craving goes away. CLINICIAN. How will you make sure you get to it in time? PATIENT. I'll keep one on my nightstand, one in my car, and one in my pocket.

Homework Helps

The realities of the clinic visit sometimes limit the amount of time or attention the clinician and patient can devote to cognitive management. But here is the good news: it is best if the majority of the cognitive work is performed by the patient, alone, outside the visit, surrounded by their environmental routines. How does a good coach motivate athletes to practice on their own? By breaking down game play into specific component sequences and giving specific direction in pursuit of specific goals. How does a good teacher solidify the pupil's newfound insight? By using the lessons learned during classroom time to solve a specific set of related problems later that night. That's right—homework.

To help accomplish cognitive management goals, it is often useful to employ worksheets or other handout tools to encourage patients to unfreeze formed associations while developing new ones. After dedicating a few minutes to establishing cognitive management goals during the visit, it is helpful to assign the patient specific at-home tasks that will help set up new, more adaptive responses to the impulse to smoke (Table 11.4).

Table 11.4. Using "homework" assignments to help solidify new skills between interventions.

Cognitive Management Objective	Suggestions for Homework Assignment
Defining the problem	Patients have been taught to approach the problem from a "character flaw" perspective, but we want them to adopt the more therapeutic "environmental influence" perspective (see also Chapter 12). To accomplish this frame shift, it is sometimes useful to anthropomorphize the neurobiology of addiction. Once explained, encourage the patient to give the biological influence of nicotine (that is, the disorder of learning and memory, the treacherous second brain) a human name. By conceptualizing addiction as a villainous "other," the components of addictive behavior that exist outside the cognitive "self" can be more easily identified and addressed.
	Suggest the patient search the internet for a suitable picture representing the new bad character. Have them print it out and hang it in a visible location within the home—perhaps on the refrigerator door. Assign them the task of writing a letter to the rogue antihero, describing the destructive nature of their relationship, the emotional toll it has taken, their intention to bring the relationship to an end, and the steps they will take to ensure this will happen. Ask the patient to anticipate the excuses the offender will make when reading the letter and the pleadings the malefactor may employ in the effort to forestall change. Have them prethink their response to each argument.
Making it cognitive	The objective here is to facilitate an awareness of automatic behaviors and patterns related to smoking. These routines can be so automatic as to be virtually invisible to smokers themselves. Begin by setting up a three-column worksheet for the patient, with the first column heading being "When do I smoke?" In this column, instruct the patient to identify one predictable cue to smoke—"with my morning coffee," for example. In the second column, ask the patient to identify their routines surrounding this instance. Suggest they work with a family member or friend to begin identifying, in as much detail as possible, components of their routine. For example, "I program the coffee

maker so it is already made when I wake up. I grab my mug from the cabinet and pour. I take my coffee black and drink it at the kitchen table while I read the paper."

The goal for the third column is to challenge the patients to imagine small changes to the ritual that, on balance, won't require that they forgo their coffee, but instead will make them more aware of each step in the routine. For example, "I could change the location of the coffee maker. I could brew the coffee after I get downstairs. I could use a different mug each day of the week. I could drink the coffee at the counter. I could leave reading the paper for the evening."

Depletion	Making patients aware that depletion happens, and providing them with the vocabulary for identifying it when it does, is an important first step. Helping them manage it effectively is the next. After reviewing the need for proper rest, exercise, and nutrition during recovery, have your patients prepare a support team—a list of at least three people in their life with whom they can discuss the work they are putting into quitting. Caution patients to avoid choosing people who will apply undue pressure or who will simply cheerlead. Since just acknowledging the depleting effects of recovery can be restorative all by itself, the most effective support teams consist of people with the ability to listen without judgment—not people who will reiterate the goal or feel compelled to give direction. Encourage the patient to broaden their scope when identifying support team members. Sometimes an acquaintance can be more effective in this role than a partner or close relative. Someone younger or older may be better suited than someone the same age. Coach the patient to ask their prospective support team members for their commitment before help is needed. Ask that they record the date the conversation happened and have the patient bring their notes about their encounter to the next visit.
Decatastrophizing	Addressing affective forecasting errors in person can be easy, if the clinician remembers to ask questions instead of giving answers. At home, though, dependence has a way of regenerating the patient's panic and magnifying their negative emotions. It is possible to promote continued attention to the connection between emotions, thoughts, and behaviors by offering a three-column worksheet, similar to the one described above. For instance, the first column heading might be, "When I think about breaking up with my cigarettes, I feel . . ." Patients should be encouraged to identify both the positive and negative associated emotions in this column. In the second column, patients might respond to the prompt, "What are the thoughts that typically follow this emotion?" If the patient has already

	anthropomorphized the problem, consider heading the column, "What does [name] try to tell you when you feel this way?" Finally, in column three, "What are some ways you respond to these thoughts and feelings when cigarettes are not around?" When reviewing the completed worksheet with patients, be sure to point out that each of the listed emotions is natural and occurs many times daily. Also be prepared to point out that simply living with the emotion for a little while, without necessarily responding to it, might feel bad momentarily but in fact causes no harm.
Implementation intention	The key to successful implementation thinking is specificity. While all implementation intention is of the form, "When ____, I will ____," the goal is to have the patients consider more than one contingency. Specificity is important in both blank spots of the plan. For example, Have the patient generate ten to fifteen specific implementation statements and write each of them on an index card. Encourage the patient to find a private location to read the cards aloud at least once each day. The small stack of index cards can also be carried in a pocket or purse and reviewed quietly several additional times daily, reinforcing the automatic nature of the target response.

Nonspecific	Semispecific	Specific
When I feel like smoking, I will distract myself.	When I feel like smoking, I will use my inhaler until the cravings disappear.	When I finish my coffee, I will use eight puffs of inhaler, and another eight when I wash the cup.

Note: Remember . . . Escape

One of the signs that patients recognize their thinking is changing is the realization that abstinence is, in fact, possible. As fewer obstacles stand in the way, the threat-detection system in the brain is forced to reckon with the notion that quitting is coming. Consequently, escape becomes more likely.

> *Validate, reframe, repeat.*
> *For as long as it takes.*

Chapter 11 Learning Points

- In the tobacco-dependence clinic, counseling becomes cognitive management—a set of tactics the clinician uses to guide the patient toward a self-realized new way of thinking.
- Begin by defining the problem(s) as opposed to simply stating the goal. Look for ambivalence statements in the patient's narrative. This is a good place to explain the neurobiology of nicotine's effect.
- Slow down the trigger-to-reaction process. Make it cognitive. Ask questions. Give the patient sufficient time to find the proper words to express their experience.
- Making it cognitive will often bring two simultaneously held but discordant ideas to light. This is good. A first-person experience of incongruence is an effective facilitator of change. Do not confuse making it cognitive with creating "gotcha" moments.
- Emotional triggers are also powerful; look for opportunities to connect emotions to automatic smoking behaviors, and help patients notice their own inherent ability to manage emotions without smoking.
- Quitting takes work. Work takes energy. Help patients avoid depletion.
- Affective forecasting errors lead to panic and catastrophization. Clinicians can decatastrophize through questions that guide the patient toward more realistic predictions.
- Prethinking specific steps for managing threats to abstinence before they arise significantly increases the odds that patients will respond to threats in adaptive rather than risky ways.
- Listen for goal-intention speech. Ask questions in search of specific implementation steps. Prethink ways to avoid triggers wherever possible and ways to manage temptation when impossible.
- Use homework assignments to unfreeze old thinking patterns and reinforce the new thinking patterns introduced in the clinic.
- Be prepared for escape. Validate. Reframe. Repeat.

Chapter 12
Influence

Quitting really changed my life.

—Elizabeth M., 90 years old

"OK, Helen. What can I say to get you to put your cigarettes down? I don't really want to keep convincing you that you need to do this," David heard himself saying to Helen one afternoon, with just enough frustration in his voice to make him feel a little bad about it. His day had been busy—too many patients, too much paperwork, not enough time to think. And to top it all off, another patient, Ralph, had really got him going earlier that morning. It seems that David's very first encounter of the day was with a patient who was not at all interested in talking about his smoking—not at all. David prides himself on having a friendly relationship with all of his patients, but he couldn't help feeling like the morning's encounter with Ralph ended the wrong way. Ralph was visibly upset, pushy, and a little rude. To his surprise, David actually felt angry at Ralph for being so stubborn. The visit ended a bit awkwardly, as David thought to himself, "Let him smoke if he wants to. I can't help him if he doesn't care about getting sick." Now he felt himself developing the same sense of frustration with Helen, even before she had a chance to speak. He decided to add a little sternness to his voice, hoping that Helen would finally respond to his directions. "Doctor's order," he said.

———

It is safe to say that clinicians who are great at what they do get that way, in part, by excelling at the human-to-human part of their job. This is likely to be particularly true when dealing with "emotionally charged" conditions like tobacco dependence. Understanding the hidden meaning behind a subtle smile or a shift of weight in the chair can mean the difference between a therapeutic relationship and an acquaintance. Call it emotional intelligence, bedside manner, people skills, whatever. These "soft skills" have been associated with improved clinical performance and higher levels of patient satisfaction.

So what are these soft skills? At various points this book has addressed the importance of getting to the patient's backstory, of empathy and validation, and of paying careful attention to both verbal and nonverbal communication pathways. These are important components of interpersonal skill, but in our experience, the one component that can make or break a tobacco-treatment visit is the ability to project a sense of "sameness" with the patient.

Homophily, or literally "love of the same," refers to the tendency among humans to bond more strongly with people they perceive as being similar to themselves. Homophily is not the same thing as love of self (narcissism) or loyalty to a particular ethnographic group (tribalism). It is simply the idea that people tend to feel most comfortable associating with other people they perceive as sharing similar points of view or life experience. It is the idea that two strangers are more likely to have a better understanding of each other from the outset if they share past challenges. There is at least the possibility of mutual understanding that can facilitate the process of getting to know each other better if the initial "sameness" level is high. If it is low, it takes longer to develop a truly therapeutic relationship.

As important as homophily is to the first impression, clinicians cannot create sameness. Clinicians should never feel like they have to pretend to be someone they are not; honesty and genuineness are essential when establishing trust. But clinicians can and should do more to minimize "not-sameness," or the sense of other that may derive from the experience of being a nonsmoker. Clinicians have been exposed to the same messages of smoking marginalization, ridicule, and delegitimization and may be most comfortable with this perspective. Is it a wonder that clinicians might harbor unconscious negative attitudes about patients who smoke? Even worse, is it a wonder that smokers themselves might harbor the same?

Be prepared for the "Have you ever smoked?" question. It is not a challenge; it is a search for "sameness." Statements that maximize the sense of sameness are more than simple empathy statements. Felicitous sameness statements have the power to diminish out-group identity and emphasize a shared in-group experience. Sameness statements do not just communicate a recognition of the experience; they communicate an ownership of the experience (Table 12.1).

Table 12.1. Language choices and their effect on homophily. Choosing words carefully can facilitate a sense of sameness between patient and clinician.

Bad Answers	Better Answers
"No. Why?"	"No, I haven't. But I understand why that could be an important question."
"No. Have you ever been a clinician?"	"I know sometimes clinicians find it hard to understand. I will try to do better."
"No, but I don't need to have had lung cancer to know how to treat it."	"It's impossible for me to know exactly what you're going through, but I promise I will try. If I am off-base, you have to promise you will let me know."
"No. I would never."	"No. I was lucky it never came my way when I was young."
"Yes, but that's not important right now."	"I have (or "My [family/friend] has), and it is terrible how other people made [me/him/her/them] feel. I'm sorry that happens."
"Yes. I loved it. I would go back if I could."	"Yes. I remember how important it was to me, how confusing it was. I'm glad that's behind me now."

Cognitive Biases and Heuristics

It is obvious that both warm clothing and a supply of food are necessary for survival. When faced with limited financial resources, one might expect the purely rational decision-maker to find the most utilitarian compromise, maximizing the balance of resources to best meet both needs. But if that sweater is amazing—well, then the calculus changes, even though "amazing" is not necessary for survival. When it comes to tobacco dependence, neither patients nor clinicians may be purely rational actors. If they were, given the social, economic, and biologic consequences of smoking, neither would spend time focused on anything else. Fortunately, social psychologists have described the subconscious undercurrents that influence decision-making in ways that on the surface seem to be irrational.

Behavioral economics studies how commonly held beliefs and mental shortcuts affect our decision-making in profound ways. These shortcuts, or heuristics, combine lessons of past experience with prediction of the future to quickly come to a "good enough" decision. Heuristics do not require the same cognitive load as more deductive reasoning might and as a consequence tend to frequently guide our decision-making. Generally, that is OK. Most times, "good enough" answers are, well, good enough. But a good enough answer is not always the same thing as the correct answer. So, by definition, there is at least a chance that overreliance on common heuristics can bring clinicians to the wrong conclusion about the patient in front of them—unless they are careful.

When thinking specifically about the way heuristics affect tobacco-dependence practice, probably the most important thing to be aware of is the influence of availability bias. When an event is dramatic or recent, it can distort the clinician's impression of the probability the same circumstances are operational the next time that event arises. For example, imagine the first patient on David's clinic schedule is Ralph. When asked about smoking, Ralph uses colorful language and aggressive tones to communicate his unwillingness to engage in conversation. Because this event is unusual, emotional, dramatic, and recent, it is highly available to David when Helen, the next patient on the schedule, arrives for her visit. The availability of the "Ralph event" in David's mind has a tendency to bias his estimation of how likely Helen will be willing to engage in a similar conversation, and it may lead to a decision to leave the problem of tobacco for another day. Availability bias can have a negative impact on a clinicians' estimation of (1) a patient's willingness to engage in treatment, (2) the likelihood of achieving a specific clinical outcome, (3) the time investment required to make an impact on patient care, and (4) the suitability of tobacco conversations in the face of other life-threatening or debilitating conditions. The point is not that availability bias always makes clinical judgment wrong; the point is clinical judgment is not always right.

> *Sometimes patients who receive a diagnosis of lung cancer really want to talk about smoking.*

Representative bias is the tendency to overestimate the likelihood that individuals within a group will share all the characteristics stereotypically assigned to that group. Because English majors are stereotypically more bookish, we are likely to overestimate the probability that the English major we just met is also a bookish person. In the event our English major truly turns out to be bookish, we are at risk of underestimating the likelihood he also plays football for the school team. In the tobacco clinic, stereotypes are easily available to the mind and can therefore have a disproportionate influence on decisions. For example, since people who smoke are stereotypically unwilling to pursue abstinence, clinicians are at risk of overestimating the probability that the patient in front of them is also unwilling. Since abstinence is stereotypically difficult to achieve, clinicians may underestimate the probability their new patient will achieve abstinence easily. While clinicians often initially rely on general patterns to help focus thinking, they always sharpen their patient-level thinking through careful incorporation of individuating information about the patient—combined with an awareness of the relevant evidence. Clinicians should vigorously avoid reliance on perilous assumptions and stereotypes.

Focusing Effect Bias in the Clinic: The Acute Myocardial Infarction

Gordon W., a 76-year-old, long-standing patient of the Tobacco Dependence Service, with a known history of cardiovascular disease and systolic heart failure, presents to Perdition University Hospital with a two-day complaint of waxing and waning substernal chest pressure. His symptoms were initially brought on by exertion while walking his dog but were not reliably relieved by rest. He did experience temporary relief from his nitroglycerin tablets but called emergency services once the medication ceased having an effect. His electrocardiogram and laboratory values were consistent with an ST-elevation myocardial infarction. Evaluation of cardiac function suggested he suffered a further decline in myocardial contractility and was expected to have a difficult recovery. Before his discharge home, Mr. W.'s clinicians discussed plans for his medical management as an outpatient:

Clinician 1. Nice save. That guy doesn't know how close he came. What is the plan from here?

Clinician 2. He did well with balloon revascularization. I started him on a beta-blocker, aspirin, and clopidogrel for his vascular heart disease, and an ACE inhibitor and diuretic for his heart failure. I'll follow up with him in a month and make sure his echocardiogram remains unchanged.

Clinician 1. OK. I'd like to start him on a patch to help him quit smoking. Can you take care of ordering that?

Clinician 2. I wouldn't. Way too much going on right now. He is on five new medications, and I just gave him a boatload of instructions on a salt-free diet and cardiac rehabilitation exercises. I think adding one more thing is going to be just too much for him to handle.

Clinician 1. Right, but helping him stop smoking will have a huge impact on his mortality—about the same impact as the balloon catheterization and the beta-blocker—and using the patch does not increase his risk of a postinfarction cardiac event. I think we should start him on something.

Clinician 2. All that's true, sure. But . . . I don't know. It just feels like it would be too much, all at once. I do not want anything to mess up his medical management. The guy's condition is tenuous. Let's leave it alone for now, and I'll reevaluate the issue on the next visit.

The focusing effect bias is operational when clinicians place emphasis on selected details of the patient's current condition, excluding or diminishing consideration for the overall picture. A tendency to prefer "first things first" may lead to errors in estimation of future outcome probabilities. Clinicians should be wary of the human tendency to treat the problem in front of them—without paying sufficient attention to the problem sneaking up behind them.

The Hardest Thing

In a misguided attempt to affirm the difficulties that patients face when abstaining, it is not uncommon to hear people refer to quitting in superlative terms: "It is the most important thing you can do for your health," or "Cigarette smoke is the most dangerous thing you can put in your body." Among the familiar hyperbolic statements is one that is unique in its potentially counterproductive influence: "Quitting is the hardest thing you will ever do, but it is totally worth it."

Whether this was initially derived from some Spartan work ethic where the pain is the gain is unclear, but it is clear that most non-Spartans tend to avoid engaging in their hardest things—ever. This may be particularly true if they have recently had their confidence shaken, say, by relapsing after a period of hard-won abstinence. Besides the illogic of overstating the pain to a person who is by definition uncertain of the gain, there are also subtle cognitive biases in effect when clinicians present quitting in tough terms. Comparison bias is the human tendency to evaluate options relative to each other rather than as individual possibilities. The most familiar example of this happens in the morning.

Suppose the local coffee shop offered two sizes to choose from, small and large (Figure 12.1). In this first example, the mind is unconsciously evaluating the two options against each other, calculating whether the extra coffee is worth the extra cost. While it is certainly possible that some consumers would prefer the larger volume and be willing to pay more, the majority tend to see the extra few ounces as "not worth" the additional $4 cost.

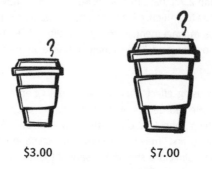

$3.00 $7.00

Figure 12.1. Comparison framed as two options.

The shop owner, on the other hand, would prefer that customers saw it differently. Since most of the costs of preparing and serving the coffee have already been incurred regardless of which size the customer orders, the extra $4 would represent a much nicer profit. Anyone who has ever been to a coffee shop recognizes the decoy effect—adding a third medium size option, strategically priced so that it is not very different from the large, changes the consumers' decisional balance dramatically (Figure 12.2).

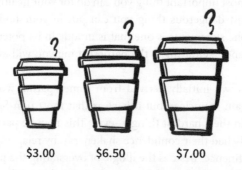

$3.00 $6.50 $7.00

Figure 12.2. Comparison framed as three options.

Because it is hard to evaluate three options at one time, this second decision calculation is actually processed as an evaluation of two sets of two options. On the left, the small bit of extra coffee hardly seems worth the difference of $3.50. But on the right, a large increase in caffeinated volume only costs an extra 50 cents. That is a lot more benefit for a very small increase in cost. In other words, the shop owner has created a situation where the apparent marginal cost of getting the large coffee is minimal. The entrepreneur creates a circumstance where the consumer's most likely visceral response is "sure, why not?" Perhaps this has happened to you. Not surprisingly, the number of shoppers who opt for the large tub of coffee rises dramatically when the right comparator is presented (Figure 12.3). Everyone is happy.

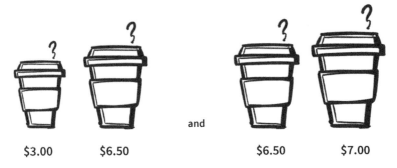

$3.00 $6.50   and $6.50 $7.00

Figure 12.3. Comparison framing: three options evaluated as two sets of two options.

Despite being well-intentioned, comparison bias can sometimes work against the clinical goals (Table 12.2).

Table 12.2. Influence of comparison bias on treatment engagement.

Example	Effect
"Quitting is the hardest thing you will ever do, but it is totally worth it."	• Emphasizes the large marginal difference in "cost" of quitting • Forces temporal discounting of potential gains by focusing attention on long-term health consequences • Highlights preeminence of clinicians' values
"Learning to not smoke is a skill that you can practice, just like a lot of other skills you've learned in life."	• Emphasizes the relatively minimal marginal cost of achieving abstinence goals • Anchored to previous patient experience, wherein benefit may have been more clearly worth the cost • Increases homophily; shift from smoking to other behaviors creates opportunity for sameness statements

Stigma

A few short decades ago, smoking cigarettes was viewed as "cool" or "glamorous." These days, things are very different. One of the most successful aspects of modern-era attempts to curtail smoking rates has been their absolute effectiveness at decreasing the social acceptability of this behavior. While the general unacceptability of smoking has led to dramatic declines in tobacco use, the problem has always been that it is too easy to conflate the behavior itself with a character statement about the person displaying the behavior. Today, it seems nearly all people who smoke are acutely aware of the negative characterization of smoking, and nearly all the stereotypes associated with the smokers themselves are negative.

About 40% of current smokers living in the United States are on the receiving end of significant family pressure to stop, and about 30% report being discriminated against because of their smoking status. Coercive pressure is so ubiquitous that it is not at all uncommon for smokers themselves to have confused threats and bullying with "support." In our practice, it is not unusual to hear patients describe their spouse's supportiveness using terms a divorce lawyer would find more familiar. Smokers know that nonsmokers think less of them. Forty percent of smoking respondents report perceiving high stigma within their environment and agree with the statement, "Most people think less of a person who smokes."

From a strictly clinical perspective, this level of stigmatization raises several important alarms. Foremost among them is the impact stigma has on willingness to present to the clinic for help. People respond very differently to mortification or embarrassment than they do to discomfort or anxiety. In addition, as much as 8% of current smokers conceal their smoking status from their primary care provider. It is not hard to imagine that number being quite a bit higher in circumstances where trust in the clinical relationship has not yet matured—for example, when the clinician is perceived as judgmental or when the presenting illness is caused by smoking. Other important negative consequences of stigma include an increased risk for relapse, unwillingness to disclose relapse, increased resistance to pharmacotherapy, and increase in experienced stress. It also remains unclear how smoking stigma affects clinical outcomes for other conditions. For example, lung cancer survivors do not experience the same length or quality of life as other cancer survivors. Because of the strong association with smoking, lung cancer patients who perceive higher smoking stigma also experience worse depression symptoms compared with those who have other types of cancer, regardless of whether they themselves have ever actually smoked.

Pregnant women also report strong social pressures to stop smoking. They are often subject to "pregnancy policing," the background social norms that make it acceptable for others to express their negative judgments to a degree that might otherwise be culturally inappropriate. This leaves women who smoke in a position where they have to prove their qualifications as good mothers, which in turn makes it harder for them to disclose their smoking status, remain adherent to tobacco pharmacotherapy, and achieve control over their compulsion.

One of the worst unintended effects of stigma is that it may actually increase the likelihood of smoking within some otherwise stigmatized groups. For example, LGBTQ youth start smoking at younger ages, and LGBTQ adults smoke cigarettes at nearly twice the rate of their heterosexual counterparts. The theory is that social disparities, such as higher rates of discrimination and social rejection, create a fertile social backdrop for targeted marketing, emphasizing themes of liberation, pride, individualism, social success, and acceptance. Though less well studied, it is easy to imagine the same framework applies to other marginalized groups, such as adolescents, African Americans, and Indigenous Americans.

Becoming Aware of Being Unaware

Imagine you are in line behind five other customers at your favorite coffee shop, waiting patiently to order your 40-ounce coffee. Suddenly, someone enters the queue—directly in front of you. Ignore the ways you were taught to act, and focus instead on how you feel. Generally, when confronted with another person's problematic behavior, humans are predisposed to overemphasize the dispositional traits, or character flaws, that may have led to the affront. The effect is an underestimation of the impact environmental and situational factors had on the event. We may not initially be inclined to consider the loud background noise or chaotic surroundings as the true underlying cause. However, the opposite is true if the line-cutter happens to be a friend. Because the friend's behavior is interpreted through the lens of "sameness," the mind tends to overemphasize the circumstantial contributions to the situation.

This tendency to weigh dispositional versus situational factors differently depending on the degree of perceived sameness is so deep that psychologists have postulated that it is a central characteristic of human thought. For clinicians, the fundamental attribution error is especially treacherous because smoking can seem like a particularly egregious behavior with potential life-or-death consequences. In the setting of such urgency, smoking has the potential to generate very powerful emotions among clinicians, even if they're not exactly aware of them.

Albeit subliminally, when the clinician attributes smoking to the patient's flawed disposition, the resulting emotions are always negative, similar to the [expletive] emotions experienced when that stranger cut the coffee line. Anger, frustration, and even combativeness are the inevitable results. However, when clinicians recognize the environmental variables that perpetuate smoking—the cigarette's universal availability, its addictive design, the ubiquitous advertisements, the high community prevalence, and the prevailing normative signaling in popular culture—it is possible for clinicians to manage their error-prone attribution. For example, in our practice, the average patient is exposed to one tobacco retailer every twenty-five yards every time they leave their home. At the top end, that number goes up to once every twenty-five feet. That is an enormous situational influence. And that does not count the loose cigarettes illegally sold at the corner stores.

There are a few important heuristics that derive from the fundamental attribution error. Even when aware of the environmental-situational variables that promote ongoing smoking, humans still tend to attribute failure to character flaw if they perceive insufficient effort has been invested in controlling the behavior—even if that expectation is unreasonable. Causal controllability bias makes David feel like Helen needs to be doing more to quit, even if he is intellectually aware of the addictive capacity of free-base nicotine and knows that she passes a tobacco retailer every twenty-five feet on her way to the bus stop.

Another derivative heuristic is the just-world fallacy. This is the tendency to assume that people get what they deserve and deserve what they get. In a just-world mindset, the assignment of blame allows an observer to experience a sense of control over events, even when they are intellectually aware that such events are uncontrollable. Unfortunately, the consequence of the just-world fallacy is that patients who smoke tend to get blamed for their smoking-related disease. It is easy to imagine the sense of security and the psychological benefit this tendency engenders for the observer; it is harder to imagine the impact of blame on the person being judged. It is bad enough when Helen gets lung cancer; it is worse when her clinician blames her for it. And it is heartbreaking when Helen believes she deserves it.

So far, mental shortcuts have created a dark path. Let's review. Not-sameness tends the mind toward predictable "character flaw" attribution error. Character flaw is confirmed when the patient is interpreted as a "slackard." Just-world bias provides the comfort of a straightforward explanation and allows us to ignore the stuff that is harder to control. But here's where it gets really dark. Culpability bias is the tendency to be less willing to give help to people perceived as blameworthy. In circumstances where the affront is attributed to social, environmental, or biological factors (that is, situational), the clinician's judgment of responsibility for the illness is more synonymous with the idea of "ownership." That is, the patient "owns" the disease and is therefore only responsible for doing their best to secure the help they need. This is sometimes referred to as the sickness condition. Sickness engenders a positive emotional response among caregivers, including sympathy and empathy, and results in high willingness to invest effort into help-giving. On the other hand, if the behavior is attributed to a character flaw (that is, dispositional), the clinician's judgment of responsibility is more in line with its "culpability" connotation. That is, the patient is to "blame" for the disease and is facing the inevitable consequences of their decisions. This is the sin condition. Sin, in turn, engenders a very different emotional response; instead of a positive, warm reaction, sin results in frustration and anger and a willingness to invest effort into help-giving is very low.

> *All this is happening below the level of conscious awareness.*

Time and again, when clinicians are surveyed, they report a good understanding of their potential role in helping people stop smoking. They also have a solid foundation in the principles laid out in published guidelines. They care deeply. Yet, despite the enormous number of annual interactions between people who smoke and their health care providers, the rate at which clinicians engage in tobacco-dependence treatment remains remarkably low. Why? The total answer is complex, but the extent to which these heuristics trap clinicians into maladaptive patterns of thinking is a growing area of scientific inquiry. The University of Pennsylvania Comprehensive Smoking Treatment Program was able to first confirm the influence of these cognitive biases on tobacco decision-making in 2015 and documented that clinicians change their behaviors in positive ways after being made aware of these counterproductive influences.

In 2019, the research team also documented a strong culpability bias among clinicians who care for smokers by asking subjects from across the United States to participate in computer-based implicit association testing (IAT). Implicit associations are the instinctive undercurrents, adopted over a lifetime of subtle inputs, that create a subconscious framework for our conscious thoughts. They are neither a reflection of a person's character nor of their deeply held beliefs. Rather, they are associations that have been implanted beneath consciousness such that some pairs of ideas simply seem to go together better than others, even though we may consciously (even intensely) disagree. To the subconscious, the notion of "spider" may align better with expressions of evil intent than with those of kindness, even though we rationally understand the spider's behavior carries neither meaning.

The IAT revealed a strong incompatibility between images of smoking and words conveying "innocence." When compared to sorting images of smoking with words meaning "guilt," clinicians took nearly twice as long to sort pictures of smoking alongside synonyms for innocence. In IAT latency times, this is a huge discrepancy. To make sure this was implicit, and not a reflection of otherwise explicit attributions to a character flaw, our subjects completed a series of closed- and open-ended questionnaire items exploring their explicit attitudes about patients with tobacco dependence or hypertension. On the explicit scales, there was absolutely no difference in response patterns between conditions—except for items on the emotional subscale. Between the two conditions, they saw no difference in utility to the patient, their technical abilities to carry out treatment, or the degree of professional fulfillment. However, themes of frustration cropped up often within tobacco responses but didn't appear at all in the hypertension controls. The regular occurrence of frustration themes suggested to us that the sin-versus-sickness framework may be relevant to tobacco-dependence treatment and, if so, may be particularly dangerous because of the impact on willingness to help. At minimum, it is reasonable to assume that very complex, subconscious, social motivations may be operational in the care of tobacco dependence, even among dedicated and informed clinicians. Understanding this should motivate clinicians to continuously self-assess their decision-making assumptions.

Persuasion Basics

Next time a commercial touting a new pharmaceutical miracle comes on the television, watch it with the sound turned off. The underlying visual storyline is often very different from the words that simultaneously reach your ears. The visual inputs create a warm feeling about the handsome man playing fetch with his beautiful dog or the adoring grandmother pushing a laughing grandchild on a swing. Why? Marketers know that the feelings created by the ad will be transformed by heuristics into the consumer's judgment of their product. It does not matter that the narrator is warning of vomiting and hair loss if there are sailboats and sunshine in the foreground. Marketers know that what the audience understands is different from how the message makes them feel, and their feelings will eventually influence how they understand what they come to know. Advertisers always deliver a central message, which is composed of the cognitive stuff, alongside a peripheral message, which carries the instinctive stuff, because central messages are by definition much less influential. First, central messages require cognitive resources; they represent a cognitive load that requires energy to process. The denser the central message, the bigger the cognitive load, and the less willing the audience member is to incorporate the message. Peripheral messages, on the other hand, do not require cognitive processing and therefore do not represent a load. These messages are easy to deliver and are incorporated easily. It does not matter if the central and peripheral messages align: what does a cute cartoon animal mascot have to do with medical miracles anyway? As long as the peripheral message creates a positive feeling, the majority of the audience will receive the central message positively.

There are several common heuristics that are fundamental to peripheral messaging. Of primary importance is the attractiveness heuristic, or halo effect: the receiver automatically assigns the overall attractiveness of the ad (that is, youthful models, awe-inspiring settings, artistic composition) to their judgment of the message. The familiarity heuristic is related. Famous faces, cultural themes, or events can transfer the same sense of familiarity to the juxtaposed central idea. Because the mind equates familiar with friendly, the safety and security experienced with familiarity are transferred onto the whole message. Celebrity endorsements of politicians are valuable not because celebrities are intrinsically more capable of making political decisions but because their familiar faces and attractive smiles make it more likely that the receiver will incorporate the celebrities' point of view into their own. Mood misattribution occurs when the mood engendered by the background is subconsciously assigned to the central message. It is the reason why sitcoms are accompanied by a laugh track and shark movies have a bass-intensive music score. It is also why tobacco advertisers will often employ images of the flag or symbols of liberty.

None of this is to say that the audience is made up of passive robots, ready to accept whatever message comes their way as long as it feels good. Instead, the receivers are active—unconsciously estimating the degree to which the message is appropriate for their consumption. Confirmation bias is the tendency for messages that align with our preconceptions to be more easily accepted than messages that challenge our established ideas. If a new message does not line up with the old, it is more likely to be selectively avoided. The more often the idea that quitting is hard is repeated, the less likely people are to accept that it should be made easy. Forewarning refers to the degree to which the persuasive intent of the message is apparent. If the persuasive intent is obvious, it is easier for the message to be ignored. Use of serial exclamation points, capital letters, or other histrionics to convey a sense of urgency should be UTTERLY AVOIDED!!! Obvious persuasive intent leads to reactance, the negative emotion produced when the message is perceived as limiting the receiver's freedom of choice.

Most clinicians can't afford models or television ads. But knowing what the advertisers know is important to reaching an audience effectively, regardless of what medium or vehicle is used. Begin by acknowledging that for every patient who contacts the clinic, there are probably hundreds more who will need a little persuading to do so. In many ways, the narrative available to these soon-to-be patients is critical to establishing the therapeutic foundations of care after they arrive. Rethink every communication tool used in daily practice, including websites, printed materials, and promotional gadgets. Even nontraditional tools like patient education materials, after-visit summaries, clinical letters, and the like can have a peripheral impact. Check to be sure peripheral inputs are promoting rather than preventing patient engagement. In all cases, first ensure messaging promotes trust (Chapter 7), then pay as much attention to the feel of the material as to the content (Table 12.3). For proof, google a few tobacco industry ads.

Table 12.3. Analyzing different approaches to persuasive messaging.

Peripheral Route	Theirs	Ours
Attractiveness		
Familiarity		
Mood attribution		
Forewarning	Low	High

Chapter 12 Learning Points

- Homophily is the human tendency to bond more meaningfully with people perceived as having a similar life experience. Though clinicians can't create "sameness," they can minimize the impact of "not-sameness."
- Smoking status can be a very powerful symbol of "not-sameness" that clinicians find difficult or even undesirable to overcome because of ubiquitous delegitimization messages in the public sphere. Instead, purposeful attention to the social, cultural, and biological similarities between patient and clinician can help minimize "not-sameness" during the clinical encounter.
- Be prepared for the "have you ever smoked" question. Well-placed and timely sameness statements decrease the patient's out-group marginalization and increase their sense of in-group solidarity.
- A variety of mental shortcuts, or heuristics, make it more likely that clinicians will come to the wrong conclusion about their patient. Awareness of and attention to these biases can result in important, positive changes in clinical behaviors.
- Understanding the impact of comparison bias is important to promoting patient engagement. Minimizing the apparent marginal cost of engagement is critical to facilitating adaptive decision-making.
- Smoking stigma is a significant barrier to tobacco-dependence treatment. Clinicians should be aware of the potential impact stigma may have on the therapeutic needs of the patient.
- Fundamental attribution error is treacherous and can lead clinicians to overemphasize dispositional (character flaw) contributions to behavior and underappreciate the role of social, environmental, and biological contributors.
- A variety of heuristics derived from the fundamental attribution error can easily lead to a reduced willingness to provide care. The impact of blame (that is, sin versus sickness) on clinical decision-making can be profound and is an implicit bias that can be operational even when the clinician strongly holds the opposite explicit opinions.
- Persuasion relies on peripheral messaging more than central (logical) arguments. Reactions to messages are more important than the messages themselves. Facility with the common heuristics that provide access to patient decision-making through the peripheral route can help clinicians set the proper feel of their communication materials in support of their central message.

Part III

Knowing "Who"

Chapter 13
Organization

Why should I trust you?

—Louis C., 52 years old

On most days, David encounters the complete spectrum of "success" with patients. For some patients, everything goes correctly—strong family support, effective medications, positive outcome. For other patients, everything seems to go wrong—insurance issues, poor response to medications, difficulty managing appointments. Whether it was recommending the flu shot, managing diabetes, or discussing when antibiotics are indicated, David could only have so many debates or offer so many words of encouragement before feeling defeated. He was learning that helping patients to manage their tobacco dependence was no different. As soon as they leave his office, environmental cues abound and often prove to be more powerful than his words. "There must be a better way to help these patients," he thought. Insurance companies, pharmacists, other physicians, advertisers, family, and friends all had opinions about the importance of quitting, but there was no unified system available.

It wasn't just his patients he worried about; David was also growing more concerned about his brother's smoking. Helen had taught him a lot about her struggles, and he knew his brother was not getting the help he needed. His brother had the support of his wife, but he also needed the support of the larger health care system. David took a deep breath before he knocked on the door of the department chair. He told his boss about his experience trying to manage tobacco dependence within his busy practice and in his personal life. "For too many years I thought that my brother and patients like Helen were stuck in their ways, unable to commit to making a change, regardless of the consequences," he explained to his boss. "But ironically, I was somewhat stuck in my ways—accepting the status quo, believing that there was only so much I could do to change a person's behaviors. I owe it to my brother and to Helen to try to make a change in a system that is stuck in its ways." David's goal was to see what changes his department could make in order to alter the path of destiny for his patients.

———

Fifth Vital Sign

Most clinicians, regardless of discipline, are familiar with the centuries-old concept of the vital sign. Taken together, vital signs represent a set of four simple assessments that give clinicians insight into the current health of the patient and provide clues as to the risk of future illness or events. For example, a high temperature may indicate the early stages of infection and suggest a risk of severe illness in the near future if not adequately addressed. Though unsensed by the patient, a sustained high blood pressure can represent a significant risk of early death in the distant future. Of all the signs available to the clinician in the course of practice, the vital signs remain special because they are easy to assess and are consequential while being directly actionable: the perfect combination.

Beginning in the early 1990s, the idea of expanding the classic tetrad of signs to include other important measures started to take hold. The medical literature is chock-full of suggestions for a "fifth vital sign," including things like pain score, menstrual cycle, depression, and travel status. All these measures are important, but few had been shown to reliably change clinician behaviors. Early on, recording smoking status was recognized as an exception to that rule.

For context, remember that in the early 1990s, nicotine patches had only recently become available, and concerns over cardiovascular toxicity remained paramount. The complex molecular effects of nicotine on the brain had not yet been worked out. Tobacco use was still considered a lifestyle choice, an interesting component of the social history that remained outside any meaningful clinical intervention. An occasional stern warning might carry weight with some patients, prompting them to stop smoking, but for the most part there was a prevailing therapeutic nihilism—a feeling that patients were going to do whatever they were going to do. Then a groundbreaking demonstration showed that it was possible for a simple workflow change to make a substantial difference in what patients were going to do. Integrating a routine assessment of smoking status— categorizing the patient as either a "never," "former," or "current" smoker—and placing the information in a prominent position as the fifth vital sign significantly increased the rate at which clinicians asked about smoking and offered advice to quit during the visit. That was big news because clinician advice to quit is a powerful motivator. The thinking went that even if absolute quit rates were low, if every clinician brought it up at every visit, the population-level impact of a universal assessment strategy applied to billions of clinical visits every year could eventually be huge. Looking back, there were a couple of unanticipated issues.

Start by stipulating that clinician advice and support can help patients achieve abstinence rates of 5% to 10% with minimal interventions. In relative terms, that is a huge difference when compared with spontaneous background rates of about 3%. The problem is that in the clinic it is most likely to be the absolute numbers that inform judgment. Even if every clinician could achieve that 10% mark, our understanding of the availability heuristic makes plain the idea that the ten out of a hundred patients who actually do stop smoking are likely to have far less impact on the future judgment of clinicians than the ninety out of one hundred patients who do not. Imagine the potential negative impact of ninety instances of frustration and learned helplessness, even if positive gains are demonstrable. Things only get worse if the stipulation turn out to be a best-case assumption.

In addition, the universal assessment approach is premised on motivational deficit. In the best case, all current smokers are identified at every visit, and for those unwilling to attempt abstinence initially, clinicians have to rely on the cumulative impact of repetitive messaging at subsequent visits to influence the patient's future willingness. However, repetitive messaging relies solely on the frequency of messaging and ignores the role of emotion on influence. Because repetitive messaging is constructed from the clinician's perspective, a natural emphasis on central messages about risk of ill health is likely. As with all other central messages, for it to be effective, patients must (1) pay attention to the message (it must be noticed to be effective), (2) be able to understand the message (incomprehensible or misunderstood messages will have no effect), and (3) be willing to accept the message (reactance to the obvious persuasive intent may cause a boomerang effect). While there is no denying that some patients benefit from repeat motivational messaging, there is equally no doubt that repetitive messaging can create a nontherapeutic obstacle for others.

To be clear, the point is not that universal assessment and repetitive messaging are intrinsically bad ideas but rather that they can be counterproductive if that is all that is offered. Both tactics should be seen as a means to an end, not an end in themselves. To illustrate this, imagine that the clinical problem being addressed is diabetes. Given its high prevalence and the demonstrated impact glucose control can have on both morbidity and mortality, many clinicians have advocated for the fifth position of the vital sign set to be occupied by routine blood sugar measurements. If a simple workflow adjustment would result in more early diabetes being identified and more early conversations about diet modification and the risks of unchecked blood glucose levels were the consequence, it might readily be seen as a significant boost to public health. However, what is unlikely is that clinical norms would allow providers to remain content with only 10% of patients achieving blood sugar control, regardless of how large the relative improvement. It is hard to imagine clinicians remaining satisfied in the hope that repetitive messaging would have its intended effect someday. If the problem being addressed were diabetes, universal assessment and repetitive messaging would be intermediate tactics in service of a larger goal, not the goal itself. They would function in concert with other practices employed and the resources we demand of health systems, aligning patients who need care with the care they need—no more, but no less.

> *Tobacco dependence isn't actually different;*
> *it has just been framed that way.*

Everyone's Responsibility Becomes No One's Responsibility

A clinician's individual responsibility in the approach to disease is derived from the skill set that guides that person's actions and decisions in the course of patient care. In patients with diabetes, each discipline involved in the care has its own unique and circumscribed set of individual responsibilities. It is clear to everyone that the primary care provider, the diabetes nurse educator, the vascular surgeon, and the endocrinologist have overlapping and complementary roles. Each is responsible for making the best decisions possible, within the limits of their practice, to maximize the patient's benefit.

To make those disparate skills work together effectively, systems have to be put in place to facilitate collaborative care. Organizational responsibility extends beyond the boundary of "self" and refers to the relationships we expect clinicians to engage in while in service to their patients. We expect the consulting endocrinologist to communicate with the primary care clinician and the diabetes educator to respond to requests for counseling services. We expect the nephrologist to coordinate access to dialysis services when necessary. Clinical organizations have a responsibility to ensure that all resources are at least available to the patient and that coordination among clinicians is driven by the need to exactly match the patient needs to the services provided. No single element of the organization is responsible for the whole of diabetes care nor is every element expected to perform the same role: it is the functional relationship between clinicians that defines the comprehensive nature of care.

The set of professional norms and expectations—the mechanism of social order that reflects our professional values—are a direct expression of our clinical culture and our social purpose. As such, clinicians have a set of institutional responsibilities that transcend individual or organizational needs and form the basis for long-established customs that define the professional role. When a patient arrives in the emergency department with life-threatening low blood sugar, institutional responsibility creates the moral imperative to respond regardless of ability to pay. Imagine how profoundly contrary to the clinical culture it would be if the emergency room staff began asking patients with diabetes to affirm a particular belief before initiating care. Similarly, if that same patient were found to require dialysis for renal failure, it would strike us as antithetical to our standards if the nephrologist chose to forgo the recommendation because it was personally inconvenient. Institutional responsibility compels the professional community to (1) create evidence-based clinical systems that use insights into pathophysiology, not common sense, to address the problem; (2) identify the unique role of various individuals making up the healthcare team and create functional organizations that maximize effectiveness; (3) ensure that resources and services are in some manner available to the people who need them; (4) transmit accumulated knowledge from one generation to the next to ensure permanence; and (5) continuously refine systems of care to improve outcomes.

> *The care of tobacco dependence has not yet*
> *reached this level of integration.*
> *Why not?*

Vertical Integration of Care

Imagine a set of cultural norms around tobacco-use treatment that exactly mirrors the norms of care for other chronic illnesses. Perhaps the primary care clinician is responsible for diagnosing tobacco dependence and initiating care. Perhaps there is a coordinated, comprehensive care plan that includes input from a variety of related disciplines, including behavioral health, social work, pharmacy, and others. Perhaps there is an easy way to refer particularly complex patients to specialty providers who are prepared with resources specifically aimed at the longitudinal control of tobacco dependence. Perhaps the care plan involves community-based peer resources for education, monitoring, and support. Perhaps systems would be in place for determining which level of care is most appropriate to meet an individual patient's needs at any given time and for ensuring that those patients could gain access to that care regardless of their initial point of contact with the system. Perhaps norms would discourage clinicians from relying on seemingly common-sense interventions and instead promote fidelity to the available evidence. Perhaps trainees would be engaged in developing a formal understanding of principles and practice. A model of vertical integration might look something like Figure 13.1.

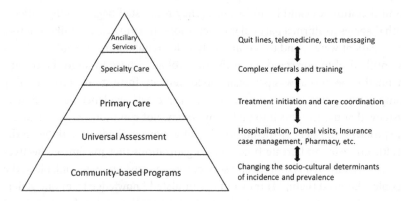

Figure 13.1. Vertical integration of tobacco-dependence treatment into current healthcare structure.

Integration Is Innovation

In our current, fragmented system of managing tobacco dependence, the overall goal of cessation is distributed across all levels of the pyramid. The levels function independently, with only minimal harmonization and no central site of coordination. Patients engage these levels randomly, interchangeably, based on their level of interest or their general healthcare experience, or both. The overall strategy is predicated on the motivational value of repetitive messaging—additive rather than synergistic. In contrast, a vertically integrated system relies on the interaction between levels. How might community-based programs and social policies be constructed to amplify the impact of universal assessment efforts? How can assessment protocols be tailored so as not to end in a full stop once the patient expresses ambivalence? How can systems be in place for identified smokers to be connected directly to their primary care clinicians, and how can those clinicians then feasibly structure a visit so that tobacco dependence is the primary, not secondary, reason for the service? Imagine if every health system had an identified source for specialty care of tobacco dependence, meeting the needs of the most complicated patients and providing a backup source of expertise for primary care clinicians who want to do more. It is easy to imagine the specialty clinic as a source of informal knowledge dissemination to the practice community, as well as a source of formal education for trainees. Can we imagine a cooperative arrangement between health systems and third-party vendors that fully integrate the care goals of the primary care clinician with the care goals of community counselors, telephone quit lines, and text-messaging services?

> *The first step in building such a vertically integrated system of care is the recognition that tobacco dependence is a chronic illness. The second step is recognizing that our individual, organizational, and institutional responsibilities apply to this chronic disease just the same as they do to all the other diseases.*

Review the aspirational model shown in Table 13.1.

Constructionism

A clinician who has read this book, internalized its message, and visualized a way to be most effective with tobacco-dependent patients faces a reality in which these integrated resources are not yet available. Perhaps it is because there are precious few like-minded individuals with whom to collaborate. Perhaps it is because the surrounding clinical culture is so deeply invested in the cessation mind-set that it is difficult for colleagues to share the vision. It is easy to get discouraged and imagine oneself powerless in creating change. However, keep in mind that lessons learned about helping individual patients with change are equally applicable to efforts at system change. Remember three important points:

1. Change often happens incrementally, as barriers to change are sequentially resolved.

2. Efforts are directed at altering the probability of change, not guaranteeing it.

3. Efforts that appear to have no impact today are cumulative and may facilitate change tomorrow.

Instead of thinking about system building from scratch, a constructionist approach uses the information, the motivations, and the resources already in place within an organization and puts them into novel alignment so that the

Table 13.1. Future-oriented model of a vertically integrated systematic approach to the tobacco dependence epidemic.

Level	Description	Current Example	Future Tobacco Analogy
Community-based programs	Includes outreach strategies and public health policies that extend the way diverse organizations contribute to health improvement.	As part of the National Diabetes Education Program, the Centers for Disease Control and Prevention promote community involvement by recognizing a variety of organizations engaged in helping people spot the signs of prediabetes, make healthy food choices, participate in aerobic activities, and connect with community healthcare resources.	Includes policy initiatives promoting deeper awareness of nicotine addiction and approach to treatment. Advocacy groups work to minimize restrictions on care. Synchronized messaging and toolkits reduce culpability bias and stigma. Payment adjustments for home health organizations using community healthcare navigators trained to address the problem.
Universal assessment	Promote awareness of and attention to tobacco dependence as a solvable problem.	The U.S. Agency for Healthcare Research and Quality published a set of questions, answered by patients, that assesses personal behaviors and risks. The program helps clinicians guide patients toward goal identification, agenda setting, and navigation through a complex healthcare system.	Health workers, including dentists, case managers, and pharmacists, trained in nonjudgmental assessment of tobacco smoke exposure, help smoke-exposed patients identify goals and set an agenda for care. Providers assist with system navigation and facilitate engagement of appropriate services.
Primary care	Includes health promotion, disease prevention, patient counseling, and education—in addition to diagnosis and	The American Academy of Family Practice defines primary care as the discipline responsible for skilled comprehensive first contact and ongoing care for any patient, regardless of problem origin,	Exquisitely positioned to shift philosophy from cessation model to longitudinal management of chronic relapsing illness. Central point of coordination between all levels of vertical

treatment of acute and chronic illness. Central point of collaboration between health professionals.	responsibilities of primary care include advocating for cost-effective and coordinated care systems, promoting effective communication with patients, and encouraging the role of the patient as a partner in health care.	integration. Payment models modified to account for shift from brief counseling to more complex coordination and ongoing care. Front-line advocates for comprehensive resources to meet patient needs based on illness severity and complexity.
Specialty care		
Advanced care and treatment using skills and procedures specific to the condition. Specialty clinics may integrate inputs from a variety of related disciplines.	National Cancer Institute Designated Comprehensive Cancer Centers provide patient-centered care, informed by cutting-edge research and evidence-based guidelines. They work to identify better treatments through multidisciplinary collaborations and participation in clinical trials. They train future generations of cancer care experts and disseminate an understanding of cancer into the community.	Regional healthcare organizations provide matrix structure for transdisciplinary tobacco dependence treatment services—coordinated interventions by prescribing clinicians, behavioral health providers, social work, certified counselors, etc. Referral destination for primary care provider network. Participation in generation and dissemination of new knowledge. Recruit and train future clinicians and researchers.
Ancillary services		
Refers to a wide range of services provided in support of primary and specialty care. Includes both diagnostic and therapeutic services, provided either in person or remotely.	The American Thoracic Society promotes an integrated model of chronic obstructive pulmonary disease (COPD) care that involves self-management training, pulmonary rehabilitation, home nursing, sleep testing, community support groups (e.g., Better Breathers Club), and interactive web-based instruction programs to support self-management decision-making. Integrated services can improve quality of life and exercise capacity and can reduce hospital admissions.	Computerized record systems and information-sharing agreements allow for integration of multiple community-based services, employed in support of the overall goal of reducing tobacco dependence morbidity and relapse to uncontrolled smoking. As with COPD care, ancillary services are complementary, not interchangeable. Balance of primary care, specialty, and ancillary service utilization shifts based on specific patient needs.

preexisting parts may now serve a new purpose. Constructionists start with an established mental model and work to help others understand how the services they currently provide can fit into that vision with only minor alteration. Constructionism involves incremental discovery of new methods—learning which processes work and using those successes to build a growing set of services. For example, the clinician who works to figure out how tobacco-dependence treatment principles can efficiently fit within established practice routines is soon in a position to offer those same services to other colleagues. The clinician who figures out how to effectively offer referral services is soon in a position to offer tailored services to meet the needs of specific care areas (for example, oncology or cardiology). As the clinician's network grows, caregivers with overlapping skill sets and priorities become visible. Over and over, constructionists work to refine health system policies and protocols until an integrated care model begins to take shape. There are a number of excellent examples of integrated tobacco-treatment systems across the country. Take a look around and find the models that incorporate resources similar to those most readily available. Then, steal the ideas that work and leave the rest behind.

With diligence and patience, the constructionist clinician can achieve systematic change by keeping a few important tips in mind (Table 13.2).

Table 13.2. Constructionist tips for achieving tobacco goals.

Stop calling it cessation. Use all opportunities to reinforce the idea that patients may cease smoking but clinicians treat tobacco dependence.
Start with small, easy goals. Set aside a few hours in your weekly schedule to dedicate to tobacco-related activities (see patients, prepare lectures, review hospital policies, etc.)
Identify a single patient care policy that could work better. Maybe it is a care goal that's on the books but doesn't actually get done. Maybe it is a regulatory requirement that is currently subject to satisficing. Whatever it is, coordinate with the responsible parties to make it work a little better.
Volunteer to educate. Perhaps it is a lunch-and-learn, or maybe it is Grand Rounds. Either way, find a vehicle for telling your colleagues what you know about tobacco dependence and its treatment.
Become a member of the tobacco dependence professional community. There are several professional societies dedicated exclusively to furthering the care of tobacco-dependent patients. Alternatively, many specialty societies have policy, treatment, or education committees that concern themselves with tobacco dependence. Get involved and take advantage of the collective experience of the group.
Identify colleagues within your organization who share your mindset. Share news articles, research reports, system announcements, and other communications that are relevant to tobacco dependence.

Identify your deficits, then find local personnel to help fill the gaps. If you're not a billing provider, find someone who is willing to use your services to bill for incident care. If you are a physical health provider, identify a behavioral health colleague who is willing to consult with you when you have concerns about mental illness. If you're a psychiatrist, find a social worker who can help patients engage social services, including the drug and alcohol recovery services available in your area.

If you are a billing provider, do not let anyone tell you that you can't bill for the tobacco services you provide. There's a functional difference between smoking cessation and the treatment of tobacco dependence. There are a few good resources to help you understand the documentation and coding requirements for billing based on your specialty. Find them and share them with your business manager.

Remember that you understand tobacco dependence better than 99% of people on Earth. Whenever someone begins a sentence with "You can't . . . ," it is usually because they are still struggling to understand. Be patient with them, and work to help them come along.

Chapter 13 Learning Points

- Because relatively small numbers of tobacco-dependent patients stop smoking spontaneously, simple process changes, like including tobacco-use status as a fifth vital sign, can result in a large relative impact.
- The tendency for recent and accessible events to bias judgment means that clinicians are likely to be more strongly influenced by the large absolute number of patients for whom simple interventions do not achieve the desired effect.
- Universal assessment and repetitive messaging tactics are based on assumptions of motivational deficit. They should instead be employed in service of larger treatment goals, including facilitation of integrated and sophisticated care.
- The obvious persuasive intent of repetitive messaging risks reactance, a negative emotional reaction that may affect a result opposite to that which was intended.
- Clinicians, and the healthcare systems they populate, have overlapping individual, organizational, and institutional responsibilities to their tobacco-dependent patients.
- Tobacco dependence is currently an outlier among complex chronic illnesses. Care systems and clinical norms have yet to reach the level of integration otherwise afforded to other morbid conditions.
- A vertically integrated model of care can take many final forms, but all rely on multiple distinct but complementary levels of care to achieve complex and long-lasting treatment objectives.

- The first step in building a vertically integrated system is recognizing to-bacco dependence as a chronic illness. The second is applying individual, organizational, and institutional responsibilities to this chronic illness.
- Multiple models of vertical integration already exist across healthcare. Future tobacco treatment systems should emulate these services.
- A constructionist approach uses existing motivations and resources in creative ways so that services already in place may serve an expanded purpose.

Chapter 14
Twenty Questions

By now, astute clinicians have come to recognize that the truth about tobacco dependence and its treatment sometimes runs counter to the patient's prevalent, commonsense understandings of smoking. "You have to be ready to quit" is one example. "It is better to quit without a crutch" is another. When the clinician says something that seemingly contradicts a patient's closely held dogmatic beliefs, previously learned from other trusted sources, predictable questions arise. To the artful clinician, this a decisive moment. When answered skillfully, patients' questions represent a crucial opportunity to deliver a persuasive message. But when approached clumsily, answers become de facto proof that the clinician is out of touch.

Engaging patient questions effectively is an opportunity to build new ideas from scratch. Questions most commonly arise at two distinct junctures in care. Very early in the course of treatment, typically within the first or second visit, patients may be assessing the trustworthiness of the clinical advice. Later, but typically not long after treatment has been initiated, patients begin to assess the requirements for long-term change in behavior. The clinical response to patients' questions should follow the same rhythm of cognitive management established in Chapter 11; validate, reframe, repeat. Effective preparation for unpredictable, time-pressured, and sometimes confusing encounters in the clinic involves thinking through the insights necessary to answer the most common patient questions and prethinking the response structure most likely to achieve therapeutic goals.

Patients are not the only ones who benefit from implementation-oriented thinking when changing the course of tobacco dependence.

Questions Asked Early in the Course of Treatment

Question: *Were you ever a smoker?*
Clinical insight: Probably one of the most commonly asked questions.
                   In most cases, patients who ask this are assessing the
                   clinician's ability to empathize with their ambivalence.
                   In some cases, patients have come to believe, either
                   through common doctrine or from unfortunate past
                   encounters with other clinicians, that only someone with
                   the same life experience can identify with their position.
                   Less commonly, patients will ask this question when the
                   clinician's evident understanding of the experience of
                   smoking does not align with their assumption that med-
                   ical people do not smoke.
Response elements: Reaffirm the importance of empathy. Validate the notion
                   that a patient's previous clinical encounters may have
                   been different. Emphasize the universal nature of am-
                   bivalence. Admit the limits of your understanding, and
                   reiterate your desire to learn. Invite the patient to cor-
                   rect your understanding if you have it wrong. (Optional:
                   disclose a personal experience that closely resembles
                   tobacco dependence in structure.)

Question: *Do I have to quit today?*
Clinical insight: This is often an expression of threat. Remember that the
                   approach-avoidance behavior pattern is characterized by
                   retreat from the goal as steps toward the goal begin to
                   threaten the status quo. Patients who deeply desire fu-
                   ture abstinence are likely to be, by definition, reluctant to
                   engage in an abstinence attempt in the present.
Response elements: A derivative of the cessation mind-set, this question of-
                   fers opportunity to refocus the patient on the impulse to
                   smoke (rather than on just the smoking) and to establish
                   the basis of a dependence mind-set instead. There is of-
                   ten a palpable sense of great relief when the clinician de-
                   fuses this expectation, using a joining statement, such as
                   "No—not today. I don't want you to try to quit smoking
                   until we are ready to go there."

Question:	*Can I quit today?*
Clinical insight:	The subtext of this patient request is obviously an urgency to relegate smoking to the past. At times, the patient has identified today as a quit day for practical reasons, such as upcoming surgery or travel. More likely, the question is an expression of emotional exigency, frustration, annoyance, or even disgust with smoking. It is important that the clinician explore the specific motivation behind the question before setting a premature quit date.
Response elements:	For urgencies based on emotions, the approach should validate the patient's desire to "put all this in the rearview mirror." Reframe the process of unlearning, the initiation of pharmacotherapy, or both, as the preparatory steps necessary for maintaining comfort and equanimity when the patient eventually takes the desired step forward. For urgencies truly related to practical deadlines, clinicians should prioritize educating the patient on the proper use of a controller-reliever combination with rapid onset of action.

Question:	*Can't you just scare me out of smoking?*
Clinical insight:	Again, an expression of urgency. However, this question also implies the patient perceives continued smoking as a character flaw. Within the premise of the question lies the common assumption that continued smoking is a matter of insufficient motivation to stop.
Response elements:	Scare tactics do not reliably work with addiction. It is important to maintain a positive affective presence. Acknowledge that the patient clearly already knows enough about the ill effects of smoking to provide sufficient motivation, and resist the temptation to sneak in a list of reasons why smoking is bad. One example might be, "I'm not going to try to scare you because you already know smoking causes [insert favorite scary illnesses]." Reframe the point of treatment away from increasing motivation; focus instead on reducing abnormally amplified drive signals originating from survival structures hijacked by nicotine.

Question: *I could just gradually cut down?*

Clinical insight: Perhaps an expression of escape, but equally likely to be an expression of the desire to avoid the deep sense of unease produced by forced abstinence.

Response elements: Clinicians should probe to assess the genesis of this question. The desire to avoid the dysphoria of abstinence provides an opportunity to reframe or reiterate the goals of pharmacotherapy. The clinical goal should be to eliminate the struggle inherent to progressive reduction efforts.

Question: *How much weight will I gain?*

Clinical insight: Concern about weight gain is common and may be unspoken. Consider the patient's starting weight when developing a treatment plan. Use the same scale each time weight is recorded, and allow for normal annual variations (+5% of baseline is reasonable). The patient's internalized perceptions of weight change can sometimes differ from measured weight trends.

Response elements: Because nicotine abstinence can result in sustained survival activation—a generalized appetitive state—clinicians should consider weight gain to be a sign of poorly controlled compulsion, even in the absence of other reported withdrawal symptoms. Weight gain with abstinence is not inevitable; adequate pharmacotherapeutic control reliably minimizes post-cessation weight gain. Concern regarding weight gain provides an opportunity to develop shared care goals. Avoid relying on the "relative harm" approach (that is, "Weight gain is not as bad for you as smoking").

Question: *Which of these medications works best?*

Clinical insight: Another derivative of the cessation paradigm, patients have been conditioned to think of pharmacotherapies as interchangeable or, worse, as mutually exclusive of each other. While it may be possible to identify personalized treatment approaches in some research settings, it remains infeasible in the clinic at this time. The goal of pharmacotherapeutic decision-making is to optimize control over the compulsion to smoke while minimizing cost, complexity, and the likelihood of side effects.

Response elements: Validate the patient's need for certainty in effectiveness. Information derived from clinical trials or guidelines may be a useful reassurance for some patients. Most patients appreciate personalization of response, such as "In our experience . . ." or "Here's why I think this choice is best for you."

Question: *How much is the medication going to cost? Is it covered?*
Clinical insight: Details regarding the exact coverage benefits for each of the tobacco-dependence pharmacotherapies vary significantly by plan and region. Most formularies cover some available FDA-approved pharmacotherapies, but administrative restrictions may apply. Remember that medications that are available over the counter may be covered if prescribed. Be prepared to request prior authorization of the preferred intervention from the insurer, clarifying your rationale for using one intervention over others. Cost can be a significant barrier for uninsured or underinsured patients, so clinicians should become familiar with manufacturer assistance programs, municipal health clinics, and regional quit-line resources offering free or reduced-cost pharmacotherapy.

Response elements: Validate the patient's concern about expenses. Provide reassurance that out-of-pocket costs are important elements of decision-making. Reaffirm your commitment to working through systematic barriers to access. Reinforce the notion that generic products can be equally effective.

Question: *Does this stuff have side effects?*
Clinical insight: Misconceptions regarding the utility of pharmacotherapy, magnified by rampant misinformation and negative personal anecdotes, may conspire to make patients uncertain about the desirability of pharmacotherapy. Patients may express an interest in trying to achieve abstinence "cold turkey" first.

Response elements: Refer to Chapter 9 for intervention-specific side effects and the approach to management. Validate the patient's concern, and express an understanding of their interest in unassisted cessation. Ensure the patient understands that pharmacotherapy is not mandatory. However, reaffirm that the goal of pharmacotherapy is to significantly improve the probability of abstinence and to help the brain achieve the desired change in patterns of patterns.

Question: *What do you think of acupuncture? Hypnosis?*
Clinical insight: Nearly 20% of people seek complementary and alternative treatments before seeking conventional medical care. The effects of these interventions described in uncontrolled studies have been notoriously difficult to confirm in randomized controlled trials. Rigorous evidence-based reviews suggest there is no clear, generalizable benefit for either acupuncture or hypnotherapy. However, specific instruction in self-hypnosis techniques can be useful in helping the patient control impulsive responses to anxiety.
Response elements: Affirm the general attraction of hypnotherapy, and assess the specific appeal to the patient. Be open to finding ways the patient might use alternative therapies as an adjunct to care. If pursued, it is reasonable to focus the patient's attention on hypnotherapy that is aimed at controlling the emotional consequences of abstinence, while guiding them away from impersonal, mass-audience events or gadgets. Consider communicating directly with the hypnotherapist to establish shared therapeutic goals.

Question: *What do you think about using an e-cigarette to quit?*
Clinical insight: Currently, the evidence supporting use of the electronic cigarette to help people achieve abstinence is poor. Uncertainty in the anticipated beneficial effects makes it impossible to recommend e-cigarettes in a clinical setting. Additionally, a growing body of evidence suggests e-cigarette aerosol may have a unique risk profile, independent of that of cigarettes. Multiple professional societies have recommended against the use of e-cigarettes in clinical contexts. Regardless of the device used to deliver nicotine, patients suffering nicotine dependence deserve access to evidence-based pharmacotherapies.
Response elements: Validate the patient's interest in novel approaches to ces-

sation. Evaluate which aspects of e-cigarette use are most attractive to the patient, and seek ways to achieve these goals using methods with established safety records. On occasion, a patient will present having already achieved abstinence using an e-cigarette: clinicians should consider adding an approved pharmacotherapy both to address the underlying nicotine dependence and to reduce exposure to potentially harmful e-cigarette aerosol toxicants.

Question:	*Don't people get cancer/have heart attacks after they stop?*
Clinical insight:	Risk of life-threatening illness relates to cumulative smoke exposure over the patient's lifetime and begins to revert toward baseline levels of risk after cessation. The rate at which risk recedes varies based on the specific illness and depends on factors like patient age, total exposure, family history, and comorbidities.
Response elements:	Validate the concern. Reassure the patient that cigarette smoke is not protective (that is, their risk doesn't get worse after quitting; it only gets better). For patients younger than 45, it is feasible for cessation of exposure to return their long-term health risk back to their baseline, pre-smoking levels.
Question:	*I'm not addicted. I need help with the habit. What can you do to help me?*
Clinical insight:	Clinically, addiction refers to an induced disorder of motivational control and is not defined by the presence of euphoria or withdrawal drama. This distinction may be confusing, particularly to patients who have adopted outdated concepts of distinct physical and psychological addictions. Alternatively, patients sometimes harbor negative feelings about the word "addiction," usually stemming from the associated social stigma.
Response elements:	Assess the patient's understanding of addiction. Identify and correct educational deficits as needed, but avoid forcing a specific vocabulary, particularly if the patient expressed concerns about the social consequences of labeling their problem as addiction. In either case, consider shifting the frame of pharmacotherapy decisions

away from withdrawal management and toward a means
of reducing the automaticity of habitual behaviors.

Questions That Patients Ask Later in the Course of Treatment

Question: *I'm smoking more now than I was before. Is that normal?*
Clinical insight: The threat of impending abstinence can sometimes am-
                      plify the anticipatory drive to smoke. This pattern is of
                      no therapeutic consequence and should not imply the
                      established plan will be ineffective. On occasion, patients
                      started on pharmacotherapy may smoke more because
                      the reinforcing effects of cigarette nicotine have been
                      undermined by the medication's pharmacodynamics.
                      Patients may temporarily experience a paradoxical in-
                      crease in smoking when the medications are working
                      well.
Response elements: Reassure the patient the increase in tobacco use is tem-
                      porary and not a sign of waning commitment. Consider
                      increasing the frequency of as-needed reliever use to
                      compensate for the increase in nicotine requirements
                      produced by anticipatory pressure.

Question: *I'm coughing more than I was before. Is that normal?*
Clinical insight: Accumulation of mucus in the small airways results from
                      the lung's protective response to smoke-induced inflam-
                      mation. Cigarette smoke increases both the production
                      and viscosity of mucus and has an inhibitory effect on
                      ciliated airway epithelial cells. Absent effective airway
                      clearance, the smallest airways may become laden with
                      inflammatory debris and clogged. As smoke exposure
                      decreases, ciliary beat frequency increases, improving
                      airway clearance and sometimes resulting in increased
                      cough and sputum production.
Response elements: Reassure the patient that this is not a pathological effect
                      but rather a sign that the lungs are restoring their nat-
                      ural protective mechanisms following the elimination
                      of smoke irritants. Clinicians should advise patients
                      to maintain adequate hydration and avoid over-the-
                      counter cough suppressants. Pulmonary hygiene can be

accelerated by teaching the patient to breathe deeply to total lung capacity, followed by "huffing" exercises (exhaling forcefully in short, sharp breaths).

Question:	*Am I hopeless?*
Clinical insight:	Learned hopelessness is a common derivative of the cessation paradigm. Patients have often been previously taught to frame their recovery in terms of success or failure—often to the detriment of progress toward recovery. On occasion, the interrogative "Am I hopeless?" is used as proxy for the declarative "I am hopeless," which can be an expression of depressed mood or escape.
Response elements:	Language choices are critical in the face of learned helplessness. Clinicians should avoid focusing the patient on "quitting" and should refrain from terms-of-art, such as cessation, quit rates, and success or failure. Recall the four magic words of interaction style: empathy, joining, validation, and hope (Chapter 7). Remember to reframe the problem into a problem that's solvable and to reaffirm the commitment to work tirelessly to find the right solutions. Accept responsibility for the system's role in limiting progress: "We're going to get there. If we haven't found the right answer yet, I will just need to work harder to get it done."

Question:	*How long do I have to be on this medication?*
Clinical insight:	In addition to the natural variation in effect that is expected within a diverse population of patients, there is also a wide array of social-environmental factors that may influence the discontinuation decision. For example, patients who suffer a trauma just before the six-month follow-up visit may be ill positioned to consider discontinuation because of the emotional milieu of the moment. In all cases, decisions regarding duration of therapy should be based on the achievement of desired clinical outcomes rather than on calendar days.
Response elements:	Early in the course of treatment, clinicians should establish an expectation of maintenance therapy that extends well beyond the date of cessation. Though it is difficult to offer a precise anticipated duration at the outset, it is

helpful to establish the expectation of prolonged therapy (for example, "at least six months"). Assess the patient's perceived vulnerability to relapse before discontinuation. For patients on combination regimens, it can be very useful to discontinue one medication at a time to avoid sudden shifts in control.

Question: *The patch caused red welts on my skin. What should I do?*

Clinical insight: Most often, dermatologic reactions to the nicotine patch are the result of direct mast cell activation within the skin rather than an allergic event. Nicotine causes mast cells to release histamine, causing a localized reaction characterized by swelling, reddening, and itchiness. On occasion, the welt will be accompanied by a dull muscle ache in the associated area. The effect is local, so it often manifests as a well-circumscribed area of redness immediately under the patch application site. In contradistinction, the very rare "true" allergic reaction is characterized by rash that can extend to areas distant to the application site.

Response elements: This local reaction can be very uncomfortable and can result in skin "staining" that lasts several weeks, but it does not constitute an absolute contraindication to continued patch use. Clinicians may alleviate the problem by counseling the patient to apply over-the-counter hydrocortisone cream to the area of skin intended for the patch—before the patch is applied. Persistent or painful reactions can be treated with a once-daily, over-the-counter, nonsedating antihistamine. In circumstances where the clinician suspects a true allergic reaction, immediate discontinuation of the offending agent is warranted, and reuse should be avoided unless monitored by a trained professional.

Question: *I have a friend who got addicted to the gum and used it for years. Will I be able to stop using it when I'm done?*

Clinical insight: Because of the pharmacokinetics of delivery, pharmaceutical nicotine products using nicotine salt preparations (not free-base nicotine) have extremely low addiction liabilities. With the exception of nicotine nasal spray users, most patients treated with nicotine will not develop dependence on the pharmacotherapeutic. Refer to Chapter 6 for a review of the device characteristics that have been engineered to maximize impact. Ongoing reliance on pharmaceutical nicotine is most often a manifestation of an ongoing sense of vulnerability to relapse.

Response elements: Clinicians should first validate the observation and affirm that the rare patient continues to feel vulnerable to the allure of nicotine for several years after discontinuing the behavior. This question provides an excellent entry into discussion of the unique delivery characteristics of engineered tobacco devices and can serve as a focus for joining. Reinforce the idea that the clinical approach to achieving control over compulsion is akin to a process by which the patient "unlearns" how to be a smoker; the goal is to change the brain's pattern of patterns until the probability of relapse becomes trivial.

Chapter 15
Lessons Learned

Nothing screams "last chapter" like a chance to finally put some new ideas to work. In accordance with the well-known axiom to finish by telling them what you told them, the space below contains five fictional case vignettes, each accompanied by three essay-style challenge questions. Don't panic: it's not a test. We present our own interpretation of the answers directly below each question. Think of this challenge as an opportunity to integrate the information gained at various points in the book into a balanced and seamless articulation of your approach to common problems in the clinic.

Challenge yourself to think through the bullet points of your own answer before moving on to review ours. Use the exercise as a prompt to review any material that has become fuzzy over time. Seek additional sources of information when formulating responses (some really interesting sources are listed in Part IV), and do not be afraid to include additional elements to your own answers, even if they were omitted from ours.

> *Have fun living the experience of tobacco-*
> *dependence treatment in the privacy of your mind*
> *before taking your new skills out into practice.*
> *Your patients will directly benefit from your investment.*

Case #1: "I just can't put them down"

Walter S. is a 59-year-old, self-employed machinist from Allentown, Pennsylvania. He began smoking cigarettes at age 14 and reached his maximum daily intake of twenty to twenty-five cigarettes per day by age 17. He served in the U.S. Navy as a young man and has an extensive travel history as a result. He is married, with three adult children and four young grandchildren. He was an avid soccer player as a young man, more recently serving as a referee for the youth soccer league in which his grandson plays. Lately, he has begun to forgo soccer assignments because of an increasing sense of shortness of breath on exertion. His business is failing, and he worries about losing his health insurance.

Mr. S. has attempted cessation on a number of occasions in the past. He has used both the nicotine patch and varenicline with limited success. His longest period of abstinence was eight months, occurring five years earlier. A few months ago, he bought a box of nicotine gum with the intention of using it as a cessation aid but has not found the courage to try it. He was referred to you by his cardiologist for assistance with treating his tobacco dependence.

Question 1.1: Describe your approach to assessing Mr. S. Discuss your strategy for gaining control over his compulsion to smoke. List your anticipated treatment contingencies, and briefly outline your chosen approach should they occur.

- Begin with conversation aimed at getting to know the person behind the tobacco dependence. Remember the importance of understanding the patient's backstory—the frame through which Mr. S. has experienced tobacco dependence—for developing true empathy and establishing trust. Remember that the backstory is revealed only slowly and sometimes in pieces. Don't rush this part of the assessment.
- Take a careful tobacco-use history. Make sure your probing extends well beyond the superficial pack-year assessment. Use a note-taking template that facilitates structured questioning. Refer to Chapter 7 for a list of potential conversation-starter questions. Assess the clinical severity of dependence using several key qualitative indicators, such as time to first cigarette in the morning, minimum number of daily cigarettes consumed, relight frequency, subjective agitation during forced abstinence, anticipatory anxiety when considering abstinence, embarrassment-causing episodes related to smoking urgency.
- Complete your assessment using the U*P*P*S*S framework (Chapter 7), cataloging insights from past quit attempts, evaluating the potential moderating effects

of psychiatric comorbidities, weighing the potential relevance of other substance use history, and gauging the impact of household smoking. Assess intrinsic and extrinsic motivators of change. Estimate the patient's confidence in their ability to achieve abstinence.

- The overall strategic approach to controlling the compulsion to smoke requires working to minimize the threat salience of abstinence. Conversationally, this means divorcing the idea of managing tobacco dependence from the clinical goal of cessation. Minimizing threat salience also involves (1) building trust; (2) paying attention to interaction style (that is, four magic words, positive affective presence); (3) gain framing by emphasizing the benefits of resolved ambivalence (instead of the benefits of quitting); and (4) relying on proven pharmacotherapies to improve transition probabilities through the process of change (Chapter 9).

- Specific contingencies are derived from the details of the tobacco-use history and backstory. Generally, clinicians can anticipate predictable roadblocks when initiating care. Extrinsic roadblocks, such as coverage barriers, lack of pharmacy inventory, or misinformation from external sources, can generally be managed easily. We recommend clinicians establish the expectation of extrinsic roadblocks and conclude each visit with a specific return instruction: for example, "Come back to see me in ___ weeks to give me a report, no matter what happens." Roadblocks may also originate intrinsically and may be an expression of escape. The rhythm for managing escape (validate, reframe, repeat) is discussed in detail in Chapter 8. Remember to reframe the problem into a problem that is solvable.

Question 1.2: Characterize the distortions in neurophysiology that led to Mr. S's reluctance to abstain.

- Nicotine acts as an exogenous ligand (agonist) of the nicotinic acetylcholine receptors in the central nervous system. The receptor set implicated in the development of dependence is located primarily within the mesolimbic (survival) system. Densely concentrated α4β2 receptors in the ventral tegmental area (VTA) of the midbrain are highly sensitive and imbue otherwise irrelevant environmental signals with survival salience. Activation of the VTA leads to activation of the dopaminergic nucleus accumbens, resulting in a generalized appetitive state and an increased drive to react. Failure to respond results in negative prediction error signaling, which turns on negative affect and frames cognition so that action is rationalized (Chapter 2).

- Smoking is not a monolithic behavior. There is a great deal of variability in the expression of compulsion within the population of affected individuals. Biologic phenotypes, such as the nicotine metabolite ratio, influence smoking topography as well as response to therapy. Clinical phenotypes are useful in matching intervention intensity to patient needs (Chapter 10).

Question 1.3: Describe the biologic basis for the chronic relapsing and remitting nature of tobacco dependence.

- Receptor stimulation results in a series of predictable molecular changes within the neuron (Chapter 3). These intracellular changes result in distorted neurotransmitter production, arborization patterns, and receptor density and sensitivity. CREB and ΔFosB within the cell regulate the strength of long-term connections within motor activation pathways and confer longevity to the abnormal pattern of patterns (Chapter 5).
- Chapter 4 discusses the impact nicotine exposure has on stress resolution and allostatic load. Nicotine exposure makes it hard for the brain's allostatic mechanisms to return to a low-energy, comfortable, neutral homeostasis. Allostatic load creates an inefficiency in shifting the brain from neutral to drive and back again and can limit the body's response to stress in the long run. Disinhibition of automatic responses is experienced as the "screw it!" phenomenon —an instinctive release from the disincentives to smoking.

Case #2: "Why quit now?"

Mrs. Denise B. is a 70-year-old, widowed, African American woman. She lives alone in a West Philadelphia apartment, unable to work because of severe chronic obstructive pulmonary disease. She has two adult daughters with whom she has what she describes as a good relationship. She doesn't see them as much as she would like because of her disability. In addition to her respiratory illness, her past medical history includes ischemic heart disease, type 2 diabetes, hypertension, and hypercholesterolemia. She is on a number of different medications and at times finds herself confused about which pills to take and when.

Mrs. B. uses oxygen delivered by nasal cannula. She also smokes ten to twelve cigarettes per day. On two past occasions, the oxygen supply company has refused to complete her delivery, citing safety concerns over evidence of cigarette ashes in the vicinity of her tanks. On both occasions, Mrs. B. has chosen to relinquish her oxygen rather than her cigarettes. She has never made a serious quit attempt nor does she plan to. Her position is "the damage is already done, leave me alone."

Question 2.1: Describe some of the maladaptive cognitive patterns that may be influencing Mrs. B.'s disposition toward abstinence.

- Learned helplessness, hopelessness, and frustration are common among people who have experienced the soft power of nicotine's draw, especially among those who have internalized the notion that continued smoking is a function of deficit in willpower and strength of character. In Mrs. B.'s particular case, it is important to notice that her smoking and the disability it has caused have potentially resulted in significant isolation. It is clear that she experiences less contact with her daughters than she would like, and it is easy to imagine that she also lacks for otherwise day-to-day social interactions within the community.
- For many patients, the restrictive consequences of requiring supplemental oxygen can result in a sense of frustration and disability and may serve as an outward symbol of "lack of resolve" to those who are so inclined. Given Mrs. B.'s several tobacco-related comorbidities, it is also easy to imagine that her life is occupied in part by visits to healthcare providers who may have unwittingly emphasized the need for motivation to quit. Recall that culpability bias (Chapter 12) is often operational during clinical encounters and may be unintentionally communicated nonverbally during the visit (Chapter 7).
- Chronic hypoxemia is associated with an increased risk for cognitive decline and dementia. Early stages of dementia are often associated with depression and anxiety, which in turn exacerbate isolation and frustration.
- COPD is often described as a disease characterized by "irreversible airflow obstruction." This statement is often misunderstood to mean that patients with COPD have irreversible deficits. In truth, patients with COPD who are helped to stop smoking enjoy significant improvements in symptoms, frequency of exacerbations, longevity, and quality of life. Misplaced nihilism may unfairly bias Mrs. B.'s utility estimate and may prevent her from engaging help.
- Contrary to popular misconceptions, oxygen does not explode. Like any compressed gas, if a cylinder of oxygen is exposed to an external heat source, the cylinder may indeed fail if the heated gas expands to produce an internal pressure that exceeds the containment threshold of the cylinder. But the oxygen is not exploding. While oxygen does not independently ignite, it does accelerate combustion when in contact with an open flame. This truism leads to concerns over bringing the burning coal of the cigarette into proximity of the oxygen discharge port of the nasal cannula. However, the high oxygen concentration at the nasal cannula becomes quickly diluted by the surrounding air and equilibrates to the ambient oxygen concentration within a few inches of discharge. Concerns over increased fire hazards in homes with supplemental oxygen are overstated and should never limit a hypoxemic patient's access to much-needed oxygen.

Nevertheless, patients with COPD who smoke often face the humiliation of having oxygen deliveries denied and used as leverage to motivate cessation (that is, oxygen hostage-taking).

Question 2.2: Discuss the social norms or traditions that might affect your approach to Mrs. B.'s care. Explain your assumptions. Describe how you might alter your approach as a result.

- Circumstances in which patients face the complications of chronic illness can lead to the loss of social capital. Engagement with the healthcare system can be confusing. Patients forced to navigate confusing systems without the assistance of social networks that can help develop a shared understanding and trust suffer worse outcomes. Particularly when managing mistaken notions of tobacco dependence, it may be important to slow down and focus on developing trust before making recommendations for therapy.
- It is clear Mrs. B. has a strong family orientation. Engaging her daughters in a networked-care approach can be helpful in establishing new norms and improving the social support required for achieving abstinence.
- Multiunit housing complexes are increasingly becoming smoke-free. Given Mrs. B.'s disability, this may present an insurmountable problem for her. Explore her relationship to neighbors, as well as to the landlord. Find out if there are designated areas for smoking while waiting for treatment to work. Offer to act as an arbiter if relationships with the landlord have been compromised.
- Mrs. B. lives in a densely packed urban area of Philadelphia. Proximity to tobacco sources is high. Remember to assess the influence of both typical (grocery stores, pharmacies) and atypical (neighbors, loosie sales, takeout restaurants) sources of tobacco, as well as the practicality of altering procurement routines.

Question 2.3: Describe your approach to cognitive management. Specifically, discuss your approach to overcoming Mrs. B.'s resistance to change.

- Remember that reluctance to stop using the substance of addiction is the hallmark of dependence. However, resistance is a particularly aggressive pattern of reluctance in which the patient is characteristically closed to new ideas or discussion and may sabotage the encounter. As with all expressions of reluctance, the clinician's objective is to maintain a positive affective presence and to engage the patient in conversation using the validate-reframe-repeat framework for counseling. Validation emphasizes the patient's autonomy. The clinician's conversation remains focused on whichever topic the patient prioritizes (for example, their backstory, avocation, or goals), rolling with the resistance while trying to understand its source. The conversation proceeds long enough to find a toehold, providing an opportunity to adopt one of the patient's own goals.

- It is important to build trust—and trust in this situation depends on joining. Change will not happen through force, coercion, or persuasion. With the resistant patient, the only persuasive tool the clinician has is interaction style. Remember the four magic words: empathy, joining, validation, hope.

- Minimize threat salience by searching for detailed elements of routine and asking for an easy change—preferably one that does not require the patient to forfeit critical parts of the smoking ritual. Listen for clues regarding what changes were successful in the past.

- Consider offering pharmacotherapy without obligation to change smoking routines. Set a follow-up interval of four to six weeks to assess the impact of medication. Assess threat salience rather than number of cigarettes consumed when determining whether the strategy has been effective.

Case #3: "It must be better, right?"

Ms. Gloria M. is a 42-year-old African American woman who has been in your care for over one year. She has been desperate to stop smoking and has successfully decreased her daily intake from twenty to four cigarettes per day since you began treating her. She has no significant medical history and is on no other medications. With respect to tobacco use, she has variously tried the 21-milligram nicotine patch, 4-milligram nicotine lozenge, and varenicline, 1 milligram twice daily. Each has resulted in side effects, which have limited their continued use. She presents today still smoking the same amount as at the past four visits and has several questions regarding the use of the e-cigarette.

Question 3.1: Describe the cigarette's properties as a nicotine delivery device.

- There are a variety of mechanical properties of the cigarette that make it uniquely capable of delivering nicotine, including

  - density of the tobacco rod;
  - density (porosity) of the tobacco paper;
  - burn rate and combustion temperature of the coal;
  - filter paper characteristics, including embossed ventilation channels and porosity;

and

   ◦ microperforations in the tipping paper, facilitating side-wall ventilation.

- The chemical properties of the cigarette are also engineered to maximize the impact of nicotine, including

   ◦ ammonization of the tobacco during processing;
   ◦ the acid-base balance (pH) of the smoke;
   ◦ the free-base nicotine content of the smoke;
   ◦ the availability of minor alkaloids; and
   ◦ mentholation.

- By virtue of delivery directly to the lungs, the nicotine carried by cigarette smoke comes into close contact with a very large blood volume that, because of the anatomy of the cardiopulmonary system, will return directly to the left ventricle, ready to carry the highly concentrated nicotine bolus to the main effector organ, the brain.

Question 3.2: Incorporate guideline recommendations for pharmacotherapy into practical treatment recommendations for Ms. M. Consider her previous experience when formulating your plan.

- 2020 guidelines published by the American Thoracic Society have evaluated the impact of pretreatment strategies—that is, beginning pharmacotherapy in patients before they are ready to stop smoking. The guideline panel calculated that clinicians could expect to help more than three hundred additional patients to stop smoking per one thousand treated, just by starting varenicline well before the patient expresses a readiness to quit.
- Despite Ms. M.'s unfulfilling past experience with pharmacotherapy, there are a number of ways in which effectiveness may be improved while minimizing side effects. To the clinician, details about past therapeutic failures can provide important insight into educational needs and dosing modifications. Here are some examples:

   ◦ Lack of therapeutic effect of varenicline is frequently a function of an inadequate pretreatment period or of an unreasonable expectation setting. If patients expect the medication to result in complete abstinence within a week, a partial effect or delayed onset of action may be prematurely interpreted as "failure."

- ○ Combination medications work better than monotherapies.
- ○ Combining controller medications to reduce the frequency and intensity of cravings with a reliever designed to give the patient an active means by which they can address a craving may give the patient a more robust sense of control and allows for more precise titration of pharmacologic support.
- ○ Therapeutic failures are sometimes the result of treatment periods that are too short. Check to be sure Ms. M. understands the need to continue therapy well past the quit date, establish the expectation of prolonged treatment per guideline recommendations, and frame the decision to modify or discontinue dosing as a joint responsibility.

- Though there are very few well-done studies evaluating the relative value of electronic cigarettes compared with regulated pharmacotherapies, there is little doubt that the rate of serious adverse events and the long-term potential harms of e-cigarette aerosol outweigh those of pharmacotherapy. Though there are anecdotes of patients successfully eschewing cigarettes in favor of e-cigarettes, neither reliability nor safety have reached the level of certainty necessary for them to be considered a clinical intervention. Finally, remember that the clinician's role is not solely to eliminate smoke exposure but to manage the underlying addiction to nicotine.

Question 3.3: Anticipate and address some of the more common questions about the use of nonapproved cessation support that Ms. M. is likely to bring up during the visit.

- For Ms. M., as for many patients, the electronic cigarette may represent a means of compromise (escape), allowing her to continue to gratify her dependence without using a cigarette to do it. Consumers are likely to view e-cigarettes as relatively safe but are generally unaware of the potential ill effects of aerosolized propylene glycol, organic flavorants, aldehydes, and contaminants.
- A significant number of patients consider use of hypnosis, acupuncture, and auricular clips or magnets when approaching cessation. Unfortunately, the evidence supporting these interventions is of poor quality. Though unlikely to be physically harmful, the financial costs and the potential deleterious effects of misplaced hope should be considered when discussing these modalities with Ms. M.
- Some patients still seem to harbor a desire to be punished into quitting. This may be a remnant of early behavioral studies on smoking, where a variety of aversive techniques were used in attempts to extinguish the learned associations of

smoking. Strategies designed to make people really uncomfortable, such as rapid smoking, rapid puffing, and electric shock, were paired with smoking behaviors, images of smoking, even imagined smoking—Clockwork Orange style—in the hopes of making it so distasteful that people would be encouraged to stop smoking. Aversive therapies do not seem to work and became unethical once pharmacotherapies were developed. Put the car battery back in the car.

Case #4: "Gotta be ready"

Sean J. is a 27-year-old male college student who is home for summer break. He has come to see you for assistance with tobacco dependence treatment on the advice of his mother. Mr. J. has smoked approximately twenty cigarettes per day since age 19 and has never made a serious quit attempt. In addition to tobacco use, he admits to using both alcohol ("two to three beers per day") and marijuana ("one, maybe two joints per day") on a routine basis. His summer job is in housing construction and feels like his coworkers would be hard pressed to accommodate any change to their smoking routines around him. About three months ago, Mr. J. developed an intermittent cough productive of purulent sputum. His symptoms have his mother extremely upset, and her concern is starting to make him worry that something may be wrong. When he presented to his primary care office for evaluation, he was told his symptoms were most likely due to chronic bronchitis and was counseled to stop smoking. He was offered a packet of self-help materials with instructions to "call the number when you're ready to quit." On the advice of his mother, he presents to your tobacco treatment clinic for further guidance.

Question 4.1: Identify the common biases, heuristics, and cultural norms that may be affecting Mr. J.'s tobacco-related decision-making. Be sure to include the assumptions that are likely influencing each of the several people directly impacting his case. What points might you make to counteract these social influences?

- The societal approach to tobacco dependence has traditionally been informed by a number of counterproductive cultural norms and assumptions regarding behavior change. One of the most damaging has been the dogmatic belief that patients must be "ready" for change before clinicians can be effective. In our view, patients must indeed be ready (and willing) to participate in their care, but it is the clinician's responsibility to create the conditions in which change becomes possible.
- Generic self-help materials that simply encourage cessation and offer access to

therapeutic resources are unlikely to produce the desired result; like all other types of dependence interventions, the effectiveness of self-help materials depends on intensity of contact (single versus serial), degree to which they offer specific behavioral advice (generic versus tailored), and integration of pharmacotherapy into the intervention.

- Traditionally, substances of addiction have been considered separately, from the perspective of the major neurotransmitter system involved in developing dependence. More recently, there is a growing awareness that the underlying physiology of addiction shares common functional elements across substance categories. Mr. J.'s alcohol and marijuana use may be a confounding factor in achieving abstinence.
- The potentially significant impact of the following common cognitive biases should be considered:

  o Availability bias: A recent or memorable quit attempt may be unfairly influencing Mr. J.'s perception of success probability.
  o Impact bias: He may have an excessively high estimation of the strain or effort required of him or his construction crew, or of the emotional disruption that abstinence may cause.
  o Focusing effect bias: Remember to explore any competing life concerns that may be distracting Mr. J. from prioritizing an abstinence attempt.
  o Omission bias: Having heard rumors about unpleasant side effects, Mr. J. may simply find it more appropriate to avoid discussion of pharmacotherapy rather than take a chance on experiencing complications.

Question 4.2: Describe the importance of "causal controllability" assumptions as they relate to Mr. J.

- Because his chronic bronchitis is most likely the direct result of smoking, Mr. J.'s problem may be implicitly interpreted as causally controllable. If the clinician overestimates the role of character while underestimating the role of environmental influences on the smoking behavior, it is possible for the assessment of responsibility to be biased in favor of "culpability" rather than "ownership." An implicit bias toward culpability leads to a reduced investment in help-giving.
- Remember to spend some time evaluating the contours of his mother's recommendation. Was it coercive? If so, vexation, stigmatization, and shame may be important undercurrents coloring Mr. J.'s receptivity to suggestion and may need to be addressed.

Question 4.3: Imagine your organization has decided to develop a program aimed at reaching a demographic group much like Mr. J's. Distinguish between effective and ineffective methods of attracting such an audience to the tobacco treatment message.

- The audience expects negative imagery and threatening messages. However, effective materials aimed at attracting an audience to the tobacco-dependence treatment message require a positive affective presence, just like in the clinical encounter.
- Messages with obvious or overdrawn persuasive intent are more likely to result in reactance and selective avoidance.
- Effective methods pay attention to matters affecting the reader's sense of homophily.
- Persuasion basics (Chapter 12) include the use of peripheral messaging, using the attractiveness, familiarity, and/or mood attribution heuristics.

Case #5: "Systematic system change"

Perdition University Hospital has asked you to consult on an initiative to improve inpatient-to-outpatient transitional care services. The initiative is part of an overall effort to reduce readmissions to the hospital and improve the flow of critical information to outpatient staff. System administrators have identified tobacco treatment as a high priority, given its inclusion in the Joint Commission (JCAHO) quality standards. Unfortunately, there are no health system staff currently treating tobacco dependence in any department. As a consequence, system administrators have very little experience with the care of tobacco-dependent patients and need a clinician's help in identifying a system-based tobacco intervention that is both feasible and effective. Assume that you have a "small" annual budget to work with but that the ideal proposal would be one that keeps costs low.

Question 5.1: What does your ideal systems-based tobacco intervention look like? Describe your process for implementing such an intervention program.

- A systems-based intervention can be any idea that seems plausible, given the idiosyncratic constraints of the local environment. Whatever the planned intervention, remember to articulate the individual, organizational, and institutional responsibilities that drive this change (Chapter 13).

- A constructionist approach starts with an established mental model, and then works to incrementally bring others to an understanding of how their services can fit into that model, with only minor alterations in workflow or priorities. Use the information, the motivations, and the resources already in place within an organization, and put them into alignment around tobacco treatment. Learn which processes work, and use those successes to build a growing set of services.
- Identify the relationships in a vertically integrated model of care, and develop reasonable timeline expectations. Liberally use models of vertical integration that already exist across the healthcare system to develop an organizational schema that emulates them, and rely on the familiarity heuristic to make your ideas more available to decision-makers.

Question 5.2: What outcome measures would you employ to prove intervention effectiveness? How would you collect this data? Using "dummy data," build one representative graph illustrating your point.

- When it comes to tobacco evaluations, it is common for the field of view to be constrained to clinical response rates at predetermined intervals. However, when thinking about program evaluation, it is important to also identify measures that give insight into structural growth, efficiency of workflow, and overall impact on the system. Structural metrics relate to the components of care delivery and might include measures of staff involvement, funding sources, or number of locations served across the health system. Process measures provide insight on the interaction between patients and clinicians. These might include the number of patients cared for, proportion of total referrals successfully engaged, levels of service provided, or average delay between phone contact and appointment date. Finally, outcome measures might reflect the impact your program is having on the overall delivery of healthcare. These might include rates of readmission for key indicator illnesses like COPD or cardiovascular disease, impact on disparities in care, rate of pharmacotherapy prescription, or rate of seamless transition from inpatient to outpatient care (Figure 15.1).

Question 5.3: Assume your recommendations are approved and implementation is under way. Describe your plan for educating the target audience regarding the availability of the intervention, including any logistical information (how to access the service, what to expect, and so on).

- Referring clinicians often start off anchored to the same assumptions about "smoking cessation" as prospective patients. Initial educational efforts should

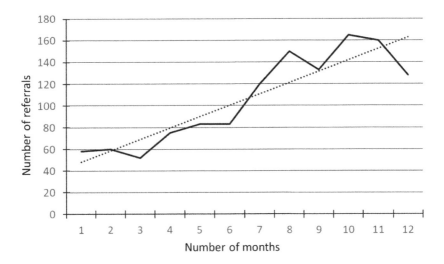

Figure 15.1. New patient referrals by month, 2020. An example of important outcome measures that reflect the impact your program (Question 5.2).

focus on distinguishing the program's tobacco-dependence theory of care from common assumptions. A toll-free phone number or a catchy vanity web address can be very useful to ensure that access to your clinic is easy—and easy to remember. Begin disseminating your ideas through readily available channels (for example, lectures, emails, brochures), but consider expanding to include websites, social media sites, and paid advertising when appropriate. Remember to use automated patient education materials, after-visit summaries, and letters to referring clinicians as a means of amplifying your narrative.

Part IV

Knowing "More"

Part IV

Knowing "More"

Bibliography
Additional Reading and Useful References

Is that really how it works? I didn't know that.

—Susan V., 63 years old

Chapter 1. Ambivalence

The Patient's Experience

Armitage, C. J. (2016). Evidence that implementation intentions can overcome the effects of smoking habits. *Health Psychology, 35*(9), 935–943. https://doi.org/10.1037/hea0000344.

Armitage, C. J., & Conner, M. (2000). Attitudinal ambivalence: A test of three key hypotheses. *Personality and Social Psychology Bulletin, 26*(11), 1421–1432. https://doi.org/10.1177/0146167200263009.

Conner, M., & Armitage, C. J. (2008). Attitudinal ambivalence. In *Attitudes and attitude change* (pp. 261–286). Psychology Press.

Harrist, S. (2006). A phenomenological investigation of the experience of ambivalence. *Journal of Phenomenological Psychology, 37*(1), 85–114. https://doi.org/10.1163/15691624-90000006.

Jonas, K., Broemer, P., & Diehl, M. (2000). Attitudinal ambivalence. *European Review of Social Psychology, 11*(1), 35–74. https://doi.org/10.1080/14792779943000125.

Nordgren, L. F., van Harreveld, F., & van der Pligt, J. (2006). Ambivalence, discomfort, and motivated information processing. *Journal of Experimental Social Psychology, 42*(2), 252–258. https://doi.org/10.1016/j.jesp.2005.04.004.

Schneider, I. K., & Schwarz, N. (2017). Mixed feelings: The case of ambivalence. *Current Opinion in Behavioral Sciences, 15*, 39–45. https://doi.org/10.1016/j.cobeha.2017.05.012.

Thompson, M. M., Zanna, M. P., & Griffin, D. W. (1995). Let's not be indifferent about (attitudinal) ambivalence. In *Attitude strength: Antecedents and consequences* (pp. 361–386). Lawrence Erlbaum Associates.

Williams, S., & Reid, M. (2010). Understanding the experience of ambivalence in anorexia nervosa: The maintainer's perspective. *Psychology & Health, 25(5), 551–567.* https://doi.org/10.1080/08870440802617629.

The Triune Brain

Cory, G. A. (1999). MacLean's triune brain concept: In praise and appraisal. In G. A. Cory (Ed.), *The reciprocal modular brain in economics and politics: Shaping the rational and moral basis of organization, exchange, and choice* (pp. 13–27). Springer US. https://doi.org/10.1007/978-1-4615-4747-1_3.

Farris, S. M. (2008). Evolutionary convergence of higher brain centers spanning the protostome-deuterostome boundary. *Brain, Behavior and Evolution, 72(2), 106–122.* https://doi.org/10.1159/000151471.

MacLean, P. D. (1973). The brain's generation gap: Some human implications. *Zygon, 8(2), 113–127.* https://doi.org/10.1111/j.1467-9744.1973.tb00218.x.

MacLean, P. D. (1977). The triune brain in conflict. *Psychotherapy and Psychosomatics, 28(1/4), 207–220.* https://doi.org/10.1159/000287065.

MacLean, P. D., & George, M. S. (1992). The triune brain in evolution: Role in paleocerebral functions. *Cognitive and Behavioral Neurology, 5(1), 68.*

Ploog, D. W. (2003). The place of the triune brain in psychiatry. *Physiology & Behavior, 79(3), 487–493.* https://doi.org/10.1016/S0031-9384(03)00154-9.

Pogliano, C. (2017). Lucky triune brain: Chronicles of Paul D. MacLean's neuro-catchword. *Nuncius, 32(2), 330–375.* https://doi.org/10.1163/18253911-03202004.

Smith, C. U. M. (Chris). (2010). The triune brain in antiquity: Plato, Aristotle, Erasistratus. *Journal of the History of the Neurosciences, 19(1), 1–14.* https://doi.org/10.1080/09647040802601605.

Nicotine as Soft Power

Botti, S., Orfali, K., & Iyengar, S. S. (2009). Tragic choices: Autonomy and emotional responses to medical decisions. *Journal of Consumer Research, 36(3), 337–352.* https://doi.org/10.1086/598969.

Carmody, T. P., Vieten, C., & Astin, J. A. (2007). Negative affect, emotional acceptance, and smoking cessation. *Journal of Psychoactive Drugs, 39(4), 499–508.* https://doi.org/10.1080/02791072.2007.10399889.

Cinciripini, P. M., Robinson, J. D., Carter, B. L., Lam, C., Wu, X., de Moor, C. A., Baile, W. F., & Wetter, D. W. (2006). The effects of smoking deprivation and nicotine administration on emotional reactivity. *Nicotine & Tobacco Research, 8(3), 379–392.* https://doi.org/10.1080/14622200600670272.

Koch, S. B. J., Mars, R. B., Toni, I., & Roelofs, K. (2018). Emotional control, reappraised. *Neuroscience & Biobehavioral Reviews, 95, 528–534.* https://doi.org/10.1016/j.neubiorev.2018.11.003.

Molas, S., DeGroot, S. R., Zhao-Shea, R., & Tapper, A. R. (2017). Anxiety and nicotine dependence: Emerging role of the habenulo-interpeduncular axis. *Trends in Pharmacological Sciences, 38(2), 169–180.* https://doi.org/10.1016/j.tips.2016.11.001.

Shiv, B., Loewenstein, G., & Bechara, A. (2005). The dark side of emotion in deci-sion-making: When individuals with decreased emotional reactions make more advantageous decisions. *Cognitive Brain Research, 23*(1), 85–92. https://doi.org/10.1016/j.cogbrainres.2005.01.006.

Spillane, N. S., Combs, J., Kahler, C., & Smith, G. T. (2013). Emotion-based impulsiv-ity, smoking expectancies, and nicotine dependence in college students. *Addiction Research & Theory, 21*(6), 489–495. https://doi.org/10.3109/16066359.2012.748894.

Tucker, D. M., Luu, P., Desmond, R. E., Jr., Hartry-Speiser, A., Davey, C., & Flaisch, T. (2003). Corticolimbic mechanisms in emotional decisions. *Emotion, 3*(2), 127–149. https://doi.org/10.1037/1528-3542.3.2.127.

Weinberg, P. (1995). Emotional aspects of decision behavior: A comparison of explana-tion concepts. In Flemming Hansen (Ed.), *European advances in consumer research* (Vol. 2, pp. 246–250). Association for Consumer Research. https://www.acrwebsite.org/volumes/11520/volumes/e02/E-02/full.

Young, M. C., & O'Neil, B. M. (1992). Mind over money: The emotional aspects of financial decisions. *Journal of Financial Planning, 5(1), 32.*

Loss Salience

Koca-Atabey, M., & Oner-Özkan, B. (2014). Loss anxiety: An alternative explanation for the fundamental fears in human beings. *Death Studies, 38*(6–10), 662–671. https://doi.org/10.1080/07481187.2013.844748.

Kwak, Y., & Huettel, S. (2018). The order of information processing alters economic gain-loss framing effects. *Acta Psychologica, 182,* 46–54. https://doi.org/10.1016/j.actpsy.2017.11.013.

Luo, S., Wu, B., Fan, X., Zhu, Y., Wu, X., & Han, S. (2019). Thoughts of death affect reward learning by modulating salience network activity. *NeuroImage, 202,* 116068. https://doi.org/10.1016/j.neuroimage.2019.116068.

Markett, S., Heeren, G., Montag, C., Weber, B., & Reuter, M. (2016). Loss aversion is associated with bilateral insula volume: A voxel based morphometry study. *Neuro-science Letters, 619,* 172–176. https://doi.org/10.1016/j.neulet.2016.03.029.

Montford, W. J., Leary, R. B., & Nagel, D. M. (2019). The impact of implicit self-theories and loss salience on financial risk. *Journal of Business Research, 99,* 1–11. https://doi.org/10.1016/j.jbusres.2019.02.015.

Reisbig, A. M. J., Hafen, M., Siqueira Drake, A. A., Girard, D., & Breunig, Z. B. (2017). Companion animal death. *Omega, 75*(2), 124–150. https://doi.org/10.1177/0030222815612607.

Shear, M. K., & Skritskaya, N. A. (2012). Bereavement and anxiety. *Current Psychiatry Reports, 14*(3), 169–175. https://doi.org/10.1007/s11920-012-0270-2.

Vignapiano, A., Mucci, A., Merlotti, E., Giordano, G. M., Amodio, A., Palumbo, D., & Galderisi, S. (2018). Impact of reward and loss anticipation on cogni-tive control: An event-related potential study in subjects with schizophrenia and healthy controls. *Clinical EEG and Neuroscience, 49*(1), 46–54. https://doi.org/10.1177/1550059417745935.

Chapter 2. Structure

The Mesolimbic System in Survival and Appetitive Behavior

Brown, C. R. H., Forster, S., & Duka, T. (2018). Goal-driven attentional capture by appetitive and aversive smoking-related cues in nicotine-dependent smokers. *Drug and Alcohol Dependence, 190,* 209–215. https://doi.org/10.1016/j.drugalcdep.2018.06.011.

Feltenstein, M. W., & See, R. E. (2008). The neurocircuitry of addiction: An overview. *British Journal of Pharmacology, 154*(2), 261–274. https://doi.org/10.1038/bjp.2008.51.

Gardner, E. L. (2011). Addiction and brain reward and antireward pathways. *Advances in Psychosomatic Medicine, 30,* 22–60. https://doi.org/10.1159/000324065.

Henningfield, J. E., Smith, T. T., Kleykamp, B. A., Fant, R. V., & Donny, E. C. (2016). Nicotine self-administration research: The legacy of Steven R. Goldberg and implications for regulation, health policy, and research. *Psychopharmacology, 233*(23–24), 3829–3848. https://doi.org/10.1007/s00213-016-4441-4.

Hyman, S. E. (2005). Addiction: A disease of learning and memory. *American Journal of Psychiatry, 162*(8), 1414–1422. https://doi.org/10.1176/appi.ajp.162.8.1414.

Koob, G. F., & Volkow, N. D. (2016). Neurobiology of addiction: A neurocircuitry analysis. *Lancet, Psychiatry, 3*(8), 760–773. https://doi.org/10.1016/S2215-0366(16)00104-8.

Kostowski, W. (2002). Drug addiction as drive satisfaction ("antidrive") dysfunction. *Acta Neurobiologiae Experimentalis, 62*(2), 111–117.

Mojica, C. Y., Belluzzi, J. D., & Leslie, F. M. (2014). Age-dependent alterations in reward-seeking behavior after brief nicotine exposure. *Psychopharmacology, 231*(8), 1763–1773. https://doi.org/10.1007/s00213-013-3266-7.

Quintero Garzola, G. C. (2019). Review: Brain neurobiology of gambling disorder based on rodent models. *Neuropsychiatric Disease and Treatment, 15,* 1751–1770. https://doi.org/10.2147/NDT.S192746.

Stott, S. R. W., & Ang, S.-L. (2013). Chapter 23—The generation of midbrain dopaminergic neurons. In J. L. R. Rubenstein & P. Rakic (Eds.), *Patterning and cell type specification in the developing CNS and PNS* (pp. 435–453). Academic Press. https://doi.org/10.1016/B978-0-12-397265-1.00099-X.

Szechtman, H., Ahmari, S. E., Beninger, R. J., Eilam, D., Harvey, B. H., Edemann-Callesen, H., & Winter, C. (2017). Obsessive-compulsive disorder: Insights from animal models. *Neuroscience & Biobehavioral Reviews, 76,* 254–279. https://doi.org/10.1016/j.neubiorev.2016.04.019.

U.S. Department of Health and Human Services. (2020). Neurobiology of nicotine addiction. In *Smoking cessation: A report of the surgeon general* (pp. 125–129). https://www.cdc.gov/tobacco/data_statistics/sgr/2020-smoking-cessation/index.html.

Willis, M. A., & Haines, D. E. (2018). Chapter 31—The limbic system. In D. E. Haines & G. A. Mihailoff (Eds.), *Fundamental neuroscience for basic and clinical applications* (5th ed., pp. 457–467.e1). Elsevier. https://doi.org/10.1016/B978-0-323-39632-5.00031-1.

The Thalamus and Sensory Integration

Ahissar, E., & Oram, T. (2015). Thalamic relay or cortico-thalamic processing? Old question, new answers. *Cerebral Cortex, 25*(4), 845–848. https://doi.org/10.1093/cercor/bht296.

Hwang, K., Bertolero, M. A., Liu, W. B., & D'Esposito, M. (2017). The human thalamus is an integrative hub for functional brain networks. *Journal of Neuroscience, 37*(23), 5594–5607. https://doi.org/10.1523/JNEUROSCI.0067-17.2017.

McCormick, D. A., & Bal, T. (1994). Sensory gating mechanisms of the thalamus. *Current Opinion in Neurobiology, 4*(4), 550–556. https://doi.org/10.1016/0959-4388(94)90056-6.

Mitchell, A. S., Sherman, S. M., Sommer, M. A., Mair, R. G., Vertes, R. P., & Chudasama, Y. (2014). Advances in understanding mechanisms of thalamic relays in cognition and behavior. *Journal of Neuroscience, 34*(46), 15340–15346. https://doi.org/10.1523/JNEUROSCI.3289-14.2014.

Ventral Tegmental Area

Corrigall, W. A., Coen, K. M., & Adamson, K. L. (1994). Self-administered nicotine activates the mesolimbic dopamine system through the ventral tegmental area. *Brain Research, 653*(1–2), 278–284. https://doi.org/10.1016/0006-8993(94)90401-4.

Ikemoto, S., Qin, M., & Liu, Z.-H. (2006). Primary reinforcing effects of nicotine are triggered from multiple regions both inside and outside the ventral tegmental area. *Journal of Neuroscience, 26*(3), 723–730. https://doi.org/10.1523/JNEUROSCI.4542-05.2006.

Mao, D., Gallagher, K., & McGehee, D. S. (2011). Nicotine potentiation of excitatory inputs to ventral tegmental area dopamine neurons. *Journal of Neuroscience, 31*(18), 6710–6720. https://doi.org/10.1523/JNEUROSCI.5671-10.2011.

Yeomans, J., & Baptista, M. (1997). Both nicotinic and muscarinic receptors in ventral tegmental area contribute to brain-stimulation reward. *Pharmacology Biochemistry and Behavior, 57*(4), 915–921. https://doi.org/10.1016/S0091-3057(96)00467-4.

The Striatum and Activation

Flannery, J. S., Riedel, M. C., Poudel, R., Laird, A. R., Ross, T. J., Salmeron, B. J., Stein, E. A., & Sutherland, M. T. (2019). Habenular and striatal activity during performance feedback are differentially linked with state-like and trait-like aspects of tobacco use disorder. *Science Advances, 5*(10), eaax2084. https://doi.org/10.1126/sciadv.aax2084.

Fung, Y. K., & Lau, Y.-S. (1989). Effects of prenatal nicotine exposure on rat striatal dopaminergic and nicotinic systems. *Pharmacology Biochemistry and Behavior, 33*(1), 1–6. https://doi.org/10.1016/0091-3057(89)90419-X.

Giorguieff-Chesselet, M. F., Kemel, M. L., Wandscheer, D., & Glowinski, J. (1979). Regulation of dopamine release by presynaptic nicotinic receptors in rat striatal slices: Effect of nicotine in a low concentration. *Life Sciences, 25*(14), 1257–1261. https://doi.org/10.1016/0024-3205(79)90469-7.

214   Bibliography

Hopkins, P. M. (2006). Chapter 35—Voluntary motor systems: Skeletal muscle, reflexes, and control of movement. In H. C. Hemmings & P. M. Hopkins (Eds.), *Foundations of anesthesia* (2nd ed., pp. 421–433). Mosby. https://doi.org/10.1016/B978-0-323-03707-5.50041-3.

Rice, M. E., & Cragg, S. J. (2004). Nicotine amplifies reward-related dopamine signals in striatum. *Nature Neuroscience, 7*(6), 583–584. https://doi.org/10.1038/nn1244.

Schott, B. H., Minuzzi, L., Krebs, R. M., Elmenhorst, D., Lang, M., Winz, O. H., Seidenbecher, C. I., Coenen, H. H., Heinze, H.-J., Zilles, K., Düzel, E., & Bauer, A. (2008). Mesolimbic functional magnetic resonance imaging activations during reward anticipation correlate with reward-related ventral striatal dopamine release. *Journal of Neuroscience, 28*(52), 14311–14319. https://doi.org/10.1523/JNEUROSCI.2058-08.2008.

Nucleus Accumbens and Negative Prediction Error Signaling

Baldwin, P. R., Alanis, R., & Salas, R. (2011). The role of the habenula in nicotine addiction. *Journal of Addiction Research & Therapy, Suppl. 1*(2). https://doi.org/10.4172/2155-6105.S1-002.

Beyeler, A., Eckhardt, C. A., & Tye, K. M. (2014). Chapter 12—Deciphering memory function with optogenetics. In Z. U. Khan & E. C. Muly (Eds.), *Progress in molecular biology and translational science* (Vol. 122, pp. 341–390). Academic Press. https://doi.org/10.1016/B978-0-12-420170-5.00012-X.

Cadoni, C., Muto, T., & Di Chiara, G. (2009). Nicotine differentially affects dopamine transmission in the nucleus accumbens shell and core of Lewis and Fischer 344 rats. *Neuropharmacology, 57*(5–6), 496–501. https://doi.org/10.1016/j.neuropharm.2009.07.033.

Deperrois, N., & Gutkin, B. (2018). Nicotinic and cholinergic modulation of reward prediction error computations in the ventral tegmental area: A minimal circuit model. *BioRxiv,* 423806. https://doi.org/10.1101/423806

Gould, T. J., & Davis, J. A. (2008). Associative learning, the hippocampus, and nicotine addiction. *Current Drug Abuse Reviews, 1*(1), 9–19.

Hanlon, C. A., Dowdle, L. T., & Jones, J. L. (2016). Chapter 6—Biomarkers for success: Using neuroimaging to predict relapse and develop brain stimulation treatments for cocaine-dependent individuals. In N. M. Zahr & E. T. Peterson (Eds.), *International review of* neurobiology (Vol. 129, pp. 125–156). Academic Press. https://doi.org/10.1016/bs.irn.2016.06.006.

Nisell, M., Marcus, M., Nomikos, G. G., & Svensson, T. H. (1997). Differential effects of acute and chronic nicotine on dopamine output in the core and shell of the rat nucleus accumbens. *Journal of Neural Transmission, 104*(1), 1–10. https://doi.org/10.1007/BF01271290.

Rebec, G. V., Grabner, C. P., Johnson, M., Pierce, R. C., & Bardo, M. T. (1996). Transient increases in catecholaminergic activity in medial prefrontal cortex and nucleus accumbens shell during novelty. *Neuroscience, 76*(3), 707–714. https://doi.org/10.1016/S0306-4522(96)00382-X.

Schultz, W. (2016). Dopamine reward prediction error coding. *Dialogues in Clinical Neuroscience, 18*(1), 23–32.

Amygdala and Hippocampus

Ferry, B., Roozendaal, B., & McGaugh, J. L. (1999). Role of norepinephrine in mediating stress hormone regulation of long-term memory storage: A critical involvement of the amygdala. *Biological Psychiatry, 46*(9), 1140–1152. https://doi.org/10.1016/S0006-3223(99)00157-2.

Fu, Y., Matta, S. G., James, T. J., & Sharp, B. M. (1998). Nicotine-induced norepinephrine release in the rat amygdala and hippocampus is mediated through brainstem nicotinic cholinergic receptors. *Journal of Pharmacology and Experimental Therapeutics, 284*(3), 1188–1196.

Isaacson, R. L. (2004). Hippocampus. In L. R. Squire (Ed.), *Encyclopedia of neuroscience* (pp. 1119–1127). Academic Press. https://doi.org/10.1016/B978-008045046-9.02026-X.

Jones, S., Hyde, A., & Davidson, T. L. (2020). Reframing appetitive reinforcement learning and reward valuation as effects mediated by hippocampal-dependent behavioral inhibition. *Nutrition Research, 79*, 1–12. https://doi.org/10.1016/j.nutres.2020.05.001.

Kenney, J. W., & Gould, T. J. (2008). Modulation of hippocampus-dependent learning and synaptic plasticity by nicotine. *Molecular Neurobiology, 38*(1), 101–121. https://doi.org/10.1007/s12035-008-8037-9.

McDonald, A. J. (2014). Amygdala. In M. J. Aminoff & R. B. Daroff (Eds.), *Encyclopedia of the neurological sciences* (2nd ed., pp. 153–156). Academic Press. https://doi.org/10.1016/B978-0-12-385157-4.01113-1.

Olucha-Bordonau, F. E., Fortes-Marco, L., Otero-García, M., Lanuza, E., & Martínez-García, F. (2015). Chapter 18—Amygdala: Structure and function. In G. Paxinos (Ed.), *The rat nervous system* (4th ed., pp. 441–490). Academic Press. https://doi.org/10.1016/B978-0-12-374245-2.00018-8.

Quirarte, G. L., Galvez, R., Roozendaal, B., & McGaugh, J. L. (1998). Norepinephrine release in the amygdala in response to footshock and opioid peptidergic drugs. *Brain Research, 808*(2), 134–140. https://doi.org/10.1016/S0006-8993(98)00795-1.

Tully, K., Li, Y., Tsvetkov, E., & Bolshakov, V. Y. (2007). Norepinephrine enables the induction of associative long-term potentiation at thalamo-amygdala synapses. *Proceedings of the National Academy of Sciences, 104*(35), 14146–14150. https://doi.org/10.1073/pnas.0704621104.

Zeki, S., Kandel, E. R., & Pittenger, C. (1999). The past, the future and the biology of memory storage. *Philosophical Transactions of the Royal Society of London. Series B: Biological Sciences, 354*(1392), 2027–2052. https://doi.org/10.1098/rstb.1999.0542.

Pre-frontal and Fronto-orbital Cortex

Lucantonio, F., Stalnaker, T. A., Shaham, Y., Niv, Y., & Schoenbaum, G. (2012). The impact of orbitofrontal dysfunction on cocaine addiction. *Nature Neuroscience, 15*(3), 358–366. https://doi.org/10.1038/nn.3014.

Mansvelder, H., & Goriounova, N. (2012). Nicotine exposure during adolescence alters the rules for prefrontal cortical synaptic plasticity during adulthood. *Frontiers in Synaptic Neuroscience, 4*. https://doi.org/10.3389/fnsyn.2012.00003.

Mashhoon, Y., Betts, J., Farmer, S. L., & Lukas, S. E. (2018). Early onset tobacco cigarette smokers exhibit deficits in response inhibition and sustained attention. *Drug and Alcohol Dependence, 184*, 48–56. https://doi.org/10.1016/j.drugalcdep.2017.11.020.

Pelchat, M. L. (2002). Of human bondage: Food craving, obsession, compulsion, and addiction. *Physiology & Behavior, 76*(3), 347–352. https://doi.org/10.1016/S0031-9384(02)00757-6.

Schoenbaum, G., Roesch, M. R., & Stalnaker, T. A. (2006). Orbitofrontal cortex, decision-making and drug addiction. *Trends in Neurosciences, 29*(2), 116–124. https://doi.org/10.1016/j.tins.2005.12.006.

Schoenbaum, G., & Shaham, Y. (2008). The role of orbitofrontal cortex in drug addiction: A review of preclinical studies. *Biological Psychiatry, 63*(3), 256–262. https://doi.org/10.1016/j.biopsych.2007.06.003.

Spinella, M. (2002). Correlations between orbitofrontal dysfunction and tobacco smoking. *Addiction Biology, 7*(4), 381–384. https://doi.org/10.1080/1355621021000005964.

Spinella, M. (2003). Relationship between drug use and prefrontal-associated traits. *Addiction Biology, 8*(1), 67–74. https://doi.org/10.1080/1355621031000069909.

Spinella, M. (2004). Neurobehavioral correlates of impulsivity: Evidence of prefrontal involvement. *International Journal of Neuroscience, 114*(1), 95–104. https://doi.org/10.1080/00207450490249347.

Torregrossa, M. M., Quinn, J. J., & Taylor, J. R. (2008). Impulsivity, compulsivity, and habit: The role of orbitofrontal cortex revisited. *Biological Psychiatry, 63*(3), 253–255. https://doi.org/10.1016/j.biopsych.2007.11.014.

Chapter 3. Function

Cholinergic Receptors

Cole, R. D., Poole, R. L., Guzman, D. M., Gould, T. J., & Parikh, V. (2015). Contributions of β2 subunit-containing nAChRs to chronic nicotine-induced alterations in cognitive flexibility in mice. *Psychopharmacology, 232*(7), 1207–1217. https://doi.org/10.1007/s00213-014-3754-4.

de Kloet, S. F., Mansvelder, H. D., & De Vries, T. J. (2015). Cholinergic modulation of dopamine pathways through nicotinic acetylcholine receptors. *Biochemical Pharmacology, 97*(4), 425–438. https://doi.org/10.1016/j.bcp.2015.07.014.

Drenan, R. M., Grady, S. R., Whiteaker, P., McClure-Begley, T., McKinney, S., Miwa, J. M., Bupp, S., Heintz, N., McIntosh, J. M., Bencherif, M., Marks, M. J., & Lester, H. A. (2008). In vivo activation of midbrain dopamine neurons via sensitized, high-affinity α6* nicotinic acetylcholine receptors. *Neuron, 60*(1), 123–136. https://doi.org/10.1016/j.neuron.2008.09.009.

Exley, R., & Cragg, S. J. (2008). Presynaptic nicotinic receptors: A dynamic and diverse cholinergic filter of striatal dopamine neurotransmission. *British Journal of Pharmacology, 153*(Suppl. 1), S283–S297. https://doi.org/10.1038/sj.bjp.0707510.

Greenbaum, L., & Lerer, B. (2009). Differential contribution of genetic variation in multiple brain nicotinic cholinergic receptors to nicotine dependence: Recent progress and emerging open questions. *Molecular Psychiatry, 14*(10), 912–945. https://doi. org/10.1038/mp.2009.59.

Ksir, C., Hakan, R., Hall, D. P., & Kellar, K. J. (1985). Exposure to nicotine enhances the behavioral stimulant effect of nicotine and increases binding of [3H]acetyl-choline to nicotinic receptors. *Neuropharmacology, 24*(6), 527–531. https://doi. org/10.1016/0028-3908(85)90058-9.

McKay, B. E., Placzek, A. N., & Dani, J. A. (2007). Regulation of synaptic transmission and plasticity by neuronal nicotinic acetylcholine receptors. *Biochemical Pharmacology, 74*(8), 1120–1133. https://doi.org/10.1016/j.bcp.2007.07.001.

Perry, E., Smith, C., Perry, R., Whitford, C., Johnson, M., & Birdsall, N. (1989). Regional distribution of muscarinic and nicotinic cholinergic receptor binding activities in the human brain. *Journal of Chemical Neuroanatomy, 2*(4), 189–199.

Trauth, J. A., Seidler, F. J., McCook, E. C., & Slotkin, T. A. (1999). Adolescent nicotine exposure causes persistent upregulation of nicotinic cholinergic receptors in rat brain regions. *Brain Research, 851*(1), 9–19. https://doi.org/10.1016/S0006-8993(99)01994-0.

Yanai, J., Pick, C. G., Rogel-Fuchs, Y., & Zahalka, E. A. (1992). Alterations in hippocampal cholinergic receptors and hippocampal behaviors after early exposure to nicotine. *Brain Research Bulletin, 29*(3), 363–368. https://doi.org/10.1016/0361-9230(92)90069-A.

Zhou, F.-M., Liang, Y., & Dani, J. A. (2001). Endogenous nicotinic cholinergic activity regulates dopamine release in the striatum. *Nature Neuroscience, 4*(12), 1224–1229. https://doi.org/10.1038/nn769.

Role of Dopamine in Reinforcement

Le Foll, B., Wertheim, C., & Goldberg, S. R. (2007). High reinforcing efficacy of nicotine in non-human primates. *PLOS One, 2*(2), e230. https://doi.org/10.1371/journal. pone.0000230.

Mansvelder, H. D., & McGehee, D. S. (2000). Long-term potentiation of excitatory inputs to brain reward areas by nicotine. *Neuron, 27*(2), 349–357. https://doi. org/10.1016/S0896-6273(00)00042-8.

Olds, J., & Milner, P. (1954). Positive reinforcement produced by electrical stimulation of septal area and other regions of rat brain. *Journal of Comparative and Physiological Psychology, 47*(6), 419–427. https://doi.org/10.1037/h0058775.

Rice, M. E., & Cragg, S. J. (2004). Nicotine amplifies reward-related dopamine signals in striatum. *Nature Neuroscience, 7*(6), 583–584. https://doi.org/10.1038/nn1244.

Subramaniyan, M., & Dani, J. A. (2015). Dopaminergic and cholinergic learning mechanisms in nicotine addiction. *Annals of the New York Academy of Sciences, 1349*, 46–63. https://doi.org/10.1111/nyas.12871.

Wightman, R. M., & Robinson, D. L. (2002). Transient changes in mesolimbic dopamine and their association with "reward." *Journal of Neurochemistry, 82*(4), 721–735. https://doi.org/10.1046/j.1471-4159.2002.01005.x.

Zhang, H., & Sulzer, D. (2004). Frequency-dependent modulation of dopamine release by nicotine. *Nature Neuroscience, 7*(6), 581–582. https://doi.org/10.1038/nn1243.

ΔFosB and CREB

Brunzell, D. H., Mineur, Y. S., Neve, R. L., & Picciotto, M. R. (2009). Nucleus accumbens CREB activity is necessary for nicotine conditioned place preference. *Neuropsychopharmacology, 34*(8), 1993–2001. https://doi.org/10.1038/npp.2009.11.

Eagle, A. L., Gajewski, P. A., Yang, M., Kechner, M. E., Masraf, B. S. A., Kennedy, P. J., Wang, H., Mazei-Robison, M. S., & Robison, A. J. (2015). Experience-dependent induction of hippocampal ΔFosB controls learning. *Journal of Neuroscience, 35*(40), 13773–13783. https://doi.org/10.1523/JNEUROSCI.2083-15.2015.

Gonzalez-Nunez, V., & Rodríguez, R. E. (2017). Chapter 12—Cocaine and transcription factors. In V. R. Preedy (Ed.), *The neuroscience of cocaine* (pp. 107–124). Academic Press. https://doi.org/10.1016/B978-0-12-803750-8.00012-9.

Grueter, B. A., Robison, A. J., Neve, R. L., Nestler, E. J., & Malenka, R. C. (2013). ΔFosB differentially modulates nucleus accumbens direct and indirect pathway function. *Proceedings of the National Academy of Sciences, 110*(5), 1923–1928. https://doi.org/10.1073/pnas.1221742110.

Isola, R., Zhang, H., Tejwani, G. A., Neff, N. H., & Hadjiconstantinou, M. (2008). Dynorphin and prodynorphin mRNA changes in the striatum during nicotine withdrawal. *Synapse, 62*(6), 448–455. https://doi.org/10.1002/syn.20515.

Kaste, K. (2009). Transcription factors ΔFosB and CREB in drug addiction: Studies in models of alcohol preference and chronic nicotine exposure. [Doctoral dissertation, University of Helsinki, Finland]. https://helda.helsinki.fi/handle/10138/19112.

Leshner, A. I. (1997). Addiction is a brain disease, and it matters. *Science, 278*(5335), 45–47. https://doi.org/10.1126/science.278.5335.45.

Marttila, K., Raattamaa, H., & Ahtee, L. (2006). Effects of chronic nicotine administration and its withdrawal on striatal FosB/ΔFosB and c-Fos expression in rats and mice. *Neuropharmacology, 51*(1), 44–51. https://doi.org/10.1016/j.neuropharm.2006.02.014.

Nestler, E. J., & Aghajanian, G. K. (1997). Molecular and cellular basis of addiction. *Science, 278*(5335), 58–63. https://doi.org/10.1126/science.278.5335.58.

Nestler, E. J., Barrot, M., & Self, D. W. (2001). ΔFosB: A sustained molecular switch for addiction. *Proceedings of the National Academy of Sciences, 98*(20), 11042–11046. https://doi.org/10.1073/pnas.191352698.

Pagliusi, S. R., Tessari, M., DeVevey, S., Chiamulera, C., & Pich, E. M. (1996). The reinforcing properties of nicotine are associated with a specific patterning of c-fos expression in the rat brain. *European Journal of Neuroscience, 8*(11), 2247–2256. https://doi.org/10.1111/j.1460-9568.1996.tb01188.x.

Picciotto, M. R., & Kenny, P. J. (2013). Molecular mechanisms underlying behaviors related to nicotine addiction. *Cold Spring Harbor Perspectives in Medicine, 3*(1), a012112. https://doi.org/10.1101/cshperspect.a012112.

Ruffle, J. K. (2014). Molecular neurobiology of addiction: What's all the (Δ)FosB about? *American Journal of Drug and Alcohol Abuse, 40*(6), 428–437. https://doi.org/10.3109/00952990.2014.933840.

Singh, T. G., Sharma, S., & Dhiman, S. (2016). Chapter 19—Neurotransmitter systems and the nicotine dependence-induced withdrawal syndrome: Dopamine, glutamate, GABA, endogenous opioids, endocannabinoids, noradrenaline, arginine vasopressin, neuropeptide Y, MAO, CREB, and corticotropin-releasing factor. In V. R. Preedy (Ed.), *Neuropathology of drug addictions and substance misuse* (pp.

201–208). Academic Press. https://doi.org/10.1016/B978-0-12-800213-1.00019-5.

Soderstrom, K., Qin, W., Williams, H., Taylor, D. A., & McMillen, B. A. (2007). Nicotine increases FosB expression within a subset of reward- and memory-related brain regions during both peri- and post-adolescence. *Psychopharmacology, 191*(4), 891–897. https://doi.org/10.1007/s00213-007-0744-9.

Conditioned Place Preference

Belluzzi, J. D., Lee, A. G., Oliff, H. S., & Leslie, F. M. (2004). Age-dependent effects of nicotine on locomotor activity and conditioned place preference in rats. *Psychopharmacology, 174*(3), 389–395. https://doi.org/10.1007/s00213-003-1758-6.

Le Foll, B., & Goldberg, S. R. (2005). Nicotine induces conditioned place preferences over a large range of doses in rats. *Psychopharmacology, 178*(4), 481–492. https://doi.org/10.1007/s00213-004-2021-5.

Pascual, M. M., Pastor, V., & Bernabeu, R. O. (2009). Nicotine-conditioned place preference induced CREB phosphorylation and Fos expression in the adult rat brain. *Psychopharmacology, 207*(1), 57–71. https://doi.org/10.1007/s00213-009-1630-4.

Prus, A. J., James, J. R., & Rosecrans, J. A. (2009). Conditioned place preference. In *Methods of behavioral analysis in neuroscience* (2nd ed., pp. 59–76). CRC Press/Routledge/Taylor & Francis Group.

Risinger, F. O., & Oakes, R. A. (1995). Nicotine-induced conditioned place preference and conditioned place aversion in mice. *Pharmacology Biochemistry and Behavior, 51*(2), 457–461. https://doi.org/10.1016/0091-3057(95)00007-J.

Smith, J. S., Schindler, A. G., Martinelli, E., Gustin, R. M., Bruchas, M. R., & Chavkin, C. (2012). Stress-induced activation of the dynorphin/κ-opioid receptor system in the amygdala potentiates nicotine conditioned place preference. *Journal of Neuroscience, 32*(4), 1488–1495. https://doi.org/10.1523/JNEUROSCI.2980-11.2012.

Spina, L., Fenu, S., Longoni, R., Rivas, E., & Di Chiara, G. (2006). Nicotine-conditioned single-trial place preference: Selective role of nucleus accumbens shell dopamine D1 receptors in acquisition. *Psychopharmacology, 184*(3), 447–455. https://doi.org/10.1007/s00213-005-0211-4.

Vastola, B. J., Douglas, L. A., Varlinskaya, E. I., & Spear, L. P. (2002). Nicotine-induced conditioned place preference in adolescent and adult rats. *Physiology & Behavior, 77*(1), 107–114. https://doi.org/10.1016/S0031-9384(02)00818-1.

Walters, C. L., Brown, S., Changeux, J.-P., Martin, B., & Damaj, M. I. (2006). The β2 but not α7 subunit of the nicotinic acetylcholine receptor is required for nicotine-conditioned place preference in mice. *Psychopharmacology, 184*(3), 339–344. https://doi.org/10.1007/s00213-005-0295-x.

Zarrindast, M.-R., Faraji, N., Rostami, P., Sahraei, H., & Ghoshouni, H. (2003). Cross-tolerance between morphine- and nicotine-induced conditioned place preference in mice. *Pharmacology Biochemistry and Behavior, 74*(2), 363–369. https://doi.org/10.1016/S0091-3057(02)01002-X.

Overlap with Other Dependence Syndromes

Cavazos-Rehg, P. A., Breslau, N., Hatsukami, D., Krauss, M. J., Spitznagel, E. L., Grucza, R. A., Salyer, P., Hartz, S. M., & Bierut, L. J. (2014). Smoking cessation is associated with lower rates of mood/anxiety and alcohol use disorders. *Psychological Medicine,*

44(12), 2523–2535. https://doi.org/10.1017/S0033291713003206.

Das, S., Hickman, N. J., & Prochaska, J. J. (2017). Treating smoking in adults with co-occurring acute psychiatric and addictive disorders. *Journal of Addiction Medicine, 11*(4), 273–279. https://doi.org/10.1097/ADM.0000000000000320.

Davenport, K. E., Houdi, A. A., & Van Loon, G. R. (1990). Nicotine protects against μ-opioid receptor antagonism by β-funaltrexamine: Evidence for nicotine-induced release of endogenous opioids in brain. *Neuroscience Letters, 113*(1), 40–46. https://doi.org/10.1016/0304-3940(90)90491-Q.

de Castro-Neto, A. G., Rameh-de-Albuquerque, R. C., de Medeiros, P. F. P., Uchôa, R., & Santos, B. S. (2019). Chapter 49—Neuroscience of tobacco and crack cocaine use: Metabolism, effects, and symptomatology. In V. R. Preedy (Ed.), *Neuroscience of nicotine* (pp. 403–410). Academic Press. https://doi.org/10.1016/B978-0-12-813035-3.00049-6.

Deal, H., Newcombe, D. A. L., Walker, N., & Galea, S. (2014). Smoking cessation in a community alcohol and drug service: Acceptability and feasibility. *Addictive Disorders & Their Treatment, 13*(4), 199. https://doi.org/10.1097/ADT.0000000000000037.

Dobscha, S. K., Morasco, B. J., Duckart, J. P., Macey, T., & Deyo, R. A. (2013). Correlates of prescription opioid initiation and long-term opioid use in veterans with persistent pain. *Clinical Journal of Pain, 29*(2), 102–108. https://doi.org/10.1097/AJP.0b013e3182490bdb.

Epstein, D. H., Marrone, G. F., Heishman, S. J., Schmittner, J., & Preston, K. L. (2010). Tobacco, cocaine, and heroin: Craving and use during daily life. *Addictive Behaviors, 35*(4), 318–324. https://doi.org/10.1016/j.addbeh.2009.11.003.

Fallin, A., Miller, A., & Ashford, K. (2016). Smoking among pregnant women in outpatient treatment for opioid dependence: A qualitative inquiry. *Nicotine & Tobacco Research, 18*(8), 1727–1732. https://doi.org/10.1093/ntr/ntw023.

Feduccia, A. A., Chatterjee, S., & Bartlett, S. E. (2012). Neuronal nicotinic acetylcholine receptors: Neuroplastic changes underlying alcohol and nicotine addictions. *Frontiers in Molecular Neuroscience, 5*, 83. https://doi.org/10.3389/fnmol.2012.00083.

Gajewski, P. A., Turecki, G., & Robison, A. J. (2016). Differential expression of FosB proteins and potential target genes in select brain regions of addiction and depression patients. *PLOS One, 11*(8), e0160355. https://doi.org/10.1371/journal.pone.0160355.

Gatch, M. B., Flores, E., & Forster, M. J. (2008). Nicotine and methamphetamine share discriminative stimulus effects. *Drug and Alcohol Dependence, 93*(1–2), 63–71. https://doi.org/10.1016/j.drugalcdep.2007.08.020.

Hadjiconstantinou, M., & Neff, N. H. (2011). Nicotine and endogenous opioids: Neurochemical and pharmacological evidence. *Neuropharmacology, 60*(7–8), 1209–1220. https://doi.org/10.1016/j.neuropharm.2010.11.010.

Harvey, D. M., Yasar, S., Heishman, S. J., Panlilio, L. V., Henningfield, J. E., & Goldberg, S. R. (2004). Nicotine serves as an effective reinforcer of intravenous drug-taking behavior in human cigarette smokers. *Psychopharmacology, 175*(2), 134–142. https://doi.org/10.1007/s00213-004-1818-6.

Henningfield, J. E., Clayton, R., & Pollin, W. (1990). Involvement of tobacco in alcoholism and illicit drug use. *British Journal of Addiction, 85*(2), 279–292. https://doi.org/10.1111/j.1360-0443.1990.tb03084.x.

Hooten, W. M., Townsend, C. O., Bruce, B. K., & Warner, D. O. (2009). The effects of smoking status on opioid tapering among patients with chronic pain. *Anesthesia & Analgesia, 108*(1), 308–315. https://doi.org/10.1213/ane.0b013e31818c7b99.

Hooten, W. M., & Warner, D. O. (2015). Varenicline for opioid withdrawal in patients with chronic pain: A randomized, single-blinded, placebo-controlled pilot trial. *Addictive Behaviors, 42*, 69–72. https://doi.org/10.1016/j.addbeh.2014.11.007.

Hopf, F. W., Stuber, G. D., Chen, B. T., & Bonci, A. (2010). Cellular plasticity in cocaine and alcohol addiction. In G. F. Koob, M. L. Moal, & R. F. Thompson (Eds.), *Encyclopedia of behavioral neuroscience* (pp. 236–241). Academic Press. https://doi.org/10.1016/B978-0-08-045396-5.00071-3.

Kandel, E. R., & Kandel, D. B. (2014). A molecular basis for nicotine as a gateway drug. *New England Journal of Medicine, 371*(10), 932–943. https://doi.org/10.1056/NEJMsa1405092.

Kenny, P. J. (2011). Common cellular and molecular mechanisms in obesity and drug addiction. *Nature Reviews Neuroscience, 12*(11), 638–651. https://doi.org/10.1038/nrn3105.

Levine, A., Huang, Y., Drisaldi, B., Griffin, E. A., Pollak, D. D., Xu, S., Yin, D., Schaffran, C., Kandel, D. B., & Kandel, E. R. (2011). Molecular mechanism for a gateway drug: Epigenetic changes initiated by nicotine prime gene expression by cocaine. *Science Translational Medicine, 3*(107), 107ra109. https://doi.org/10.1126/scitranslmed.3003062.

Loney, G. C., Angelyn, H., Cleary, L. M., & Meyer, P. J. (2019). Nicotine produces a high-approach, low-avoidance phenotype in response to alcohol-associated cues in male rats. *Alcoholism, Clinical and Experimental Research, 43*(6), 1284–1295. https://doi.org/10.1111/acer.14043.

Morasco, B. J., Duckart, J. P., Carr, T. P., Deyo, R. A., & Dobscha, S. K. (2010). Clinical characteristics of veterans prescribed high doses of opioid medications for chronic non-cancer pain. *PAIN®, 151*(3), 625–632. https://doi.org/10.1016/j.pain.2010.08.002.

Niehaus, J. L., Cruz-Bermudez, N. D., & Kauer, J. A. (2009). Plasticity of addiction: A mesolimbic dopamine short-circuit? *American Journal on Addictions, 18*(4), 259–271. https://doi.org/10.1080/10550490902925946.

Ostroumov, A., & Dani, J. A. (2018). Convergent neuronal plasticity and metaplasticity mechanisms of stress, nicotine, and alcohol. *Annual Review of Pharmacology and Toxicology, 58*(1), 547–566. https://doi.org/10.1146/annurev-pharmtox-010617-052735.

Powers, M. S., Broderick, H. J., Drenan, R. M., & Chester, J. A. (2013). Nicotinic acetylcholine receptors containing α6 subunits contribute to alcohol reward-related behaviours. *Genes, Brain and Behavior, 12*(5), 543–553. https://doi.org/10.1111/gbb.12042.

Prochaska, J. J., Delucchi, K., & Hall, S. M. (2004). A meta-analysis of smoking cessation interventions with individuals in substance abuse treatment or recovery. *Journal of Consulting and Clinical Psychology, 72*(6), 1144–1156. https://doi.org/10.1037/0022-006X.72.6.1144.

Randall, P. A., Fortino, B., Huynh, Y. W., Thompson, B. M., Larsen, C. E., Callen, M. P., Barrett, S. T., Murray, J. E., Bevins, R. A., & Besheer, J. (2019). Effects of nicotine conditioning history on alcohol and methamphetamine self-administration in rats. *Pharmacology, Biochemistry, and Behavior, 179*, 1–8. https://doi.org/10.1016/j.pbb.2019.01.005.

Roberts, W., Harrison, E. L. R., & McKee, S. A. (2017). Effects of varenicline on alcohol cue reactivity in heavy drinkers. *Psychopharmacology, 234*, 2737–2745. https://doi.org/10.1007/s00213-017-4667-9.

Tomasi, D., & Volkow, N. D. (2013). Striatocortical pathway dysfunction in addiction and obesity: Differences and similarities. *Critical Reviews in Biochemistry and Molecular Biology, 48*(1), 1–19. https://doi.org/10.3109/10409238.2012.735642.

Volkow, N. D., Wang, G.-J., Fowler, J. S., & Telang, F. (2008). Overlapping neuronal circuits in addiction and obesity: Evidence of systems pathology. *Philosophical Transactions of the Royal Society B: Biological Sciences, 363*(1507), 3191–3200. https://doi.org/10.1098/rstb.2008.0107.

Chapter 4. Compulsion

Impulsivity

Cardinal, R. N., Pennicott, D. R., Lakmali, C., Sugathapala, Robbins, T. W., & Everitt, B. J. (2001). Impulsive choice induced in rats by lesions of the nucleus accumbens core. *Science, 292*(5526), 2499–2501. https://doi.org/10.1126/science.1060818.

Counotte, D. S., Goriounova, N. A., Li, K. W., Loos, M., van der Schors, R. C., Schetters, D., Schoffelmeer, A. N. M., Smit, A. B., Mansvelder, H. D., Pattij, T., & Spijker, S. (2011). Lasting synaptic changes underlie attention deficits caused by nicotine exposure during adolescence. *Nature Neuroscience, 14*(4), 417–419. https://doi.org/10.1038/nn.2770.

Dallery, J., & Locey, M. L. (2005). Effects of acute and chronic nicotine on impulsive choice in rats. *Behavioural Pharmacology, 16*(1), 15–23.

Dalley, J. W., Mar, A. C., Economidou, D., & Robbins, T. W. (2008). Neurobehavioral mechanisms of impulsivity: Fronto-striatal systems and functional neurochemistry. *Pharmacology Biochemistry and Behavior, 90*(2), 250–260. https://doi.org/10.1016/j.pbb.2007.12.021.

Economidou, D., Theobald, D. E., Robbins, T. W., Everitt, B. J., & Dalley, J. W. (2012). Norepinephrine and dopamine modulate impulsivity on the five-choice serial reaction time task through opponent actions in the shell and core sub-regions of the nucleus accumbens. *Neuropsychopharmacology, 37*(9), 2057–2066. https://doi.org/10.1038/npp.2012.53.

Fernando, A. B. P., Economidou, D., Theobald, D. E., Zou, M.-F., Newman, A. H., Spoelder, M., Caprioli, D., Moreno, M., Hipólito, L., Aspinall, A. T., Robbins, T. W., & Dalley, J. W. (2012). Modulation of high impulsivity and attentional performance in rats by selective direct and indirect dopaminergic and noradrenergic receptor agonists. *Psychopharmacology, 219*(2), 341–352. https://doi.org/10.1007/s00213-011-2408-z.

Galtress, T. (2010). The role of the nucleus accumbens core in impulsive choice, timing, and reward processing. *Behavioral Neuroscience, 124*(1), 26–43. https://doi.org/10.1037/a0018464.

Kayir, H., Semenova, S., & Markou, A. (2014). Baseline impulsive choice predicts the effects of nicotine and nicotine withdrawal on impulsivity in rats. *Progress in Neuro-Psychopharmacology and Biological Psychiatry, 48,* 6–13. https://doi.org/10.1016/j.pnpbp.2013.09.007.

Kim, S., & Lee, D. (2011). Prefrontal cortex and impulsive decision making. *Biological Psychiatry, 69*(12), 1140–1146. https://doi.org/10.1016/j.biopsych.2010.07.005.

Kolokotroni, K. Z., Rodgers, R. J., & Harrison, A. A. (2011). Acute nicotine increases both impulsive choice and behavioural disinhibition in rats. *Psychopharmacology, 217*(4), 455–473. https://doi.org/10.1007/s00213-011-2296-2.

Locey, M. L., & Dallery, J. (2009). Isolating behavioral mechanisms of intertemporal choice: Nicotine effect on delay discounting and amount sensitivity. *Journal of the Experimental Analysis of Behavior, 91*(2), 213–223. https://doi.org/10.1901/jeab.2009.91-213.

Loree, A. M., Lundahl, L. H., & Ledgerwood, D. M. (2015). Impulsivity as a predictor of treatment outcome in substance use disorders: Review and synthesis. *Drug and Alcohol Review, 34*(2), 119–134. https://doi.org/10.1111/dar.12132.

Markou, A., Chiamulera, C. V., & West, R. J. (2008). Chapter 6—Contribution of animal models and preclinical human studies to medication development for nicotine dependence. In R. A. McArthur & F. Borsini (Eds.), *Animal and translational models for CNS drug discovery* (pp. 179–219). Academic Press. https://doi.org/10.1016/B978-0-12-373861-5.00026-6.

Pariyadath, V., Gowin, J. L., & Stein, E. A. (2016). Chapter 8—Resting state functional connectivity analysis for addiction medicine: From individual loci to complex networks. In H. Ekhtiari & M. P. Paulus (Eds.), *Progress in brain research* (Vol. 224, pp. 155–173). Elsevier. https://doi.org/10.1016/bs.pbr.2015.07.015.

Pezze, M.-A., Dalley, J. W., & Robbins, T. W. (2007). Differential roles of dopamine D1 and D2 receptors in the nucleus accumbens in attentional performance on the five-choice serial reaction time task. *Neuropsychopharmacology, 32*(2), 273–283. https://doi.org/10.1038/sj.npp.1301073.

Robbins, T. (2002). The 5-choice serial reaction time task: Behavioural pharmacology and functional neurochemistry. *Psychopharmacology, 163*(3), 362–380. https://doi.org/10.1007/s00213-002-1154-7.

Robbins, T. W. (2005). Chemistry of the mind: Neurochemical modulation of prefrontal cortical function. *Journal of Comparative Neurology, 493*(1), 140–146. https://doi.org/10.1002/cne.20717.

Rukstalis, M., Jepson, C., Patterson, F., & Lerman, C. (2005). Increases in hyperactive–impulsive symptoms predict relapse among smokers in nicotine replacement therapy. *Journal of Substance Abuse Treatment, 28*(4), 297–304. https://doi.org/10.1016/j.jsat.2005.02.002.

Spinella, M. (2005). Compulsive behavior in tobacco users. *Addictive Behaviors, 30*(1), 183–186. https://doi.org/10.1016/j.addbeh.2004.04.011.

Allostasis and Stress

Ashare, R. L., Lerman, C., Cao, W., Falcone, M., Bernardo, L., Ruparel, K., Hopson, R., Gur, R., Pruessner, J. C., & Loughead, J. (2016). Nicotine withdrawal alters neural responses to psychosocial stress. *Psychopharmacology, 233*(13), 2459–2467. https://doi.org/10.1007/s00213-016-4299-5.

Berntson, G. G., Cacioppo, J. T., & Bosch, J. A. (2017). From homeostasis to allodynamic regulation. In *Handbook of psychophysiology* (4th ed., pp. 401–426). Cambridge University Press.

Doncheck, E. M., & Mantsch, J. R. (2019). Chapter 11—Role of stress-associated signaling in addiction. In M. Torregrossa (Ed.), *Neural mechanisms of addiction* (pp. 157–178). Academic Press. https://doi.org/10.1016/B978-0-12-812202-0.00011-7.

Flandreau, E. I., Ressler, K. J., Owens, M. J., & Nemeroff, C. B. (2012). Chronic overexpression of corticotropin-releasing factor from the central amygdala produces HPA axis hyperactivity and behavioral anxiety associated with gene-expression changes in the hippocampus and paraventricular nucleus of the hypothalamus. *Psychoneuroendocrinology, 37*(1), 27–38. https://doi.org/10.1016/j.psyneuen.2011.04.014.

George, O., Le Moal, M., & Koob, G. F. (2012). Allostasis and addiction: Role of the dopamine and corticotropin-releasing factor systems. *Physiology & Behavior, 106*(1), 58–64. https://doi.org/10.1016/j.physbeh.2011.11.004.

Green, M. K., Barbieri, E. V., Brown, B. D., Chen, K.-W., & Devine, D. P. (2007). Roles of the bed nucleus of stria terminalis and of the amygdala in N/OFQ-mediated anxiety and HPA axis activation. *Neuropeptides, 41*(6), 399–410. https://doi.org/10.1016/j.npep.2007.09.002.

Holgate, J. Y., & Bartlett, S. E. (2015). Early life stress, nicotinic acetylcholine receptors and alcohol use disorders. *Brain Sciences, 5*(3), 258–274. https://doi.org/10.3390/brainsci5030258.

Hunter, R. G., Bloss, E. B., McCarthy, K. J., & McEwen, B. S. (2010). Regulation of the nicotinic receptor alpha7 subunit by chronic stress and corticosteroids. *Brain Research, 1325*, 141–146. https://doi.org/10.1016/j.brainres.2010.02.014.

Koob, G. F., & Le Moal, M. (1997). Drug abuse: Hedonic homeostatic dysregulation. *Science, 278*(5335), 52–58. https://doi.org/10.1126/science.278.5335.52.

Koob, G. F., & Le Moal, M. (2008). Addiction and the brain antireward system. *Annual Review of Psychology, 59*(1), 29–53. https://doi.org/10.1146/annurev.psych.59.103006.093548.

Lowell, B. B. (2019). New neuroscience of homeostasis and drives for food, water, and salt. *New England Journal of Medicine, 380*(5), 459–471. https://doi.org/10.1056/NEJMra1812053.

McEwen, B. (2010). Stress: Homeostasis, rheostasis, allostasis and allostatic load. In G. Fink (Ed.), *Stress science: Neuroendocrinology* (pp. 10–14). Oxford: Academic Press.

McEwen, B. S., & Wingfield, J. C. (2007). Allostasis and allostatic load. In G. Fink (Ed.), *Encyclopedia of stress* (2nd ed., pp. 135–141). Academic Press. https://doi.org/10.1016/B978-012373947-6.00025-8.

Sterling, P. (2012). Allostasis: A model of predictive regulation. *Physiology & Behavior, 106*(1), 5–15. https://doi.org/10.1016/j.physbeh.2011.06.004.

Yu, G., Chen, H., Wu, X., Matta, S. G., & Sharp, B. M. (2010). Nicotine self-administration differentially modulates glutamate and GABA transmission in hypothalamic paraventricular nucleus to enhance the hypothalamic–pituitary–adrenal response to stress. *Journal of Neurochemistry, 113*(4), 919–929. https://doi.org/10.1111/j.1471-4159.2010.06654.x.

Yu, G., & Sharp, B. M. (2012). Nicotine modulates multiple regions in the limbic stress network regulating activation of hypophysiotrophic neurons in hypothalamic paraventricular nucleus. *Journal of Neurochemistry, 122*(3), 628–640. https://doi.org/10.1111/j.1471-4159.2012.07785.x.

Anticipatory Anxiety and Mood

Braun, A. R., Heinz, A. J., Veilleux, J. C., Conrad, M., Weber, S., Wardle, M., Greenstein, J., Evatt, D., Drobes, D., & Kassel, J. D. (2012). The separate and combined effects of alcohol and nicotine on anticipatory anxiety: A multidimensional analysis. *Addictive Behaviors, 37*(4), 485–491. https://doi.org/10.1016/j.addbeh.2011.12.013.

DiFranza, J. R., Rigotti, N. A., McNeill, A. D., Ockene, J. K., Savageau, J. A., Cyr, D. S., & Coleman, M. (2000). Initial symptoms of nicotine dependence in adolescents. *Tobacco Control, 9*(3), 313–319. https://doi.org/10.1136/tc.9.3.313.

Hogle, J. M., Kaye, J. T., & Curtin, J. J. (2010). Nicotine withdrawal increases threat-induced anxiety but not fear: Neuroadaptation in human addiction. *Biological Psychiatry, 68*(8), 719–725. https://doi.org/10.1016/j.biopsych.2010.06.003.

Livneh, Y., Sugden, A. U., Madara, J. C., Essner, R. A., Flores, V. I., Sugden, L. A., Resch, J. M., Lowell, B. B., & Andermann, M. L. (2020). Estimation of current and future physiological states in insular cortex. *Neuron, 105*(6), 1094–1111.e10. https://doi.org/10.1016/j.neuron.2019.12.027.

Marshall, E. C., Johnson, K., Bergman, J., Gibson, L. E., & Zvolensky, M. J. (2009). Anxiety sensitivity and panic reactivity to bodily sensations: Relation to quit-day (acute) nicotine withdrawal symptom severity among daily smokers making a self-guided quit attempt. *Experimental and Clinical Psychopharmacology, 17*(5), 356–364. https://doi.org/10.1037/a0016883.

McLeish, A. C., Zvolensky, M. J., & Bucossi, M. M. (2007). Interaction between smoking rate and anxiety sensitivity: Relation to anticipatory anxiety and panic-relevant avoidance among daily smokers. *Journal of Anxiety Disorders, 21*(6), 849–859. https://doi.org/10.1016/j.janxdis.2006.11.003.

Morissette, S. B., Tull, M. T., Gulliver, S. B., Kamholz, B. W., & Zimering, R. T. (2007). Anxiety, anxiety disorders, tobacco use, and nicotine: A critical review of interrelationships. *Psychological Bulletin, 133*(2), 245–272. https://doi.org/10.1037/0033-2909.133.2.245.

Nutt, D., & Malizia, A. (2006). Anxiety and OCD: The chicken or the egg? *Journal of Psychopharmacology, 20*(6), 729–731. https://doi.org/10.1177/0269881106068424.

Picciotto, M. R., Lewis, A. S., van Schalkwyk, G. I., & Mineur, Y. S. (2015). Mood and anxiety regulation by nicotinic acetylcholine receptors: A potential pathway to modulate aggression and related behavioral states. *Neuropharmacology, 96*, 235–243. https://doi.org/10.1016/j.neuropharm.2014.12.028.

Spinella, M. (2005). Mood in relation to subclinical obsessive-compulsive symptoms. *International Journal of Neuroscience, 115*(4), 433–443. https://doi.org/10.1080/00207450590522838.

Zeelenberg, M., van Dijk, W. W., van der Pligt, J., Manstead, A. S. R., van Empelen, P., & Reinderman, D. (1998). Emotional reactions to the outcomes of decisions: The role of counterfactual thought in the experience of regret and disappointment. *Organizational Behavior and Human Decision Processes, 75*(2), 117–141. https://doi.org/10.1006/obhd.1998.2784.

Persistence of Effect

Abreu-Villaça, Y., Seidler, F. J., Qiao, D., Tate, C. A., Cousins, M. M., Thillai, I., & Slotkin, T. A. (2003). Short-term adolescent nicotine exposure has immediate and persistent effects on cholinergic systems: Critical periods, patterns of exposure, dose thresholds. *Neuropsychopharmacology, 28*(11), 1935–1949. https://doi.org/10.1038/sj.npp.1300221.

Berntson, G. G., Cacioppo, J. T., & Bosch, J. A. (2017). From homeostasis to allodynamic regulation. In *Handbook of psychophysiology* (4th ed., pp. 401–426). Cambridge University Press.

Braun, A. R., Heinz, A. J., Veilleux, J. C., Conrad, M., Weber, S., Wardle, M., Greenstein, J., Evatt, D., Drobes, D., & Kassel, J. D. (2012). The separate and combined effects of alcohol and nicotine on anticipatory anxiety: A multidimensional analysis. *Addictive Behaviors, 37*(4), 485–491. https://doi.org/10.1016/j.addbeh.2011.12.013.

Brielmaier, J. M., McDonald, C. G., & Smith, R. F. (2007). Immediate and long-term behavioral effects of a single nicotine injection in adolescent and adult rats. *Neurotoxicology and Teratology, 29*(1), 74–80. https://doi.org/10.1016/j.ntt.2006.09.023.

Cardinal, R. N., Pennicott, D. R., Lakmali, C., Sugathapala, Robbins, T. W., & Everitt, B. J. (2001). Impulsive choice induced in rats by lesions of the nucleus accumbens core. *Science, 292*(5526), 2499–2501. https://doi.org/10.1126/science.1060818.

Counotte, D. S., Goriounova, N. A., Li, K. W., Loos, M., van der Schors, R. C., Schetters, D., Schoffelmeer, A. N. M., Smit, A. B., Mansvelder, H. D., Pattij, T., & Spijker, S. (2011). Lasting synaptic changes underlie attention deficits caused by nicotine exposure during adolescence. *Nature Neuroscience, 14*(4), 417–419. https://doi.org/10.1038/nn.2770.

Dallery, J., & Locey, M. L. (2005). Effects of acute and chronic nicotine on impulsive choice in rats. *Behavioural Pharmacology, 16*(1), 15–23.

Dalley, J. W., Mar, A. C., Economidou, D., & Robbins, T. W. (2008). Neurobehavioral mechanisms of impulsivity: Fronto-striatal systems and functional neurochemistry. *Pharmacology Biochemistry and Behavior, 90*(2), 250–260. https://doi.org/10.1016/j.pbb.2007.12.021.

DiFranza, J. R., Rigotti, N. A., McNeill, A. D., Ockene, J. K., Savageau, J. A., Cyr, D. S., & Coleman, M. (2000). Initial symptoms of nicotine dependence in adolescents. *Tobacco Control, 9*(3), 313–319. https://doi.org/10.1136/tc.9.3.313.

Doncheck, E. M., & Mantsch, J. R. (2019). Chapter 11—Role of stress-associated signaling in addiction. In M. Torregrossa (Ed.), *Neural mechanisms of addiction* (pp. 157–178). Academic Press. https://doi.org/10.1016/B978-0-12-812202-0.00011-7.

Economidou, D., Theobald, D. E., Robbins, T. W., Everitt, B. J., & Dalley, J. W. (2012). Norepinephrine and dopamine modulate impulsivity on the five-choice serial reaction time task through opponent actions in the shell and core sub-regions of the nucleus accumbens. *Neuropsychopharmacology, 37*(9), 2057–2066. https://doi.org/10.1038/npp.2012.53.

Eppolito, A. K., & Smith, R. F. (2006). Long-term behavioral and developmental consequences of pre- and perinatal nicotine. *Pharmacology Biochemistry and Behavior, 85*(4), 835–841. https://doi.org/10.1016/j.pbb.2006.11.020.

Fernando, A. B. P., Economidou, D., Theobald, D. E., Zou, M.-F., Newman, A. H., Spoelder, M., Caprioli, D., Moreno, M., Hipólito, L., Aspinall, A. T., Robbins, T. W., & Dalley, J. W. (2012). Modulation of high impulsivity and attentional performance in rats by selective direct and indirect dopaminergic and noradrenergic receptor agonists. *Psychopharmacology, 219*(2), 341–352. https://doi.org/10.1007/s00213-011-2408-z.

Galtress, T. (20100208). The role of the nucleus accumbens core in impulsive choice, timing, and reward processing. *Behavioral Neuroscience, 124*(1), 26–43. https://doi.org/10.1037/a0018464.

George, O., Le Moal, M., & Koob, G. F. (2012). Allostasis and addiction: Role of the dopamine and corticotropin-releasing factor systems. *Physiology & Behavior, 106*(1), 58–64. https://doi.org/10.1016/j.physbeh.2011.11.004.

Goldberg, Spealman, R. D., & Goldberg, D. M. (1981). Persistent behavior at high rates maintained by intravenous self-administration of nicotine. *Science, 214*(4520), 573–575. https://doi.org/10.1126/science.7291998.

Hogle, J. M., Kaye, J. T., & Curtin, J. J. (2010). Nicotine withdrawal increases threat-induced anxiety but not fear: Neuroadaptation in human addiction. *Biological Psychiatry, 68*(8), 719–725. https://doi.org/10.1016/j.biopsych.2010.06.003.

Holgate, J. Y., & Bartlett, S. E. (2015). Early life stress, nicotinic acetylcholine receptors and alcohol use disorders. *Brain Sciences, 5*(3), 258–274. https://doi.org/10.3390/brainsci5030258.

Hunter, R. G., Bloss, E. B., McCarthy, K. J., & McEwen, B. S. (2010). Regulation of the nicotinic receptor alpha7 subunit by chronic stress and corticosteroids. *Brain Research, 1325*, 141–146. https://doi.org/10.1016/j.brainres.2010.02.014.

Kayir, H., Semenova, S., & Markou, A. (2014). Baseline impulsive choice predicts the effects of nicotine and nicotine withdrawal on impulsivity in rats. *Progress in Neuro-Psychopharmacology and Biological Psychiatry, 48*, 6–13. https://doi.org/10.1016/j.pnpbp.2013.09.007.

Kim, S., & Lee, D. (2011). Prefrontal cortex and impulsive decision making. *Biological Psychiatry, 69*(12), 1140–1146. https://doi.org/10.1016/j.biopsych.2010.07.005.

Kolokotroni, K. Z., Rodgers, R. J., & Harrison, A. A. (2011). Acute nicotine increases both impulsive choice and behavioural disinhibition in rats. *Psychopharmacology, 217*(4), 455–473. https://doi.org/10.1007/s00213-011-2296-2.

Koob, G. F., & Le Moal, M. (1997). Drug abuse: Hedonic homeostatic dysregulation. *Science, 278*(5335), 52–58. https://doi.org/10.1126/science.278.5335.52.

Koob, G. F., & Le Moal, M. (2008). Addiction and the brain antireward system. *Annual Review of Psychology, 59*(1), 29–53. https://doi.org/10.1146/annurev.psych.59.103006.093548.

Livneh, Y., Sugden, A. U., Madara, J. C., Essner, R. A., Flores, V. I., Sugden, L. A., Resch, J. M., Lowell, B. B., & Andermann, M. L. (2020). Estimation of current and future physiological states in insular cortex. *Neuron, 105*(6), 1094–1111.e10. https://doi.org/10.1016/j.neuron.2019.12.027.

Locey, M. L., & Dallery, J. (2009). Isolating behavioral mechanisms of intertemporal choice: Nicotine effect on delay discounting and amount sensitivity. *Journal of the Experimental Analysis of Behavior, 91*(2), 213–223. https://doi.org/10.1901/jeab.2009.91-213.

Loree, A. M., Lundahl, L. H., & Ledgerwood, D. M. (2015). Impulsivity as a predictor of treatment outcome in substance use disorders: Review and synthesis. *Drug and Alcohol Review, 34*(2), 119–134. https://doi.org/10.1111/dar.12132.

Lowell, B. B. (2019). New neuroscience of homeostasis and drives for food, water, and salt. *New England Journal of Medicine, 380*(5), 459–471. https://doi.org/10.1056/NEJMra1812053.

Marshall, E. C., Johnson, K., Bergman, J., Gibson, L. E., & Zvolensky, M. J. (2009). Anxiety sensitivity and panic reactivity to bodily sensations: Relation to quit-day (acute) nicotine withdrawal symptom severity among daily smokers making a self-guided quit attempt. *Experimental and Clinical Psychopharmacology, 17*(5), 356–364. https://doi.org/10.1037/a0016883.

McDonald, C. G., Dailey, V. K., Bergstrom, H. C., Wheeler, T. L., Eppolito, A. K., Smith, L. N., & Smith, R. F. (2005). Periadolescent nicotine administration produces enduring changes in dendritic morphology of medium spiny neurons from nucleus accumbens. *Neuroscience Letters, 385*(2), 163–167. https://doi.org/10.1016/j.neulet.2005.05.041.

McEwen, B. (2010). Stress: Homeostasis, rheostasis, allostasis and allostatic load. In G. Fink (Ed.). *Stress science: Neuroendocrinology* (pp. 10–14). Oxford: Academic Press.

McLeish, A. C., Zvolensky, M. J., & Bucossi, M. M. (2007). Interaction between smoking rate and anxiety sensitivity: Relation to anticipatory anxiety and panic-relevant avoidance among daily smokers. *Journal of Anxiety Disorders, 21*(6), 849–859. https://doi.org/10.1016/j.janxdis.2006.11.003.

Miao, H., Liu, C., Bishop, K., Gong, Z.-H., Nordberg, A., & Zhang, X. (1998). Nicotine exposure during a critical period of development leads to persistent changes in nicotinic acetylcholine receptors of adult rat brain. *Journal of Neurochemistry, 70*(2), 752–762. https://doi.org/10.1046/j.1471-4159.1998.70020752.x.

Morissette, S. B., Tull, M. T., Gulliver, S. B., Kamholz, B. W., & Zimering, R. T. (2007). Anxiety, anxiety disorders, tobacco use, and nicotine: A critical review of interrelationships. *Psychological Bulletin, 133*(2), 245–272. https://doi.org/10.1037/0033-2909.133.2.245.

Nutt, D., & Malizia, A. (2006). Anxiety and OCD: The chicken or the egg? *Journal of Psychopharmacology, 20*(6), 729–731. https://doi.org/10.1177/0269881106068424.

Pariyadath, V., Gowin, J. L., & Stein, E. A. (2016). Chapter 8—Resting state functional connectivity analysis for addiction medicine: From individual loci to complex networks. In H. Ekhtiari & M. P. Paulus (Eds.), *Progress in brain research* (Vol. 224, pp. 155–173). Elsevier. https://doi.org/10.1016/bs.pbr.2015.07.015.

Pezze, M.-A., Dalley, J. W., & Robbins, T. W. (2007). Differential roles of dopamine D1 and D2 receptors in the nucleus accumbens in attentional performance on the five-choice serial reaction time task. *Neuropsychopharmacology, 32*(2), 273–283. https://doi.org/10.1038/sj.npp.1301073.

Picciotto, M. R., Lewis, A. S., van Schalkwyk, G. I., & Mineur, Y. S. (2015). Mood and anxiety regulation by nicotinic acetylcholine receptors: A potential pathway to modulate aggression and related behavioral states. *Neuropharmacology, 96*, 235–243. https://doi.org/10.1016/j.neuropharm.2014.12.028.

Robbins, T. (2002). The 5-choice serial reaction time task: Behavioural pharmacology and functional neurochemistry. *Psychopharmacology, 163*(3), 362–380. https://doi.org/10.1007/s00213-002-1154-7.

Robbins, T. W. (2005). Chemistry of the mind: Neurochemical modulation of prefrontal cortical function. *Journal of Comparative Neurology, 493*(1), 140–146. https://doi.org/10.1002/cne.20717.

Rukstalis, M., Jepson, C., Patterson, F., & Lerman, C. (2005). Increases in hyperactive–impulsive symptoms predict relapse among smokers in nicotine replacement therapy. *Journal of Substance Abuse Treatment, 28*(4), 297–304. https://doi.org/10.1016/j.jsat.2005.02.002.

Smith, R. F., McDonald, C. G., Bergstrom, H. C., Ehlinger, D. G., & Brielmaier, J. M. (2015). Adolescent nicotine induces persisting changes in development of neural connectivity. *Neuroscience & Biobehavioral Reviews, 55*, 432–443. https://doi.org/10.1016/j.neubiorev.2015.05.019.

Spinella, M. (2005a). Compulsive behavior in tobacco users. *Addictive Behaviors, 30*(1), 183–186. https://doi.org/10.1016/j.addbeh.2004.04.011.

Spinella, M. (2005b). Mood in relation to subclinical obsessive-compulsive symptoms. *International Journal of Neuroscience, 115*(4), 433–443. https://doi.org/10.1080/00207450590522838.

Sterling, P. (2012). Allostasis: A model of predictive regulation. *Physiology & Behavior, 106*(1), 5–15. https://doi.org/10.1016/j.physbeh.2011.06.004.

Volkow, N. D., & Fowler, J. S. (2000). Addiction, a disease of compulsion and drive: Involvement of the orbitofrontal cortex. *Cerebral Cortex, 10*(3), 318–325. https://doi.org/10.1093/cercor/10.3.318.

Yu, G., Chen, H., Wu, X., Matta, S. G., & Sharp, B. M. (2010). Nicotine self-administration differentially modulates glutamate and GABA transmission in hypothalamic paraventricular nucleus to enhance the hypothalamic–pituitary–adrenal response to stress. *Journal of Neurochemistry, 113*(4), 919–929. https://doi.org/10.1111/j.1471-4159.2010.06654.x.

Yu, G., & Sharp, B. M. (2012). Nicotine modulates multiple regions in the limbic stress network regulating activation of hypophysiotrophic neurons in hypothalamic paraventricular nucleus. *Journal of Neurochemistry, 122*(3), 628–640. https://doi.org/10.1111/j.1471-4159.2012.07785.x.

Zeelenberg, M., van Dijk, W. W., van der Pligt, J., Manstead, A. S. R., van Empelen, P., & Reinderman, D. (1998). Emotional reactions to the outcomes of decisions: The role of counterfactual thought in the experience of regret and disappointment. *Organizational Behavior and Human Decision Processes, 75*(2), 117–141. https://doi.org/10.1006/obhd.1998.2784.

Chapter 5. Patterns

Awareness

Ayan, S. (2018). The brain's autopilot mechanism steers consciousness. *Scientific American.* https://www.scientificamerican.com/article/the-brains-autopilot-mechanism-steers-consciousness/.

Baars, B. (1997). In the theatre of consciousness: Global workspace theory, a rigorous scientific theory of consciousness. *Journal of Consciousness Studies, 4*(4), 292–309.

Braver, T. S., Paxton, J. L., Locke, H. S., & Barch, D. M. (2009). Flexible neural mechanisms of cognitive control within human prefrontal cortex. *Proceedings of the National Academy of Sciences, 106*(18), 7351–7356. https://doi.org/10.1073/pnas.0808187106.

Engel, A. K., & Singer, W. (2001). Temporal binding and the neural correlates of sensory awareness. *Trends in Cognitive Sciences, 5*(1), 16–25. https://doi.org/10.1016/s1364-6613(00)01568-0.

Gray, J. R., Braver, T. S., & Raichle, M. E. (2002). Integration of emotion and cognition in the lateral prefrontal cortex. *Proceedings of the National Academy of Sciences, 99*(6), 4115–4120. https://doi.org/10.1073/pnas.062381899.

Mansvelder, H. D., van Aerde, K. I., Couey, J. J., & Brussaard, A. B. (2006). Nicotinic modulation of neuronal networks: From receptors to cognition. *Psychopharmacology, 184*(3), 292–305. https://doi.org/10.1007/s00213-005-0070-z.

Naudé, J., Dongelmans, M., & Faure, P. (2015). Nicotinic alteration of decision-making. *Neuropharmacology, 96*, 244–254. https://doi.org/10.1016/j.neuropharm.2014.11.021.

Ott, T., & Nieder, A. (2019). Dopamine and cognitive control in prefrontal cortex. *Trends in Cognitive Sciences, 23*(3), 213–234. https://doi.org/10.1016/j.tics.2018.12.006.

Picton, T. W., & Stuss, D. T. (2000). Chapter 1—Consciousness. In E. E. Bittar & N. Bittar (Eds.), *Principles of medical biology* (Vol. 14, pp. 1–25). Elsevier. https://doi.org/10.1016/S1569-2582(00)80003-3.

Zeman, A. (2005). What in the world is consciousness? In S. Laureys (Ed.), *Progress in brain research* (Vol. 150, pp. 1–10). Elsevier. https://doi.org/10.1016/S0079-6123(05)50001-3.

Network (Hebbian) Learning

Caporale, N., & Dan, Y. (2008). Spike timing–dependent plasticity: A Hebbian learning rule. *Annual Review of Neuroscience, 31*(1), 25–46. https://doi.org/10.1146/annurev.neuro.31.060407.125639.

Gerstner, W. (2011). Chapter 9—Hebbian learning and plasticity. In M. Arbib and J. Bonaiuto (Eds.), *From neuron to cognition via computational neuroscience.* MIT Press.

Hebb, D. (1949). *The organization of behavior: A neuropsychological theory.* Wiley. http://www.amazon.ca/exec/obidos/redirect?tag=citeulike09-20&path=ASIN/0805843000.

Kempter, R., Gerstner, W., & van Hemmen, J. L. (1999). Hebbian learning and spiking neurons. *Physical Review E, 59*(4), 4498–4514. https://doi.org/10.1103/PhysRevE.59.4498.

Montague, P. R., Dayan, P., & Sejnowski, T. J. (1996). A framework for mesencephalic dopamine systems based on predictive Hebbian learning. *Journal of Neuroscience, 16*(5), 1936–1947. https://doi.org/10.1523/JNEUROSCI.16-05-01936.1996.

Song, S., Miller, K. D., & Abbott, L. F. (2000). Competitive Hebbian learning through spike-timing-dependent synaptic plasticity. *Nature Neuroscience, 3*(9), 919–926. https://doi.org/10.1038/78829.

Operant to Classical Transformation

Camí, J., & Farré, M. (2003). Drug addiction. *New England Journal of Medicine, 349*(10), 975–986. https://doi.org/10.1056/NEJMra023160.

Lewis, M. (2018). Brain change in addiction as learning, not disease. *New England Journal of Medicine, 379*(16), 1551–1560. https://doi.org/10.1056/NEJMra1602872.

Plasticity

Brown, T. H., Byrne, J. H., LaBar, K. S., LeDoux, J. E., Lindquist, D. H., Thompson, R. F., & Teyler, T. J. (2004). Chapter 18—Learning and memory: Basic mechanisms. In J. H. Byrne & J. L. Roberts (Eds.), *From molecules to networks* (pp. 499–574). Academic Press. https://doi.org/10.1016/B978-012148660-0/50019-6.

Corringer, P.-J., Sallette, J., & Changeux, J.-P. (2006). Nicotine enhances intracellular nicotinic receptor maturation: A novel mechanism of neural plasticity? *Journal of Physiology-Paris, 99*(2), 162–171. https://doi.org/10.1016/j.jphysparis.2005.12.012.

Couey, J. J., Meredith, R. M., Spijker, S., Poorthuis, R. B., Smit, A. B., Brussaard, A. B., & Mansvelder, H. D. (2007). Distributed network actions by nicotine increase the threshold for spike-timing-dependent plasticity in prefrontal cortex. *Neuron, 54*(1), 73–87. https://doi.org/10.1016/j.neuron.2007.03.006.

Dani, J. A., Ji, D., & Zhou, F.-M. (2001). Synaptic plasticity and nicotine addiction. *Neuron, 31*(3), 349–352. https://doi.org/10.1016/S0896-6273(01)00379-8.

Faillace, M. P., & Bernabeu, R. O. (2019). Chapter 45—Effects of nicotine and histone deacetylase inhibitors on the brain. In V. R. Preedy (Ed.), *Neuroscience of nicotine* (pp. 365–373). Academic Press. https://doi.org/10.1016/B978-0-12-813035-3.00045-9.

Koob, G. F., & Le Moal, M. (2005). Plasticity of reward neurocircuitry and the "dark side" of drug addiction. *Nature Neuroscience, 8*(11), 1442–1444. https://doi.org/10.1038/nn1105-1442.

Morrow, J. D., & Flagel, S. B. (2016). Chapter 1—Neuroscience of resilience and vulnerability for addiction medicine: From genes to behavior. In H. Ekhtiari & M. Paulus (Eds.), *Progress in brain research* (Vol. 223, pp. 3–18). Elsevier. https://doi.org/10.1016/bs.pbr.2015.09.004.

Pettorruso, M., di Giannantonio, M., De Risio, L., Martinotti, G., & Koob, G. F. (2020). A light in the darkness: Repetitive transcranial magnetic stimulation (rTMS) to treat the hedonic dysregulation of addiction. *Journal of Addiction Medicine, 14*(4), 272–274. https://doi.org/10.1097/ADM.0000000000000575.

Placzek, A. N., & Dani, J. A. (2009). Synaptic plasticity within midbrain dopamine centers contributes to nicotine addiction. In A. R. Caggiula & R. A. Bevins (Eds.), *The motivational impact of nicotine and its role in tobacco use* (pp. 5–15). Springer US. https://doi.org/10.1007/978-0-387-78748-0_2.

Placzek, A. N., Zhang, T. A., & Dani, J. A. (2009). Age dependent nicotinic influences over dopamine neuron synaptic plasticity. *Biochemical Pharmacology, 78*(7), 686–692. https://doi.org/10.1016/j.bcp.2009.05.014.

Tang, J., & Dani, J. A. (2009). Dopamine enables in vivo synaptic plasticity associated with the addictive drug nicotine. *Neuron, 63*(5), 673–682. https://doi.org/10.1016/j.neuron.2009.07.025.

Volkow, N. D., Koob, G. F., & McLellan, A. T. (2016). Neurobiologic advances from the brain disease model of addiction. *New England Journal of Medicine, 374*(4), 363–371. https://doi.org/10.1056/NEJMra1511480.

Chapter 6. Device

Optimization

Coggins, C. R. E., McKinney, W. J., Jr., & Oldham, M. J. (2013). A comprehensive evaluation of the toxicology of experimental, non-filtered cigarettes manufactured with different circumferences. *Inhalation Toxicology, 25*(Suppl. 2), 69–72. https://doi.org/10.3109/08958378.2013.854436.

Coggins, C. R. E., Merski, J. A., & Oldham, M. J. (2013). A comprehensive evaluation of the toxicology resulting from laser-generated ventilation holes in cigarette filters. *Inhalation Toxicology, 25*(Suppl. 2), 59–63. https://doi.org/10.3109/08958378.2013.854434.

Dittrich, D. J., Fieblekorn, R. T., Bevan, M. J., Rushforth, D., Murphy, J. J., Ashley, M., McAdam, K. G., Liu, C., & Proctor, C. J. (2014). Approaches for the design of reduced toxicant emission cigarettes. *SpringerPlus, 3*(1), 374. https://doi.org/10.1186/2193-1801-3-374.

Dunn, W. (1972). Motives and incentives in cigarette smoking. 1972, July 1. Philip Morris Records, Master Settlement Agreement. Truth Tobacco Industry Documents. Retrieved October 1, 2020, from https://www.industrydocuments.ucsf.edu/tobacco/docs/#id=tggp0125.

Huber, G. (1989). Physical, chemical, and biologic properties of tobacco, cigarette smoke, and other tobacco products. *Seminars in Respiratory and Critical Care Medicine, 10*(4), 297–332.

Ignacio de Granda Orive, J. (2019). Cigarette: Perfect engineering product to inhale but not safe. *Open Respiratory Archives, 1*(1–2), 5–6.

Lebert, H. A. (1960). Tobacco tar removal structure. U.S. Patent No. US2954786A. https://patents.google.com/patent/US2954786A/en.

Lindner, M. (2017). The power of tactility: Tipping paper in interaction with the consumer. Tann Group. https://www.coresta.org/sites/default/files/abstracts/2017_TSRC76_Lindner.pdf.

Muramatsu, M., Takeda, K., Futamura, Y., & Sagawa, T. (1995). Tipping paper and cigarette using the same. U.S. Patent No. US5394895A. https://patents.google.com/patent/US5394895A/en.

Oldham, M. J., Coggins, C. R. E., & McKinney W. J., Jr. (2013). A comprehensive evaluation of selected components and processes used in the manufacture of cigarettes: Approach and overview. *Inhalation Toxicology, 25*(Suppl. 2), 1–5. https://doi.org/10.3109/08958378.2013.854429.

Physicians for a Smoke-Free Canada. (1990). *Dictionary of tobacco terms.* http://www.smoke-free.ca/pdf_1/Dictionary.PDF.

Rice, M. E., & Cragg, S. J. (2004). Nicotine amplifies reward-related dopamine signals in striatum. *Nature Neuroscience, 7*(6), 583–584. https://doi.org/10.1038/nn1244.

Schur, M. O. (1965). Apparatus for perforating. U.S. Patent No. US3179025A. https://patents.google.com/patent/US3179025A/en.

Unknown. (1991). C. Thomas Littleton. 1991, March 20. Lorillard Records, Master Settlement Agreement. Truth Tobacco Industry Documents. Retrieved October 1, 2020, from https://www.industrydocuments.ucsf.edu/tobacco/docs/#id=kfck0063.

Unknown. (1989). Configuration optimization. 1989, March 28. RJ Reynolds Records, Master Settlement Agreement.Truth Tobacco Industry Documents. Retrieved October 1, 2020, from https://www.industrydocuments.ucsf.edu/tobacco/docs/#id=mrvp0097.

Unknown. (1991). Optimization approach. 1991, January 1. RJ Reynolds Records, Master Settlement Agreement. Truth Tobacco Industry Documents. Retrieved October 1, 2020, from https://www.industrydocuments.ucsf.edu/tobacco/docs/#id=znfp0230.

Wightman, R. M., & Robinson, D. L. (2002). Transient changes in mesolimbic dopamine and their association with "reward." *Journal of Neurochemistry, 82*(4), 721–735. https://doi.org/10.1046/j.1471-4159.2002.01005.x.

Zhang, H., & Sulzer, D. (2004). Frequency-dependent modulation of dopamine release by nicotine. *Nature Neuroscience, 7*(6), 581–582. https://doi.org/10.1038/nn1243.

Chemistry

Abobo, C. V., Ma, J., & Liang, D. (2012). Effect of menthol on nicotine pharmacokinetics in rats after cigarette smoke inhalation. *Nicotine & Tobacco Research, 14*(7), 801–808. https://doi.org/10.1093/ntr/ntr287.

Ahijevych, K., & Garrett, B. E. (2004). Menthol pharmacology and its potential impact on cigarette smoking behavior. *Nicotine & Tobacco Research, 6*(Suppl. 1), S17–S28. https://doi.org/10.1080/14622200310001649469.

Bates, C., Connolly, G., & Jarvis, M. (1999). Tobacco additives: Cigarette engineering and nicotine addiction. Action on Smoking and Health. https://ash.org.uk/resources/view/tobacco-additives-cigarette-engineering-and-nicotine-addiction.

Benowitz, N. L., Herrera, B., & Jacob, P. (2004). Mentholated cigarette smoking inhibits nicotine metabolism. *Journal of Pharmacology and Experimental Therapeutics, 310*(3), 1208–1215. https://doi.org/10.1124/jpet.104.066902.

Brunnemann, K. D., & Hoffmann, D. (1975). Chemical studies on tobacco smoke XXXIV: Gas chromatographic determination of ammonia in cigarette and cigar smoke. *Journal of Chromatographic Science, 13*(4), 159–163. https://doi.org/10.1093/chromsci/13.4.159.

Cisternino, S., Chapy, H., André, P., Smirnova, M., Debray, M., & Scherrmann, J.-M. (2013). Coexistence of passive and proton antiporter-mediated processes in nicotine transport at the mouse blood–brain barrier. *AAPS Journal, 15*(2), 299–307. https://doi.org/10.1208/s12248-012-9434-6.

Clark, P. I., Gautam, S., & Gerson, L. W. (1996). Effect of menthol cigarettes on biochemical markers of smoke exposure among black and white smokers. *Chest, 110*(5), 1194–1198. https://doi.org/10.1378/chest.110.5.1194.

El-Hellani, A., El-Hage, R., Baalbaki, R., Salman, R., Talih, S., Shihadeh, A., & Saliba, N. A. (2015). Free-base and protonated nicotine in electronic cigarette liquids and aerosols. *Chemical Research in Toxicology, 28*(8), 1532–1537. https://doi.org/10.1021/acs.chemrestox.5b00107.

Fong, C. W. (2015). Permeability of the blood–brain barrier: Molecular mechanism of transport of drugs and physiologically important compounds. *Journal of Membrane Biology, 248*(4), 651–669. https://doi.org/10.1007/s00232-015-9778-9.

Ha, M. A., Smith, G. J., Cichocki, J. A., Fan, L., Liu, Y.-S., Caceres, A. I., Jordt, S. E., &

Morris, J. B. (2015). Menthol attenuates respiratory irritation and elevates blood cotinine in cigarette smoke exposed mice. *PLOS One, 10*(2), e0117128. https://doi. org/10.1371/journal.pone.0117128.

Hawkins, B. T., Abbruscato, T. J., Egleton, R. D., Brown, R. C., Huber, J. D., Campos, C. R., & Davis, T. P. (2004). Nicotine increases in vivo blood–brain barrier permeability and alters cerebral microvascular tight junction protein distribution. *Brain Research, 1027*(1), 48–58. https://doi.org/10.1016/j.brainres.2004.08.043.

Henningfield, J. E., Pankow, J. F., & Garrett, B. E. (2004). Ammonia and other chemical base tobacco additives and cigarette nicotine delivery: Issues and research needs. *Nicotine & Tobacco Research, 6*(2), 199–205. https://doi.org/10.1080/14622200420 00202472.

Miller, G. E., Jarvik, M. E., Caskey, N. H., Segerstrom, S. C., Rosenblatt, M. R., & McCarthy, W. J. (1994). Cigarette mentholation increases smokers' exhaled carbon monoxide levels. *Experimental and Clinical Psychopharmacology, 2*(2), 154–160. https:// doi.org/10.1037/1064-1297.2.2.154.

Murray, C. L., Quaglia, M., Arnason, J. T., & Morris, C. E. (1994). A putative nicotine pump at the metabolic blood–brain barrier of the tobacco hornworm. *Journal of Neurobiology, 25*(1), 23–34. https://doi.org/10.1002/neu.480250103.

Pankow, J. F., Mader, B. T., Isabelle, L. M., Luo, W., Pavlick, A., & Liang, C. (1997). Conversion of nicotine in tobacco smoke to its volatile and available free-base form through the action of gaseous ammonia. *Environmental Science & Technology, 31*(8), 2428–2433. https://doi.org/10.1021/es970402f.

Pankow, J. F., Tavakoli, A. D., Luo, W., & Isabelle, L. M. (2003). Percent free base nicotine in the tobacco smoke particulate matter of selected commercial and reference cigarettes. *Chemical Research in Toxicology, 16*(8), 1014–1018. https://doi. org/10.1021/tx0340596.

Perfetti, T. A. (1983). Structural study of nicotine salts. *Beiträge zur Tabakforschung International (Contributions to Tobacco Research), 12*(2), 43–54. https://doi. org/10.2478/cttr-2013-0524.

Perfetti, T. A. (2014). The transfer of nicotine from nicotine salts to mainstream smoke. Beiträge zur Tabakforschung International (Contributions to Tobacco Research), 19(3), 141–158. https://doi.org/10.2478/cttr-2013-0702.

Seeman, J. I., Fournier, J. A., Paine, J. B., & Waymack, B. E. (1999). The form of nicotine in tobacco: Thermal transfer of nicotine and nicotine acid salts to nicotine in the gas phase. *Journal of Agricultural and Food Chemistry, 47*(12), 5133–5145.

van Amsterdam, J., Sleijffers, A., van Spiegel, P., Blom, R., Witte, M., van de Kassteele, J., Blokland, M., Steerenberg, P., & Opperhuizen, A. (2011). Effect of ammonia in cigarette tobacco on nicotine absorption in human smokers. *Food and Chemical Toxicology, 49*(12), 3025–3030. https://doi.org/10.1016/j.fct.2011.09.037.

Wang, T., Wang, B., & Chen, H. (2014). Menthol facilitates the intravenous self-administration of nicotine in rats. *Frontiers in Behavioral Neuroscience, 8*, 437. https://doi. org/10.3389/fnbeh.2014.00437.

Wayne, G. F., Connolly, G. N., & Henningfield, J. E. (2006). Brand differences of free-base nicotine delivery in cigarette smoke: The view of the tobacco industry documents. *Tobacco Control, 15*(3), 189–198. https://doi.org/10.1136/tc.2005.013805.

Zhang, H., & Sulzer, D. (2004). Frequency-dependent modulation of dopamine release by nicotine. *Nature Neuroscience, 7*(6), 581–582. https://doi.org/10.1038/nn1243.

Zhang, T., Zhang, L., Liang, Y., Siapas, A. G., Zhou, F.-M., & Dani, J. A. (2009). Dopamine signaling differences in the nucleus accumbens and dorsal striatum exploited by nicotine. *Journal of Neuroscience, 29*(13), 4035–4043. https://doi.org/10.1523/JNEUROSCI.0261-09.2009.

Alkaloids

Caine, S. B., Collins, G. T., Thomsen, M., Wright, C., IV, Lanier, R. K., & Mello, N. K. (2014). Nicotine-like behavioral effects of the minor tobacco alkaloids nornicotine, anabasine, and anatabine in male rodents. *Experimental and Clinical Psychopharmacology, 22*(1), 9–22. https://doi.org/10.1037/a0035749.

Dwoskin, L. P., Teng, L., Buxton, S. T., Ravard, A., Deo, N., & Crooks, P. A. (1995). Minor alkaloids of tobacco release [3H]dopamine from superfused rat striatal slices. *European Journal of Pharmacology, 276*(1), 195–199. https://doi.org/10.1016/0014-2999(95)00077-X.

Feldhammer, M., & Ritchie, J. C. (2017). Anabasine is a poor marker for determining smoking status of transplant patients. *Clinical Chemistry, 63*(2), 604–606. https://doi.org/10.1373/clinchem.2016.265546.

Hoffman, A. C., & Evans, S. E. (2013). Abuse potential of non-nicotine tobacco smoke components: Acetaldehyde, nornicotine, cotinine, and anabasine. *Nicotine & Tobacco Research, 15*(3), 622–632. https://doi.org/10.1093/ntr/nts192.

Hoofnagle, A. N., Laha, T. J., Rainey, P. M., & Sadrzadeh, S. M. H. (2006). Specific detection of anabasine, nicotine, and nicotine metabolites in urine by liquid chromatography–tandem mass spectrometry. *American Journal of Clinical Pathology, 126*(6), 880–887. https://doi.org/10.1309/LQ8U3UL956ET324X.

Jacob, P., Yu, L., Shulgin, A. T., & Benowitz, N. L. (1999). Minor tobacco alkaloids as biomarkers for tobacco use: Comparison of users of cigarettes, smokeless tobacco, cigars, and pipes. *American Journal of Public Health, 89*(5), 731–736. https://doi.org/10.2105/AJPH.89.5.731.

Jacob, P., Hatsukami, D., Severson, H., Hall, S., Yu, L., & Benowitz, N. L. (2002). Anabasine and anatabine as biomarkers for tobacco use during nicotine replacement therapy. *Cancer Epidemiology and Prevention Biomarkers, 11*(12), 1668–1673.

Pakhale, S. S., & Maru, G. B. (1998). Distribution of major and minor alkaloids in tobacco, mainstream and sidestream smoke of popular Indian smoking products. *Food and Chemical Toxicology, 36*(12), 1131–1138. https://doi.org/10.1016/S0278-6915(98)00071-4.

Saunders, J. A., & Blume, D. E. (1981). Quantitation of major tobacco alkaloids by high-performance liquid chromatography. *Journal of Chromatography A, 205*(1), 147–154. https://doi.org/10.1016/S0021-9673(00)81822-1.

Aerosol Physics

Anderson, P. J., Wilson, J. D., & Hiller, F. C. (1989). Particle size distribution of mainstream tobacco and marijuana smoke: Analysis using the electrical aerosol analyzer. *American Review of Respiratory Disease, 140*(1), 202–205. https://doi.org/10.1164/ajrccm/140.1.202.

Baker, R. R., & Dixon, M. (2006). The retention of tobacco smoke constituents in the human respiratory tract. *Inhalation Toxicology, 18*(4), 255–294. https://doi. org/10.1080/08958370500444163.

Bernstein, D. M. (2004). A review of the influence of particle size, puff volume, and inhalation pattern on the deposition of cigarette smoke particles in the respiratory tract. *Inhalation Toxicology, 16*(10), 675–689. https://doi. org/10.1080/08958370490476587.

Brinkman, M. C., Chuang, J. C., Gordon, S. M., Kim, H., Kroeger, R. R., Polzin, G. M., & Richter, P. A. (2012). Exposure to and deposition of fine and ultrafine particles in smokers of menthol and nonmenthol cigarettes. *Inhalation Toxicology, 24*(5), 255–269. https://doi.org/10.3109/08958378.2012.667218.

Brown, J. S., Gordon, T., Price, O., & Asgharian, B. (2013). Thoracic and respirable particle definitions for human health risk assessment. *Particle and Fibre Toxicology, 10*(1), 12. https://doi.org/10.1186/1743-8977-10-12.

Donaldson, K., Brown, D., Clouter, A., Duffin, R., MacNee, W., Renwick, L., Tran, L., & Stone, V. (2002). The pulmonary toxicology of ultrafine particles. *Journal of Aerosol Medicine, 15*(2), 213–220. https://doi.org/10.1089/089426802320282338.

Gowadia, N., & Dunn-Rankin, D. (2010). A transport model for nicotine in the tracheobronchial and pulmonary region of the lung. *Inhalation Toxicology, 22*(1), 42–48. https://doi.org/10.3109/08958370902862442.

Häger, B., & Niessner, R. (1997). On the distribution of nicotine between the gas and particle phase and its measurement. *Aerosol Science and Technology, 26*(2), 163–174. https://doi.org/10.1080/02786829708965422.

Harris, B. (2011). The intractable cigarette "filter problem." *Tobacco Control, 20*(Suppl. 1), i10–i16. https://doi.org/10.1136/tc.2010.040113.

Ingebrethsen, B. J., Cole, S. K., & Alderman, S. L. (2012). Electronic cigarette aerosol particle size distribution measurements. *Inhalation Toxicology, 24*(14), 976–984. https://doi.org/10.3109/08958378.2012.744781.

Ingebrethsen, B. J., Lyman, C. S., Risner, C. H., Martin, P., & Gordon, B. M. (2001). Particle-gas equilibria of ammonia and nicotine in mainstream cigarette smoke. *Aerosol Science and Technology, 35*(5), 874–886. https://doi.org/10.1080/02786820126850.

John, E., Coburn, S., Liu, C., McAughey, J., Mariner, D., McAdam, K. G., Sebestyén, Z., Bakos, I., & Dóbé, S. (2018). Effect of temperature and humidity on the gas–particle partitioning of nicotine in mainstream cigarette smoke: A diffusion denuder study. *Journal of Aerosol Science, 117*, 100–117. https://doi.org/10.1016/j.jaerosci.2017.12.015.

Kane, D. B., Asgharian, B., Price, O. T., Rostami, A., & Oldham, M. J. (2010). Effect of smoking parameters on the particle size distribution and predicted airway deposition of mainstream cigarette smoke. *Inhalation Toxicology, 22*(3), 199–209. https:// doi.org/10.3109/08958370903161224.

Keith, C. H. (1982). Particle size studies on tobacco smoke. *Beiträge zur Tabakforschung International (Contributions to Tobacco Research), 11*(3), 123–131. https://doi. org/10.2478/cttr-2013-0506.

Keith, C. H., & Derrick, J. C. (1960). Measurement of the particle size distribution and concentration of cigarette smoke by the "conifuge." *Journal of Colloid Science, 15*(4), 340–356. https://doi.org/10.1016/0095-8522(60)90037-4.

Kozlowski, L. T., & O'Connor, R. J. (2002). Cigarette filter ventilation is a defective design because of misleading taste, bigger puffs, and blocked vents. *Tobacco Control,*

11(Suppl. 1), i40–i50. https://doi.org/10.1136/tc.11.suppl_1.i40.

Morie, G. P., & Baggett, M. S. (1977). Observations on the distribution of certain tobacco smoke components with respect to particle size. *Beiträge zur Tabakforschung International (Contributions to Tobacco Research), 9*(2), 72–78. https://doi.org/10.2478/cttr-2013-0430.

Robinson, R. J., & Yu, C. P. (2001). Deposition of cigarette smoke particles in the human respiratory tract. *Aerosol Science and Technology, 34*(2), 202–215. https://doi.org/10.1080/027868201300034844.

Sahu, S. K., Tiwari, M., Bhangare, R. C., & Pandit, G. G. (2013). Particle size distribution of mainstream and exhaled cigarette smoke and predictive deposition in human respiratory tract. *Aerosol and Air Quality Research, 13*(1), 324–332. https://doi.org/10.4209/aaqr.2012.02.0041.

Song, M.-A., Benowitz, N. L., Berman, M., Brasky, T. M., Cummings, K. M., Hatsukami, D. K., Marian, C., O'Connor, R., Rees, V. W., Woroszylo, C., & Shields, P. G. (2017). Cigarette filter ventilation and its relationship to increasing rates of lung adenocarcinoma. *Journal of the National Cancer Institute, 109*(12). https://doi.org/10.1093/jnci/djx075.

Topography

Brauer, L. H., Hatsukami, D., Hanson, K., & Shiffman, S. (1996). Smoking topography in tobacco chippers and dependent smokers. *Addictive Behaviors, 21*(2), 233–238. https://doi.org/10.1016/0306-4603(95)00054-2.

Bridges, R. B., Combs, J. G., Humble, J. W., Turbek, J. A., Rehm, S. R., & Haley, N. J. (1990). Puffing topography as a determinant of smoke exposure. *Pharmacology Biochemistry and Behavior, 37*(1), 29–39. https://doi.org/10.1016/0091-3057(90)90037-I.

Djordjevic, M. V., Stellman, S. D., & Zang, E. (2000). Doses of nicotine and lung carcinogens delivered to cigarette smokers. *Journal of the National Cancer Institute, 92*(2), 106–111. https://doi.org/10.1093/jnci/92.2.106.

Franken, F. H., Pickworth, W. B., Epstein, D. H., & Moolchan, E. T. (2006). Smoking rates and topography predict adolescent smoking cessation following treatment with nicotine replacement therapy. *Cancer Epidemiology and Prevention Biomarkers, 15*(1), 154–157. https://doi.org/10.1158/1055-9965.EPI-05-0167.

Frederiksen, L. W., Miller, P. M., & Peterson, G. L. (1977). Topographical components of smoking behavior. *Addictive Behaviors, 2*(1), 55–61. https://doi.org/10.1016/0306-4603(77)90009-0.

Hammond, D., Fong, G. T., Cummings, K. M., & Hyland, A. (2005). Smoking topography, brand switching, and nicotine delivery: Results from an in vivo study. *Cancer Epidemiology and Prevention Biomarkers, 14*(6), 1370–1375. https://doi.org/10.1158/1055-9965.EPI-04-0498.

Hatsukami, D. K., Pickens, R. W., Svikis, D. S., & Hughes, J. R. (1988). Smoking topography and nicotine blood levels. *Addictive Behaviors, 13*(1), 91–95. https://doi.org/10.1016/0306-4603(88)90031-7.

Hatsukami, D., Morgan, S. F., Pickens, R. W., & Hughes, J. R. (1987). Smoking topography in a nonlaboratory environment. *International Journal of the Addictions, 22*(8), 719–725. https://doi.org/10.3109/10826088709027453.

Krebs, N. M., Chen, A., Zhu, J., Sun, D., Liao, J., Stennett, A. L., & Muscat, J. E. (2016). Comparison of puff volume with cigarettes per day in predicting nicotine uptake among daily smokers. *American Journal of Epidemiology, 184*(1), 48–57. https://doi.org/10.1093/aje/kwv341.

Lawrence, D., Cadman, B., & Hoffman, A. C. (2011). Sensory properties of menthol and smoking topography. *Tobacco Induced Diseases, 9*(1), S3. https://doi.org/10.1186/1617-9625-9-S1-S3.

Lee, E. M., Malson, J. L., Waters, A. J., Moolchan, E. T., & Pickworth, W. B. (2003). Smoking topography: Reliability and validity in dependent smokers. *Nicotine & Tobacco Research, 5*(5), 673–679. https://doi.org/10.1080/1462220031000158645.

McClure, E. A., Saladin, M. E., Baker, N. L., Carpenter, M. J., & Gray, K. M. (2013). Smoking topography and abstinence in adult female smokers. *Addictive Behaviors, 38*(12), 2833–2836. https://doi.org/10.1016/j.addbeh.2013.08.004.

Sepkovic, D. W., Parker, K., Axelrad, C. M., Haley, N. J., & Wynder, E. L. (1984). Cigarette smoking as a risk for cardiovascular disease V: Biochemical parameters with increased and decreased nicotine content cigarettes. *Addictive Behaviors, 9*(3), 255–263. https://doi.org/10.1016/0306-4603(84)90017-0.

Strasser, A. A., Malaiyandi, V., Hoffmann, E., Tyndale, R. F., & Lerman, C. (2007). An association of CYP2A6 genotype and smoking topography. *Nicotine & Tobacco Research, 9*(4), 511–518. https://doi.org/10.1080/14622200701239605.

Strasser, A. A., Pickworth, W. B., Patterson, F., & Lerman, C. (2004). Smoking topography predicts abstinence following treatment with nicotine replacement therapy. *Cancer Epidemiology and Prevention Biomarkers, 13*(11), 1800–1804.

Tidey, J. W., Rohsenow, D. J., Kaplan, G. B., & Swift, R. M. (2005). Cigarette smoking topography in smokers with schizophrenia and matched non-psychiatric controls. *Drug and Alcohol Dependence, 80*(2), 259–265. https://doi.org/10.1016/j.drugalcdep.2005.04.002.

Zacny, J. P., Stitzer, M. L., & Yingling, J. E. (1986). Cigarette filter vent blocking: Effects on smoking topography and carbon monoxide exposure. *Pharmacology Biochemistry and Behavior, 25*(6), 1245–1252. https://doi.org/10.1016/0091-3057(86)90119-X.

Chapter 7. Approach

Fundamentals

Bernstein, S. L., & Toll, B. A. (2019). Ask about smoking, not quitting: A chronic disease approach to assessing and treating tobacco use. *Addiction Science & Clinical Practice, 14*(1), 29. https://doi.org/10.1186/s13722-019-0159-z.

Epstein, R. M., Franks, P., Fiscella, K., Shields, C. G., Meldrum, S. C., Kravitz, R. L., & Duberstein, P. R. (2005). Measuring patient-centered communication in patient–physician consultations: Theoretical and practical issues. *Social Science & Medicine, 61*(7), 1516–1528. https://doi.org/10.1016/j.socscimed.2005.02.001.

Gelso, C. J., & Carter, J. A. (1985). The relationship in counseling and psychotherapy: Components, consequences, and theoretical antecedents. *Counseling Psychologist, 13*(2), 155–243. https://doi.org/10.1177/0011000085132001.

Ha, J. F., & Longnecker, N. (2010). Doctor-patient communication: A review. *Ochsner Journal, 10*(1), 38–43.

Hashim, M. J. (2017). Patient-centered communication: Basic skills. *American Family Physician, 95*(1), 29–34.

Kivlighan, D. M., Jr., Miles, J. R., & Paquin, J. D. (2010). Therapeutic factors in group-counseling: Asking new questions. In *The Oxford handbook of group counseling* (pp. 121–136). Oxford University Press.

Merrill, G. (1956). The essence of counseling. *Pastoral Psychology, 7*(67), 26–28.

Poskiparta, M., Kettunen, T., & Liimatainen, L. (1998). Reflective questions in health counseling. *Qualitative Health Research, 8*(5), 682–693. https://doi.org/10.1177/104973239800800508.

Strong, S. R. (1971). Experimental laboratory research in counseling. *Journal of Counseling Psychology, 18*(2), 106–110. https://doi.org/10.1037/h0030614.

Tongue, J. R., Epps, H. R., & Forese, L. L. (2005). Communication skills for patient-centered care: Research-based, easily learned techniques for medical interviews that benefit orthopaedic surgeons and their patients. *Journal of Bone and Joint Surgery, 87*(3), 652–658.

Affective Presence

Eisenkraft, N., & Elfenbein, H. A. (2010). The way you make me feel: Evidence for individual differences in affective presence. *Psychological Science, 21*(4), 505–510. https://doi.org/10.1177/0956797610364117.

Fosha, D. (2001). The dyadic regulation of affect. *Journal of Clinical Psychology, 57*(2), 227–242. https://doi.org/10.1002/1097-4679(200102)57:2<227::AID-JCLP8>3.0.CO;2-1.

Isen, A. M. (1984). The influence of positive affect on decision making and cognitive organization. In T. C. Kinnear (Ed.), *NA—Advances in consumer research* (Vol. 11, pp. 534–537). Association for Consumer Research. https://www.acrwebsite.org/volumes/6302/volumes/v11/NA-11/full.

Jiang, J., Gu, H., Dong, Y., & Tu, X. (2019). The better I feel, the better I can do: The role of leaders' positive affective presence. *International Journal of Hospitality Management, 78*, 251–260. https://doi.org/10.1016/j.ijhm.2018.09.007.

Niven, K. (2017). The four key characteristics of interpersonal emotion regulation. *Current Opinion in Psychology, 17*, 89–93. https://doi.org/10.1016/j.copsyc.2017.06.015.

Trust

Bending, Z. J. (2015). Reconceptualising the doctor–patient relationship: Recognising the role of trust in contemporary health care. *Journal of Bioethical Inquiry, 12*(2), 189–202. https://doi.org/10.1007/s11673-014-9570-z.

Benton, J. Z., Lodh, A., Watson, A. M., Tingen, M. S., Terris, M. K., Wallis, C. J. D., & Klaassen, Z. (2020). The association between physician trust and smoking cessation: Implications for motivational interviewing. *Preventive Medicine, 135*, 106075. https://doi.org/10.1016/j.ypmed.2020.106075.

Cairns, G., Andrade, M. de, & MacDonald, L. (2013). Reputation, relationships, risk communication, and the role of trust in the prevention and control of communicable disease: A review. *Journal of Health Communication, 18*(12), 1550–1565. https://doi.org/10.1080/10810730.2013.840696.

Carter, M. A. (2009). Trust, power, and vulnerability: A discourse on helping in nursing. *Nursing Clinics, 44*(4), 393–405. https://doi.org/10.1016/j.cnur.2009.07.012.

Fletcher-Tomenius, L., & Vossler, A. (2009). Trust in online therapeutic relationships: The therapist's experience. *Counselling Psychology Review, 24*(2), 24–34.

Frank, K. A. (2004). The analyst's trust and therapeutic action. *Psychoanalytic Quarterly, 73*(2), 335–378. https://doi.org/10.1002/j.2167-4086.2004.tb00161.x.

Karver, M. S., Handelsman, J. B., Fields, S., & Bickman, L. (2006). Meta-analysis of therapeutic relationship variables in youth and family therapy: The evidence for different relationship variables in the child and adolescent treatment outcome literature. *Clinical Psychology Review, 26*(1), 50–65. https://doi.org/10.1016/j.cpr.2005.09.001.

O'Malley, A. S., Sheppard, V. B., Schwartz, M., & Mandelblatt, J. (2004). The role of trust in use of preventive services among low-income African-American women. *Preventive Medicine, 38*(6), 777–785. https://doi.org/10.1016/j.ypmed.2004.01.018.

Peschken, W., & Johnson, M. (1997). Therapist and client trust in the therapeutic relationship. *Psychotherapy Research, 7*(4), 439–447. https://doi.org/10.1080/10503309712331332133.

Price, B. (2017). Developing patient rapport, trust and therapeutic relationships [text]. *Nursing Standard*, July 10, 2017. https://doi.org/10.7748/ns.2017.e10909.

Sagoff, M. (2013). Trust versus paternalism. *American Journal of Bioethics, 13*(6), 20–21. https://doi.org/10.1080/15265161.2013.781712.

Thorne, S. E., & Robinson, C. A. (1988). Reciprocal trust in health care relationships. *Journal of Advanced Nursing, 13*(6), 782–789. https://doi.org/10.1111/j.1365-2648.1988.tb00570.x.

Empathy

Davis, M. A. (2009). A perspective on cultivating clinical empathy. *Complementary Therapies in Clinical Practice, 15*(2), 76–79. https://doi.org/10.1016/j.ctcp.2009.01.001.

Hojat, M., Gonnella, J. S., Nasca, T. J., Mangione, S., Vergare, M., & Magee, M. (2002). Physician empathy: Definition, components, measurement, and relationship to gender and specialty. *American Journal of Psychiatry, 159*(9), 1563–1569. https://doi.org/10.1176/appi.ajp.159.9.1563.

Jani, B. D., Blane, D. N., & Mercer, S. W. (2012). The role of empathy in therapy and the physician-patient relationship. *Complementary Medicine Research, 19*(5), 252–257. https://doi.org/10.1159/000342998.

Krueger, T. (1997). Affective orientation, alexithymia, and multidimensional empathy in counselors-in-training. [Doctoral dissertation, Western Michigan University]. https://scholarworks.wmich.edu/dissertations/1669.

Moudatsou, M., Stavropoulou, A., Philalithis, A., & Koukouli, S. (2020). The role of empathy in health and social care professionals. *Healthcare, 8*(1), 26. https://doi.org/10.3390/healthcare8010026.

Reynolds, W. J., & Scott, B. (1999). Empathy: A crucial component of the helping relationship. *Journal of Psychiatric and Mental Health Nursing, 6*(5), 363–370. https://doi.org/10.1046/j.1365-2850.1999.00228.x.

Watson, J. C., Steckley, P. L., & McMullen, E. J. (2014). The role of empathy in promoting change. *Psychotherapy Research, 24*(3), 286–298. https://doi.org/10.1080/10503 307.2013.802823.

Adult Learning

Lieb, S. (1999). Principles of adult learning. *Arizona Department of Health Services.* https://myhero1412.files.wordpress.com/2010/10/principles-of-adult-learning.doc.

Luckner, J. L., & Nadler, R. S. (1997). *Processing the experience: Strategies to enhance and generalize learning* (2nd ed.). Kendall/Hunt Publishing Company.

Merriam, S. B. (2008). Adult learning theory for the twenty-first century. *New Directions for Adult and Continuing Education, 2008*(119), 93–98. https://doi.org/10.1002/ace.309.

Merriam, S. B., & Bierema, L. L. (2013). *Adult learning: Linking theory and practice.* John Wiley & Sons.

Mezirow, J. (1989). Personal perspective change through adult learning. In C. J. Titmus (Ed.), *Lifelong education for adults* (pp. 195–198). Pergamon. https://doi.org/10.1016/B978-0-08-030851-7.50062-X.

Shuck, B., Albornoz, C., & Winberg, M. (2007). Emotions and their effect on adult learning: A constructivist perspective. In S. M. Nielsen & M. S. Plakhotnik (Eds.), *Proceedings of the Sixth Annual College of Education Research Conference: Urban and International Education Section* (pp. 108–113). Florida International University. https://digitalcommons.fiu.edu/cgi/viewcontent.cgi?article=1270&context=sferc.

Chapter 8. Escape

General Escape

Lecca, S., Meye, F. J., Trusel, M., Tchenio, A., Harris, J., Schwarz, M. K., Burdakov, D., Georges, F., & Mameli, M. (2017). Aversive stimuli drive hypothalamus-to-habenula excitation to promote escape behavior. *ELife, 6*, e30697. https://doi.org/10.7554/eLife.30697.

Schlund, M. W., & Cataldo, M. F. (2010). Amygdala involvement in human avoidance, escape and approach behavior. *NeuroImage, 53*(2), 769–776. https://doi.org/10.1016/j.neuroimage.2010.06.058.

Sege, C. T., Bradley, M. M., & Lang, P. J. (2017). Escaping aversive exposure. *Psychophysiology, 54*(6), 857–863. https://doi.org/10.1111/psyp.12842.

Sege, C. T., Bradley, M. M., & Lang, P. J. (2018). Avoidance and escape: Defensive reactivity and trait anxiety. *Behaviour Research and Therapy, 104*, 62–68. https://doi.org/10.1016/j.brat.2018.03.002.

Seligman, M. E. P., Maier, S. F., & Solomon, R. L. (1971). Chapter 6—Unpredictable and uncontrollable aversive events. In F. R. Brush (Ed.), *Aversive conditioning and learning* (pp. 347–400). Academic Press. https://doi.org/10.1016/B978-0-12-137950-6.50011-0.

Taylor, J. A., & Maher, B. A. (1959). Escape and displacement experience as variables in the recovery from approach-avoidance conflict. *Journal of Comparative and Physiological Psychology, 52*(5), 586–590. https://doi.org/10.1037/h0048042.

Taylor, J. A., & Rennie, B. (1961). Recovery from approach-avoidance conflict as a function of escape and displacement experiences. *Journal of Comparative and Physiological Psychology, 54*(3), 275–278. https://doi.org/10.1037/h0045554.

Weiner, H. (1964). Modification of escape responding in humans by increasing the magnitude of an aversive event. *Journal of the Experimental Analysis of Behavior, 7*(3), 277–279. https://doi.org/10.1901/jeab.1964.7-277.

Approach-Avoidance

Bach, D. R., Guitart-Masip, M., Packard, P. A., Miró, J., Falip, M., Fuentemilla, L., & Dolan, R. J. (2014). Human hippocampus arbitrates approach-avoidance conflict. *Current Biology, 24*(5), 541–547. https://doi.org/10.1016/j.cub.2014.01.046.

Carver, C. S. (2006). Approach, avoidance, and the self-regulation of affect and action. *Motivation and Emotion, 30*(2), 105–110. https://doi.org/10.1007/s11031-006-9044-7.

Corr, P. J. (2013). Approach and avoidance behaviour: Multiple systems and their interactions. *Emotion Review, 5*(3), 285–290. https://doi.org/10.1177/1754073913477507.

Corr, P. J., & Krupić, D. (2017). Chapter 2—Motivating personality: Approach, avoidance, and their conflict. In A. J. Elliot (Ed.), *Advances in motivation science* (Vol. 4, pp. 39–90). Elsevier. https://doi.org/10.1016/bs.adms.2017.02.003.

Elliot, A. J. (2006). The hierarchical model of approach-avoidance motivation. *Motivation and Emotion, 30*(2), 111–116. https://doi.org/10.1007/s11031-006-9028-7.

Elliot, A. J., Eder, A. B., & Harmon-Jones, E. (2013). Approach–avoidance motivation and emotion: Convergence and divergence. *Emotion Review, 5*(3), 308–311. https://doi.org/10.1177/1754073913477517.

McNaughton, N., DeYoung, C. G., & Corr, P. J. (2016). Chapter 2—Approach/avoidance. In J. R. Absher & J. Cloutier (Eds.), *Neuroimaging personality, social cognition, and character* (pp. 25–49). Academic Press. https://doi.org/10.1016/B978-0-12-800935-2.00002-6.

Roth, S., & Cohen, L. J. (1986). Approach, avoidance, and coping with stress. *American Psychologist, 41*(7), 813–819. https://doi.org/10.1037/0003-066X.41.7.813.

Saga, Y., Ruff, C. C., & Tremblay, L. (2019). Disturbance of approach-avoidance behaviors in non-human primates by stimulation of the limbic territories of basal ganglia and anterior insula. *European Journal of Neuroscience, 49*(5), 687–700. https://doi.org/10.1111/ejn.14201.

Sabotage

Berger, D. (2005). Defenses can sabotage the therapy. *Psychiatric Times, 22*(12). https://www.psychiatrictimes.com/view/defenses-can-sabotage-therapy.

Sansone, R. A., Bohinc, R. J., & Wiederman, M. W. (2015). Healthcare adherence among patients who report the self-sabotage of their own medical care. *Innovations in Clinical Neuroscience, 12*(9–10), 10–12.

Sansone, R. A., & Sansone, L. A. (1995). Borderline personality disorder. *Postgraduate Medicine, 97*(6), 169–179. https://doi.org/10.1080/00325481.1995.11946012.

Benevolent Persuasion

Emanuel, E. J., & Emanuel, L. L. (1992). Four models of the physician-patient relationship. *Journal of the American Medical Association, 267*(16), 2221–2226. https://doi.org/10.1001/jama.1992.03480160079038.

Kaplan, S. H., Greenfield, S., & Ware, J. E. (1989). Assessing the effects of physician-patient interactions on the outcomes of chronic disease. *Medical Care, 27*(3), S110–S127.

Lazare, A., Eisenthal, S., & Frank, A. (1989). Clinician/patient relations II: Conflict and negotiation. In *Outpatient psychiatry: Diagnosis and treatment* (2nd ed., pp. 137–152). Williams & Wilkins.

Marzuk, P. M. (1985). The right kind of paternalism. *New England Journal of Medicine, 313*(23), 1474–1476. https://doi.org/10.1056/NEJM198512053132310.

Quill, T. E. (1983). Partnerships in patient care: A contractual approach. *Annals of Internal Medicine, 98*(2), 228–234. https://doi.org/10.7326/0003-4819-98-2-228.

Quill, T. E., & Brody, H. (1996). Physician recommendations and patient autonomy: Finding a balance between physician power and patient choice. *Annals of Internal Medicine, 125*(9), 763–769. https://doi.org/10.7326/0003-4819-125-9-199611010-00010.

Quill, T. E., & Cassel, C. K. (1995). Nonabandonment: A central obligation for physicians. *Annals of Internal Medicine, 122*(5), 368–374. https://doi.org/10.7326/0003-4819-122-5-199503010-00008.

Resistance

Miller, W. R., & Rose, G. S. (2009). Toward a theory of motivational interviewing. *American Psychologist, 64*(6), 527–537. https://doi.org/10.1037/a0016830.

Miller, W., & Rollnick, S. (2002). *Motivational interviewing: Preparing people to change.* Guilford Press.

Shaffer, H. J., & Simoneau, G. (2001). Reducing resistance and denial by exercising ambivalence during the treatment of addiction. *Journal of Substance Abuse Treatment, 20*(1), 99–105. https://doi.org/10.1016/S0740-5472(00)00152-5.

Walitzer, K. S., Dermen, K. H., & Connors, G. J. (1999). Strategies for preparing clients for treatment: A review. *Behavior Modification, 23*(1), 129–151. https://doi.org/10.1177/0145445599231006.

Westra, H. A., & Dozois, D. J. A. (2006). Preparing clients for cognitive behavioral therapy: A randomized pilot study of motivational interviewing for anxiety. *Cognitive Therapy and Research, 30*(4), 481–498. https://doi.org/10.1007/s10608-006-9016-y.

Chapter 9. Medication

Anxiety and Withdrawal

Ditre, J. W., Kosiba, J. D., Zale, E. L., Zvolensky, M. J., & Maisto, S. A. (2016). Chronic pain status, nicotine withdrawal, and expectancies for smoking cessation among lighter smokers. *Annals of Behavioral Medicine, 50*(3), 427–435. https://doi. org/10.1007/s12160-016-9769-9.

Hogle, J. M., Kaye, J. T., & Curtin, J. J. (2010). Nicotine withdrawal increases threat-induced anxiety but not fear: Neuroadaptation in human addiction. *Biological Psychiatry, 68*(8), 719–725. https://doi.org/10.1016/j.biopsych.2010.06.003.

Hughes, J. R., Higgins, S. T., & Bickel, W. K. (1994). Nicotine withdrawal versus other drug withdrawal syndromes: Similarities and dissimilarities. *Addiction, 89*(11), 1461–1470. https://doi.org/10.1111/j.1360-0443.1994.tb03744.x.

Johnson, K. A., Stewart, S., Rosenfield, D., Steeves, D., & Zvolensky, M. J. (2012). Prospective evaluation of the effects of anxiety sensitivity and state anxiety in predicting acute nicotine withdrawal symptoms during smoking cessation. *Psychology of Addictive Behaviors, 26*(2), 289–297. https://doi.org/10.1037/a0024133.

Keizer, I., Gex-Fabry, M., Croquette, P., Humair, J.-P., & Khan, A. N. (2019). Tobacco craving and withdrawal symptoms in psychiatric patients during a motivational enhancement intervention based on a 26-hour smoking abstinence period. *Tobacco Prevention & Cessation, 5*(June). https://doi.org/10.18332/tpc/109785.

Langdon, K. J., Leventhal, A. M., Stewart, S., Rosenfield, D., Steeves, D., & Zvolensky, M. J. (2013). Anhedonia and anxiety sensitivity: Prospective relationships to nicotine withdrawal symptoms during smoking cessation. *Journal of Studies on Alcohol and Drugs, 74*(3), 469–478. https://doi.org/10.15288/jsad.2013.74.469.

Leach, P. T., Cordero, K. A., & Gould, T. J. (2013). The effects of acute nicotine, chronic nicotine, and withdrawal from chronic nicotine on performance of a cued appetitive response. *Behavioral Neuroscience, 127*(2), 303–310. https://doi.org/10.1037/a0031913.

Lydon-Staley, D. M., Cornblath, E. J., Blevins, A. S., & Bassett, D. S. (2021). Modeling brain, symptom, and behavior in the winds of change. *Neuropsychopharmacology, 46*(1), 20–32. https://doi.org/10.1038/s41386-020-00805-6.

Lydon-Staley, D. M., Schnoll, R. A., Hitsman, B., & Bassett, D. S. (2020). The network structure of tobacco withdrawal in a community sample of smokers treated with nicotine patch and behavioral counseling. *Nicotine & Tobacco Research, 22*(3), 408–414. https://doi.org/10.1093/ntr/nty250.

Molas, S., DeGroot, S. R., Zhao-Shea, R., & Tapper, A. R. (2017). Anxiety and nicotine dependence: emerging role of the habenulo-interpeduncular axis. *Trends in Pharmacological Sciences, 38*(2), 169–180. https://doi.org/10.1016/j.tips.2016.11.001.

Pang, X., Liu, L., Ngolab, J., Zhao-Shea, R., McIntosh, J. M., Gardner, P. D., & Tapper, A. R. (2016). Habenula cholinergic neurons regulate anxiety during nicotine withdrawal via nicotinic acetylcholine receptors. *Neuropharmacology, 107*, 294–304. https://doi.org/10.1016/j.neuropharm.2016.03.039.

Shiffman, S., Patten, C., Gwaltney, C., Paty, J., Gnys, M., Kassel, J., Hickcox, M., Waters, A., & Balabanis, M. (2006). Natural history of nicotine withdrawal. *Addiction, 101*(12), 1822–1832. https://doi.org/10.1111/j.1360-0443.2006.01635.x.

Zhao-Shea, R., DeGroot, S. R., Liu, L., Vallaster, M., Pang, X., Su, Q., Gao, G., Rando, O. J., Martin, G. E., George, O., Gardner, P. D., & Tapper, A. R. (2015). Increased CRF signalling in a ventral tegmental area-interpeduncular nucleus-medial habenula circuit induces anxiety during nicotine withdrawal. *Nature Communications, 6*(1), 6770. https://doi.org/10.1038/ncomms7770.

Quit Process

Cofta-Woerpel, L., McClure, J. B., Li, Y., Urbauer, D., Cinciripini, P. M., & Wetter, D. W. (2011). Early cessation success or failure among women attempting to quit smoking: Trajectories and volatility of urge and negative mood during the first postcessation week. *Journal of Abnormal Psychology, 120*(3), 596–606. https://doi.org/10.1037/a0023755.

DiClemente, C. C., & Prochaska, J. O. (1982). Self-change and therapy change of smoking behavior: A comparison of processes of change in cessation and maintenance. *Addictive Behaviors, 7*(2), 133–142. https://doi.org/10.1016/0306-4603(82)90038-7.

Kovač, V. B., Rise, J., & Moan, I. S. (2009). From intentions to quit to the actual quitting process: The case of smoking behavior in light of the TPB. *Journal of Applied Biobehavioral Research, 14*(4), 181–197. https://doi.org/10.1111/j.1751-9861.2010.00048.x.

Mathew, A. R., Garrett-Mayer, E., Heckman, B. W., Wahlquist, A. E., & Carpenter, M. J. (2017). One-year smoking trajectories among established adult smokers with low baseline motivation to quit. *Nicotine & Tobacco Research, 20*(1), 50–57. https://doi.org/10.1093/ntr/ntw264.

McCarthy, D. E., Piasecki, T. M., Fiore, M. C., & Baker, T. B. (2006). Life before and after quitting smoking: An electronic diary study. *Journal of Abnormal Psychology, 115*(3), 454–466. https://doi.org/10.1037/0021-843X.115.3.454.

Rise, J., Kovac, V., Kraft, P., & Moan, I. S. (2008). Predicting the intention to quit smoking and quitting behaviour: Extending the theory of planned behaviour. *British Journal of Health Psychology, 13*(2), 291–310. https://doi.org/10.1348/135910707X187245.

Rogers, A. H., Bakhshaie, J., Garey, L., Piasecki, T. M., Gallagher, M. W., Schmidt, N. B., & Zvolensky, M. J. (2019). Individual differences in emotion dysregulation and trajectory of withdrawal symptoms during a quit attempt among treatment-seeking smokers. *Contemporary Issues in Behavioral Medicine, 115*, 4–11. https://doi.org/10.1016/j.brat.2018.10.007.

Schnoll, R. A., Malstrom, M., James, C., Rothman, R. L., Miller, S. M., Ridge, J. A., Movsas, B., Langer, C., Unger, M., & Goldberg, M. (2002). Processes of change related to smoking behavior among cancer patients. *Cancer Practice, 10*(1), 11–19. https://doi.org/10.1046/j.1523-5394.2002.101009.x.

Shiffman, S. (2005). Dynamic influences on smoking relapse process. *Journal of Personality, 73*(6), 1715–1748. https://doi.org/10.1111/j.0022-3506.2005.00364.x.

Shiffman, S., Engberg, J. B., Paty, J. A., Perz, W. G., Gnys, M., Kassel, J. D., & Hickcox, M. (1997). A day at a time: Predicting smoking lapse from daily urge. *Journal of Abnormal Psychology, 106*(1), 104–116. https://doi.org/10.1037/0021-843X.106.1.104.

Shiffman, S., Paty, J. A., Gnys, M., Kassel, J. A., & Hickcox, M. (1996). First lapses to smoking: Within-subjects analysis of real-time reports. *Journal of Consulting and Clinical Psychology, 64*(2), 366–379. https://doi.org/10.1037/0022-006X.64.2.366.

Shiffman, S., Scharf, D. M., Shadel, W. G., Gwaltney, C. J., Dang, Q., Paton, S. M., & Clark, D. B. (2006). Analyzing milestones in smoking cessation: Illustration in a nicotine patch trial in adult smokers. *Journal of Consulting and Clinical Psychology, 74*(2), 276–285. https://doi.org/10.1037/0022-006X.74.2.276.

Nicotine Patch

Fiore, M. C., Jorenby, D. E., Baker, T. B., & Kenford, S. L. (1992). Tobacco dependence and the nicotine patch: Clinical guidelines for effective use. *Journal of the American Medical Association*, *268*(19), 2687–2694. https://doi.org/10.1001/jama.1992.03490190087036.

Fiore, M. C., Kenford, S. L., Jorenby, D. E., Wetter, D. W., Smith, S. S., & Baker, T. B. (1994). Two studies of the clinical effectiveness of the nicotine patch with different counseling treatments. *Chest*, *105*(2), 524–533. https://doi.org/10.1378/chest.105.2.524.

Fiore, M. C., Smith, S. S., Jorenby, D. E., & Baker, T. B. (1994). The effectiveness of the nicotine patch for smoking cessation: A meta-analysis. *Journal of the American Medical Association*, *271*(24), 1940–1947. https://doi.org/10.1001/jama.1994.03510480064036.

Fiscella, K., & Franks, P. (1996). Cost-effectiveness of the transdermal nicotine patch as an adjunct to physicians' smoking cessation counseling. *Journal of the American Medical Association*, *275*(16), 1247–1251. https://doi.org/10.1001/jama.1996.03530400035035.

Greenland, S., Satterfield, M. H., & Lanes, S. F. (1998). A meta-analysis to assess the incidence of adverse effects associated with the transdermal nicotine patch. *Drug Safety*, *18*(4), 297–308. https://doi.org/10.2165/00002018-199818040-00005.

Hurt, Richard D., Dale, L. C., Fredrickson, P. A., Caldwell, C. C., Lee, G. A., Offord, K. P., Lauger, G. G., Marušić, Z., Neese, L. W., & Lundberg, T. G. (1994). Nicotine patch therapy for smoking cessation combined with physician advice and nurse follow-up: One-year outcome and percentage of nicotine replacement. *Journal of the American Medical Association*, *271*(8), 595–600. https://doi.org/10.1001/jama.1994.03510320035026.

Hurt, R. D., Lauger, G. G., Offord, K. P., Kottke, T. E., & Dale, L. C. (1990). Nicotine-replacement therapy with use of a transdermal nicotine patch—a randomized double-blind placebo-controlled trial. *Mayo Clinic Proceedings*, *65*(12), 1529–1537. https://doi.org/10.1016/S0025-6196(12)62186-7.

Imperial Cancer Research Fund General Practice Research Group. (1993). Effectiveness of a nicotine patch in helping people stop smoking: Results of a randomised trial in general practice. *British Medical Journal*, *306*(6888), 1304–1308. https://doi.org/10.1136/bmj.306.6888.1304.

Johnstone, E. C., Yudkin, P. L., Hey, K., Roberts, S. J., Welch, S. J., Murphy, M. F., Griffiths, S. E., & Walton, R. T. (2004). Genetic variation in dopaminergic pathways and short-term effectiveness of the nicotine patch. *Pharmacogenetics and Genomics*, *14*(2), 83–90.

Leischow, S. J., Muramoto, M. L., Cook, G. N., Merikle, E. P., Castellini, S. M., & Otte, P. S. (1999). OTC nicotine patch: Effectiveness alone and with brief physician intervention. *American Journal of Health Behavior*, *23*(1), 61–69. https://doi.org/10.5993/AJHB.23.1.7.

Richmond, R. L., Harris, K., & Neto, A. de A. (1994). The transdermal nicotine patch: Results of a randomised placebo-controlled trial. *Medical Journal of Australia*, *161*(2), 130–135. https://doi.org/10.5694/j.1326-5377.1994.tb127344.x.

Sachs, D. P., Säwe, U., & Leischow, S. J. (1993). Effectiveness of a 16-hour transdermal nicotine patch in a medical practice setting, without intensive group counseling. *Archives of Internal Medicine, 153*(16), 1881–1890.

Shiffman, S., Di Marino, M. E., & Pillitteri, J. L. (2005). The effectiveness of nicotine patch and nicotine lozenge in very heavy smokers. *Journal of Substance Abuse Treatment, 28*(1), 49–55. https://doi.org/10.1016/j.jsat.2004.10.006.

Shiffman, S., Gorsline, J., & Gorodetzky, C. W. (2002). Efficacy of over-the-counter nicotine patch. *Nicotine & Tobacco Research, 4*(4), 477–483. https://doi.org/10.1080/1 462220021000018416.

Shiffman, S., Sweeney, C. T., & Dresler, C. M. (2005). Nicotine patch and lozenge are effective for women. *Nicotine & Tobacco Research, 7*(1), 119–127. https://doi.org/10 .1080/14622200412331328439.

Stapleton, J. A., Russell, M. a. H., Feyerabend, C., Wiseman, S. M., Gustavsson, G., Sawe, U., & Wiseman, D. (1995). Dose effects and predictors of outcome in a randomized trial of transdermal nicotine patches in general practice. *Addiction, 90*(1), 31–42. https://doi.org/10.1046/j.1360-0443.1995.901316.x.

Wasley, M. A., McNagny, S. E., Phillips, V. L., & Ahluwalia, J. S. (1997). The cost-effectiveness of the nicotine transdermal patch for smoking cessation. *Preventive Medicine, 26*(2), 264–270. https://doi.org/10.1006/pmed.1996.0127.

Bupropion

Dale, L. C., Glover, E. D., Sachs, D. P. L., Schroeder, D. R., Offord, K. P., Croghan, I. T., & Hurt, R. D. (2001). Bupropion for smoking cessation: Predictors of successful outcome. *Chest, 119*(5), 1357–1364. https://doi.org/10.1378/chest.119.5.1357.

Hayford, K. E., Patten, C. A., Rummans, T. A., Schroeder, D. R., Offord, K. P., Croghan, I. T., Glover, E. D., Sachs, D. P. L., & Hurt, R. D. (1999). Efficacy of bupropion for smoking cessation in smokers with a former history of major depression or alcoholism. *British Journal of Psychiatry, 174*(2), 173–178. https://doi.org/10.1192/ bjp.174.2.173.

Hays, J. T., & Ebbert, J. O. (2003). Bupropion for the treatment of tobacco dependence. *CNS Drugs, 17*(2), 71–83. https://doi.org/10.2165/00023210-200317020-00001.

Holmes, S., Zwar, N., Jiménez-Ruiz, C. A., Ryan, P. J., Browning, D., Bergmann, L., & Johnston, J. A. (2004). Bupropion as an aid to smoking cessation: A review of real-life effectiveness. *International Journal of Clinical Practice, 58*(3), 285–291. https://doi.org/10.1111/j.1368-5031.2004.00153.x.

Hurt, R. D., Sachs, D. P. L., Glover, E. D., Offord, K. P., Johnston, J. A., Dale, L. C., Khayrallah, M. A., Schroeder, D. R., Glover, P. N., Sullivan, C. R., Croghan, I. T., & Sullivan, P. M. (1997). A comparison of sustained-release bupropion and placebo for smoking cessation. *New England Journal of Medicine, 337*(17), 1195–1202. https://doi.org/10.1056/NEJM199710233371703.

Jorenby, D. (2002). Clinical efficacy of bupropion in the management of smoking cessation. *Drugs, 62*(Suppl. 2), 25–35.

Lerman, C., Roth, D., Kaufmann, V., Audrain, J., Hawk, L., Liu, A., Niaura, R., & Epstein, L. (2002). Mediating mechanisms for the impact of bupropion in smoking cessation treatment. *Drug and Alcohol Dependence, 67*(2), 219–223. https://doi. org/10.1016/S0376-8716(02)00067-4.

Richmond, R., & Zwar, N. (2003). Review of bupropion for smoking cessation. *Drug and Alcohol Review, 22*(2), 203–220. https://doi.org/10.1080/09595230100100642.

Roddy, E. (2004). Bupropion and other non-nicotine pharmacotherapies. *British Medical Journal, 328*(7438), 509–511. https://doi.org/10.1136/bmj.328.7438.509.

Scharf, D., & Shiffman, S. (2004). Are there gender differences in smoking cessation, with and without bupropion? Pooled- and meta-analyses of clinical trials of bupropion SR. *Addiction, 99*(11), 1462–1469. https://doi.org/10.1111/j.1360-0443.2004.00845.x.

Smith, S. S., McCarthy, D. E., Japuntich, S. J., Christiansen, B., Piper, M. E., Jorenby, D. E., Fraser, D. L., Fiore, M. C., Baker, T. B., & Jackson, T. C. (2009). Comparative effectiveness of 5 smoking cessation pharmacotherapies in primary care clinics. *Archives of Internal Medicine, 169*(22), 2148–2155. https://doi.org/10.1001/archinternmed.2009.426.

Stapleton, J., West, R., Hajek, P., Wheeler, J., Vangeli, E., Abdi, Z., O'Gara, C., McRobbie, H., Humphrey, K., Ali, R., Strang, J., & Sutherland, G. (2013). Randomized trial of nicotine replacement therapy (NRT), bupropion and NRT plus bupropion for smoking cessation: Effectiveness in clinical practice. *Addiction, 108*(12), 2193–2201. https://doi.org/10.1111/add.12304.

Swan, G. E., Jack, L. M., Curry, S., Chorost, M., Javitz, H., McAfee, T., & Dacey, S. (2003). Bupropion SR and counseling for smoking cessation in actual practice: Predictors of outcome. *Nicotine & Tobacco Research, 5*(6), 911–921. https://doi.org/10.1080/14622200310001646903.

Swan, G. E., McAfee, T., Curry, S. J., Jack, L. M., Javitz, H., Dacey, S., & Bergman, K. (2003). Effectiveness of bupropion sustained release for smoking cessation in a health care setting: A randomized trial. *Archives of Internal Medicine, 163*(19), 2337–2344. https://doi.org/10.1001/archinte.163.19.2337.

Warner, C., & Shoaib, M. (2005). How does bupropion work as a smoking cessation aid? *Addiction Biology, 10*(3), 219–231. https://doi.org/10.1080/13556210500222670.

Wilkes, S. (2008). The use of bupropion SR in cigarette smoking cessation. *International Journal of Chronic Obstructive Pulmonary Disease, 3*(1), 45–53.

Varenicline

Andreas, S., Chenot, J.-F., Diebold, R., Peachey, S., & Mann, K. (2013). Effectiveness of varenicline as an aid to smoking cessation in primary care: An observational study. *European Addiction Research, 19*(1), 47–54. https://doi.org/10.1159/000341638.

Annemans, L., Marbaix, S., Nackaerts, K., & Bartsch, P. (2015). Cost-effectiveness of retreatment with varenicline after failure with or relapse after initial treatment for smoking cessation. *Preventive Medicine Reports, 2*, 189–195. https://doi.org/10.1016/j.pmedr.2015.03.004.

Aubin, H.-J., Bobak, A., Britton, J. R., Oncken, C., Billing, C. B., Gong, J., Williams, K. E., & Reeves, K. R. (2008). Varenicline versus transdermal nicotine patch for smoking cessation: Results from a randomised open-label trial. *Thorax, 63*(8), 717–724. https://doi.org/10.1136/thx.2007.090647.

Baker, C. L., & Pietri, G. (2018). A cost-effectiveness analysis of varenicline for smoking cessation using data from the EAGLES trial. *ClinicoEconomics and Outcomes Research, 10*, 67–74. https://doi.org/10.2147/CEOR.S153897.

Boudrez, H., Gratziou, C., Messig, M., & Metcalfe, M. (2011). Effectiveness of varenicline as an aid to smoking cessation: Results of an inter-European observational

study. *Current Medical Research and Opinion, 27*(4), 769–775. https://doi.org/10.11
85/03007995.2011.557718.

Brose, L. S., West, R., & Stapleton, J. A. (2013). Comparison of the effectiveness of varenicline and combination nicotine replacement therapy for smoking cessation in
clinical practice. *Mayo Clinic Proceedings, 88*(3), 226–233. https://doi.org/10.1016/j.
mayocp.2012.11.013.

Ebbert, J. O., Croghan, I. T., Hurt, R. T., Schroeder, D. R., & Hays, J. T. (2016). Varenicline for smoking cessation in light smokers. *Nicotine & Tobacco Research, 18*(10),
2031–2035. https://doi.org/10.1093/ntr/ntw123.

Ebbert, J. O., Hughes, J. R., West, R. J., Rennard, S. I., Russ, C., McRae, T. D., Treadow, J.,
Yu, C.-R., Dutro, M. P., & Park, P. W. (2015). Effect of varenicline on smoking cessation through smoking reduction: A randomized clinical trial. *Journal of the American Medical Association, 313*(7), 687–694. https://doi.org/10.1001/jama.2015.280.

Ebbert, J. O., Wyatt, K. D., Hays, J. T., Klee, E. W., & Hurt, R. D. (2010). Varenicline for
smoking cessation: Efficacy, safety, and treatment recommendations. *Patient Preference and Adherence, 4,* 355–362.

Garrison, G. D., & Dugan, S. E. (2009). Varenicline: A first-line treatment option for
smoking cessation. *Clinical Therapeutics, 31*(3), 463–491. https://doi.org/10.1016/j.
clinthera.2009.03.021.

Gibbons, R. D., & Mann, J. J. (2013). Varenicline, smoking cessation, and neuropsychiatric adverse events. *American Journal of Psychiatry, 170*(12), 1460–1467. https://
doi.org/10.1176/appi.ajp.2013.12121599.

Grassi, M. C., Enea, D., Ferketich, A. K., Lu, B., Pasquariello, S., & Nencini, P. (2011).
Effectiveness of varenicline for smoking cessation: A 1-year follow-up study.
Journal of Substance Abuse Treatment, 41(1), 64–70. https://doi.org/10.1016/j.
jsat.2011.01.014.

Hajek, P., McRobbie, H., Myers Smith, K., Phillips, A., Cornwall, D., & Dhanji, A.-R.
(2015). Increasing varenicline dose in smokers who do not respond to the standard
dosage: A randomized clinical trial. *JAMA Internal Medicine, 175*(2), 266–271.
https://doi.org/10.1001/jamainternmed.2014.6916.

Hajek, P., Smith, K. M., Dhanji, A. R., & McRobbie, H. (2013). Is a combination of
varenicline and nicotine patch more effective in helping smokers quit than varenicline alone? A randomised controlled trial. *BMC Medicine, 11,* 140. https://doi.
org/10.1186/1741-7015-11-140.

Hays, J. T., Ebbert, J. O., & Sood, A. (2008). Efficacy and safety of varenicline for smoking cessation. *American Journal of Medicine, 121*(4, Suppl.), S32–S42. https://doi.
org/10.1016/j.amjmed.2008.01.017.

Howard, P., Knight, C., Boler, A., & Baker, C. (2008). Cost-utility analysis of varenicline versus existing smoking cessation strategies using the BENESCO simulation
model. *PharmacoEconomics, 26*(6), 497–511. https://doi.org/10.2165/00019053-
200826060-00004.

Kaur, K., Kaushal, S., & Chopra, S. C. (2009). Varenicline for smoking cessation: A
review of the literature. *Current Therapeutic Research, 70*(1), 35–54. https://doi.
org/10.1016/j.curtheres.2009.02.004.

Keating, G. M., & Siddiqui, M. A. A. (2006). Varenicline. *CNS Drugs, 20*(11), 945–960.
https://doi.org/10.2165/00023210-200620110-00007.

Koegelenberg, C. F. N., Noor, F., Bateman, E. D., van Zyl-Smit, R. N., Bruning, A.,

O'Brien, J. A., Smith, C., Abdool-Gaffar, M. S., Emanuel, S., Esterhuizen, T. M., & Irusen, E. M. (2014). Efficacy of varenicline combined with nicotine replacement therapy vs varenicline alone for smoking cessation: A randomized clinical trial. *Journal of the American Medical Association, 312*(2), 155–161. https://doi.org/10.1001/jama.2014.7195.

Kotz, D., Brown, J., & West, R. (2014). Prospective cohort study of the effectiveness of varenicline versus nicotine replacement therapy for smoking cessation in the "real world." *BMC Public Health, 14*(1), 1163. https://doi.org/10.1186/1471-2458-14-1163.

McKee, S. A., Smith, P. H., Kaufman, M., Mazure, C. M., & Weinberger, A. H. (2016). Sex differences in varenicline efficacy for smoking cessation: A meta-analysis. *Nicotine & Tobacco Research, 18*(5), 1002–1011. https://doi.org/10.1093/ntr/ntv207.

Niaura, R., Hays, J. T., Jorenby, D. E., Leone, F. T., Pappas, J. E., Reeves, K. R., Williams, K. E., & Billing, C. B. (2008). The efficacy and safety of varenicline for smoking cessation using a flexible dosing strategy in adult smokers: A randomized controlled trial. *Current Medical Research and Opinion, 24*(7), 1931–1941. https://doi.org/10.1185/03007990802177523.

Ramon, J. M., & Bruguera, E. (2009). Real world study to evaluate the effectiveness of varenicline and cognitive-behavioural interventions for smoking cessation. *International Journal of Environmental Research and Public Health, 6*(4), 1530–1538. https://doi.org/10.3390/ijerph6041530.

Rollema, H., Chambers, L. K., Coe, J. W., Glowa, J., Hurst, R. S., Lebel, L. A., Lu, Y., Mansbach, R. S., Mather, R. J., Rovetti, C. C., Sands, S. B., Schaeffer, E., Schulz, D. W., Tingley, F. D., & Williams, K. E. (2007). Pharmacological profile of the α4β2 nicotinic acetylcholine receptor partial agonist varenicline, an effective smoking cessation aid. *Neuropharmacology, 52*(3), 985–994. https://doi.org/10.1016/j.neuropharm.2006.10.016.

Taylor, G. M., Taylor, A. E., Thomas, K. H., Jones, T., Martin, R. M., Munafò, M. R., Windmeijer, F., & Davies, N. M. (2017). The effectiveness of varenicline versus nicotine replacement therapy on long-term smoking cessation in primary care: A prospective cohort study of electronic medical records. *International Journal of Epidemiology, 46*(6), 1948–1957. https://doi.org/10.1093/ije/dyx109.

Tonstad, S., & Els, C. (2010). Varenicline: Smoking cessation in patients with medical and psychiatric comorbidity. *Clinical Medicine Insights: Therapeutics, 2*, CMT.S4012. https://doi.org/10.4137/CMT.S4012.

Tonstad, S., & Rollema, H. (2010). Varenicline in smoking cessation. *Expert Review of Respiratory Medicine, 4*(3), 291–299. https://doi.org/10.1586/ers.10.27.

Walker, N., Gainforth, H., Kiparoglou, V., Robinson, H., Woerden, H. van, & West, R. (2018). Factors moderating the relative effectiveness of varenicline and nicotine replacement therapy in clients using smoking cessation services. *Addiction, 113*(2), 313–324. https://doi.org/10.1111/add.14004.

Williams, K. E., Reeves, K. R., Jr, C. B. B., Pennington, A. M., & Gong, J. (2007). A double-blind study evaluating the long-term safety of varenicline for smoking cessation. *Current Medical Research and Opinion, 23*(4), 793–801. https://doi.org/10.1185/030079907X182185.

Wu, P., Wilson, K., Dimoulas, P., & Mills, E. J. (2006). Effectiveness of smoking cessation therapies: A systematic review and meta-analysis. *BMC Public Health, 6*(1), 300. https://doi.org/10.1186/1471-2458-6-300.

Nicotine Gum and Lozenge

Atzori, G., Lemmonds, C. A., Kotler, M. L., Durcan, M. J., & Boyle, J. (2008). Efficacy of a nicotine (4 mg)-containing lozenge on the cognitive impairment of nicotine withdrawal. *Journal of Clinical Psychopharmacology, 28*(6), 667–674. https://doi.org/10.1097/JCP.0b013e31818c9bb8.

Cepeda-Benito, A. (1993). Meta-analytical review of the efficacy of nicotine chewing gum in smoking treatment programs. *Journal of Consulting and Clinical Psychology, 61*(5), 822–830. https://doi.org/10.1037/0022-006X.61.5.822.

Choi, J. H., Dresler, C. M., Norton, M. R., & Strahs, K. R. (2003). Pharmacokinetics of a nicotine polacrilex lozenge. *Nicotine & Tobacco Research, 5*(5), 635–644. https://doi.org/10.1080/1462220031000158690.

Ebbert, J. O., Dale, L. C., Severson, H., Croghan, I. T., Rasmussen, D. F., Schroeder, D. R., Vander Weg, M. W., & Hurt, R. D. (2007). Nicotine lozenges for the treatment of smokeless tobacco use. *Nicotine & Tobacco Research, 9*(2), 233–240. https://doi.org/10.1080/14622200601080349.

Ebbert, J. O., Severson, H. H., Croghan, I. T., Danaher, B. G., & Schroeder, D. R. (2009). A randomized clinical trial of nicotine lozenge for smokeless tobacco use. *Nicotine & Tobacco Research, 11*(12), 1415–1423. https://doi.org/10.1093/ntr/ntp154.

Etter, J.-F., Huguelet, P., Perneger, T. V., & Cornuz, J. (2009). Nicotine gum treatment before smoking cessation: A randomized trial. *Archives of Internal Medicine, 169*(11), 1028–1034. https://doi.org/10.1001/archinternmed.2009.12.

Fagerström, K. O. (1984). Effects of nicotine chewing gum and follow-up appointments in physician-based smoking cessation. *Preventive Medicine, 13*(5), 517–527. https://doi.org/10.1016/0091-7435(84)90020-3.

Fagerström, K. O., Schneider, N. G., & Lunell, E. (1993). Effectiveness of nicotine patch and nicotine gum as individual versus combined treatments for tobacco withdrawal symptoms. *Psychopharmacology, 111*(3), 271–277. https://doi.org/10.1007/BF02244941.

Herrera, N., Franco, R., Herrera, L., Partidas, A., Rolando, R., & Fagerström, K. O. (1995). Nicotine gum, 2 and 4 mg, for nicotine dependence: A double-blind placebo-controlled trial within a behavior modification support program. *Chest, 108*(2), 447–451. https://doi.org/10.1378/chest.108.2.447.

Houtsmuller, E. J., Henningfield, J. E., & Stitzer, M. L. (2003). Subjective effects of the nicotine lozenge: Assessment of abuse liability. *Psychopharmacology, 167*(1), 20–27. https://doi.org/10.1007/s00213-002-1361-2.

Hughes, J. R., & Miller, S. A. (1984). Nicotine gum to help stop smoking. *Journal of the American Medical Association, 252*(20), 2855–2858. https://doi.org/10.1001/jama.1984.03350200041018.

Hughes, J. R., Wadland, W. C., Fenwick, J. W., Lewis, J., & Bickel, W. K. (1991). Effect of cost on the self-administration and efficacy of nicotine gum: A preliminary study. *Preventive Medicine, 20*(4), 486–496. https://doi.org/10.1016/0091-7435(91)90046-7.

Kozlowski, L. T., Giovino, G. A., Edwards, B., DiFranza, J., Foulds, J., Hurt, R., Niaura, R., Sachs, D. P. L., Selby, P., Dollar, K. M., Bowen, D., Cummings, K. M., Counts, M., Fox, B., Sweanor, D., & Ahern, F. (2007). Advice on using over-the-counter nicotine replacement therapy-patch, gum, or lozenge-to quit smoking. *Addictive Behaviors, 32*(10), 2140–2150. https://doi.org/10.1016/j.addbeh.2007.01.030.

Marsh, H. S., Dresler, C. M., Choi, J. H., Targett, D. A., Gamble, M. L., & Strahs, K. R. (2005). Safety profile of a nicotine lozenge compared with thatof nicotine gum in adult smokers with underlying medical conditions: A 12-week, randomized, open-label study. *Clinical Therapeutics, 27*(10), 1571–1587. https://doi.org/10.1016/j.clinthera.2005.10.008.

Muramoto, M. L., Ranger-Moore, J., & Leischow, S. J. (2003). Efficacy of oral transmucosal nicotine lozenge for suppression of withdrawal symptoms in smoking abstinence. *Nicotine & Tobacco Research, 5*(2), 223–230. https://doi.org/10.1080/1 462220031000073270.

Oster, G., Huse, D. M., Delea, T. E., & Colditz, G. A. (1986). Cost-effectiveness of nicotine gum as an adjunct to physician's advice against cigarette smoking. *Journal of the American Medical Association, 256*(10), 1315–1318. https://doi.org/10.1001/jama.1986.03380100089026.

Pack, Q. R., Jorenby, D. E., Fiore, M. C., Jackson, T., Weston, P., Piper, M. E., & Baker, T. B. (2008). A comparison of the nicotine lozenge and nicotine gum an effectiveness randomized controlled trial. *Wisconsin Medical Journal, 107*(5), 237–243.

Shiffman, S. (2005). Nicotine lozenge efficacy in light smokers. *Drug and Alcohol Dependence, 77*(3), 311–314. https://doi.org/10.1016/j.drugalcdep.2004.08.026.

Shiffman, S. (2007). Use of more nicotine lozenges leads to better success in quitting smoking. *Addiction, 102*(5), 809–814. https://doi.org/10.1111/j.1360-0443.2007.01791.x.

Shiffman, S., Di Marino, M. E., & Pillitteri, J. L. (2005). The effectiveness of nicotine patch and nicotine lozenge in very heavy smokers. *Journal of Substance Abuse Treatment, 28*(1), 49–55. https://doi.org/10.1016/j.jsat.2004.10.006.

Shiffman, S., Dresler, C. M., Hajek, P., Gilburt, S. J. A., Targett, D. A., & Strahs, K. R. (2002). Efficacy of a nicotine lozenge for smoking cessation. *Archives of Internal Medicine, 162*(11), 1267–1276.

Shiffman, S., Dresler, C. M., & Rohay, J. M. (2004). Successful treatment with a nicotine lozenge of smokers with prior failure in pharmacological therapy. *Addiction, 99*(1), 83–92. https://doi.org/10.1111/j.1360-0443.2004.00576.x.

Shiffman, S., Shadel, W. G., Niaura, R., Khayrallah, M. A., Jorenby, D. E., Ryan, C. F., & Ferguson, C. L. (2003). Efficacy of acute administration of nicotine gum in relief of cue-provoked cigarette craving. *Psychopharmacology, 166*(4), 343–350. https://doi.org/10.1007/s00213-002-1338-1.

Nicotine Inhaler

Bohadana, A., Nilsson, F., Rasmussen, T., & Martinet, Y. (2000). Nicotine inhaler and nicotine patch as a combination therapy for smoking cessation: A randomized, double-blind, placebo-controlled trial. *Archives of Internal Medicine, 160*(20), 3128–3134. https://doi.org/10.1001/archinte.160.20.3128.

Bolliger, C. T., Zellweger, J.-P., Danielsson, T., Biljon, X. van, Robidou, A., Westin, Å., Perruchoud, A. P., & Säwe, U. (2000). Smoking reduction with oral nicotine inhalers: Double blind, randomised clinical trial of efficacy and safety. *British Medical Journal, 321*(7257), 329–333. https://doi.org/10.1136/bmj.321.7257.329.

Cipolla, D., & Gonda, I. (2015). Inhaled nicotine replacement therapy. *Asian Journal of Pharmaceutical Sciences, 10*(6), 472–480. https://doi.org/10.1016/j.ajps.2015.07.004.

Croghan, I. T., Hurt, R. D., Dakhil, S. R., Croghan, G. A., Sloan, J. A., Novotny, P. J., Rowland, K. M., Bernath, A., Loots, M. L., Le-Lindqwister, N. A., Tschetter, L. K., Garneau, S. C., Flynn, K. A., Ebbert, L. P., Wender, D. B., & Loprinzi, C. L. (2007). Randomized comparison of a nicotine inhaler and bupropion for smoking cessation and relapse prevention. *Mayo Clinic Proceedings, 82*(2), 186–195. https://doi.org/10.4065/82.2.186.

Hjalmarson, A., Nilsson, F., Sjöström, L., & Wiklund, O. (1997). The nicotine inhaler in smoking cessation. *Archives of Internal Medicine, 157*(15), 1721–1728. https://doi.org/10.1001/archinte.1997.00440360143016.

Kralikova, E., Kozak, J. T., Rasmussen, T., Gustavsson, G., & Le Houezec, J. (2009). Smoking cessation or reduction with nicotine replacement therapy: A placebo-controlled double blind trial with nicotine gum and inhaler. *BMC Public Health, 9*(1), 433. https://doi.org/10.1186/1471-2458-9-433.

Leischow, S. J., Ranger-Moore, J., Muramoto, M. L., & Matthews, E. (2004). Effectiveness of the nicotine inhaler for smoking cessation in an OTC setting. *American Journal of Health Behavior, 28*(4), 291–301. https://doi.org/10.5993/AJHB.28.4.1.

Rennard, S. I., Glover, E. D., Leischow, S., Daughton, D. M., Glover, P. N., Muramoto, M., Franzon, M., Danielsson, T., Landfeldt, B., & Westin, Å. (2006). Efficacy of the nicotine inhaler in smoking reduction: A double-blind, randomized trial. *Nicotine & Tobacco Research, 8*(4), 555–564. https://doi.org/10.1080/14622200600789916.

Schneider, N. G., Olmstead, R. E., Franzon, M. A., & Lunell, E. (2001). The nicotine inhaler. *Clinical Pharmacokinetics, 40*(9), 661–684. https://doi.org/10.2165/00003088-200140090-00003.

Schneider, N. G., Olmstead, R., Nilsson, F., Mody, F. V., Franzon, M., & Doan, K. (1996). Efficacy of a nicotine inhaler in smoking cessation: A double-blind, placebo-controlled trial. *Addiction, 91*(9), 1293–1306. https://doi.org/10.1046/j.1360-0443.1996.91912935.x.

Steinberg, M. B., Zimmermann, M. H., Delnevo, C. D., Lewis, M. J., Shukla, P., Coups, E. J., & Foulds, J. (2014). E-cigarette versus nicotine inhaler: Comparing the perceptions and experiences of inhaled nicotine devices. *Journal of General Internal Medicine, 11*(29), 1444–1450. https://doi.org/10.1007/s11606-014-2889-7.

Westman, E. C., Tomlin, K. F., & Rose, J. E. (2000). Combining the nicotine inhaler and nicotine patch for smoking cessation. *American Journal of Health Behavior, 24*(2), 114–119. https://doi.org/10.5993/AJHB.24.2.4.

Electronic Cigarettes

Anderson, C., Majeste, A., Hanus, J., & Wang, S. (2016). E-cigarette aerosol exposure induces reactive oxygen species, DNA damage, and cell death in vascular endothelial cells. *Toxicological Sciences, 154*(2), 332–340. https://doi.org/10.1093/toxsci/kfw166.

Bhatta, D. N., & Glantz, S. A. (2020). Association of e-cigarette use with respiratory disease among adults: A longitudinal analysis. *American Journal of Preventive Medicine, 58*(2), 182–190. https://doi.org/10.1016/j.amepre.2019.07.028.

Chatterjee, S., Caporale, A., Tao, J. Q., Guo, W., Johncola, A., Strasser, A. A., Leone, F. T., Langham, M. C., & Wehrli, F. W. (2020). Acute e-cig inhalation impacts vascular health: A study in smoking naïve subjects. *American Journal of Physiology—Heart and Circulatory Physiology, 320*(1), H144–H158. https://doi.org/10.1152/ajpheart.00628.2020.

Chun, L. F., Moazed, F., Calfee, C. S., Matthay, M. A., & Gotts, J. E. (2017). Pulmonary toxicity of e-cigarettes. *American Journal of Physiology—Lung Cellular and Molecular Physiology, 313*(2), L193–L206. https://doi.org/10.1152/ajplung.00071.2017.

Darquenne, C. (2012). Aerosol deposition in health and disease. *Journal of Aerosol Medicine and Pulmonary Drug Delivery, 25*(3), 140–147. https://doi.org/10.1089/jamp.2011.0916.

Eissenberg, T., Bhatnagar, A., Chapman, S., Jordt, S.-E., Shihadeh, A., & Soule, E. K. (2020). Invalidity of an oft-cited estimate of the relative harms of electronic cigarettes. *American Journal of Public Health, 110*(2), 161–162. https://doi.org/10.2105/AJPH.2019.305424.

Gotts, J. E., Jordt, S.-E., McConnell, R., & Tarran, R. (2019). What are the respiratory effects of e-cigarettes? *British Medical Journal, 366*, l5275. https://doi.org/10.1136/bmj.l5275.

Historical timeline of vaping and electronic cigarettes. (n.d.). CASAA. Retrieved January 18, 2021, from https://casaa.org/education/vaping/historical-timeline-of-electronic-cigarettes/.

Hwang, J. H., Lyes, M., Sladewski, K., Enany, S., McEachern, E., Mathew, D. P., Das, S., Moshensky, A., Bapat, S., Pride, D. T., Ongkeko, W. M., & Crotty Alexander, L. E. (2016). Electronic cigarette inhalation alters innate immunity and airway cytokines while increasing the virulence of colonizing bacteria. *Journal of Molecular Medicine, 94*(6), 667–679. https://doi.org/10.1007/s00109-016-1378-3.

Khouja, J. N., Suddell, S. F., Peters, S. E., Taylor, A. E., & Munafò, M. R. (2020). Is e-cigarette use in non-smoking young adults associated with later smoking? A systematic review and meta-analysis. *Tobacco Control, 10*(30), 8–15. https://doi.org/10.1136/tobaccocontrol-2019-055433.

Leone, F. T., Carlsen, K.-H., Chooljian, D., Crotty Alexander, L. E., Detterbeck, F. C., Eakin, M. N., Evers-Casey, S., Farber, H. J., Folan, P., Kathuria, H., Latzka, K., McDermott, S., McGrath-Morrow, S., Moazed, F., Munzer, A., Neptune, E., Pakhale, S., Sachs, D. P. L., Samet, J., . . . Upson, D. (2018). Recommendations for the appropriate structure, communication, and investigation of tobacco harm reduction claims: An official American Thoracic Society policy statement. *American Journal of Respiratory and Critical Care Medicine, 198*(8), e90–e105. https://doi.org/10.1164/rccm.201808-1443ST.

Mayer, M., Reyes-Guzman, C., Grana, R., Choi, K., & Freedman, N. D. (2020). Demographic characteristics, cigarette smoking, and e-cigarette use among US adults. *JAMA Network Open, 3*(10), e2020694–e2020694. https://doi.org/10.1001/jamanetworkopen.2020.20694.

National Academies of Sciences, Engineering, and Medicine, & Board on Population Health and Public Health. (2018). *Public health consequences of e-cigarettes.* National Academies Press.

Nutt, D. J., Phillips, L. D., Balfour, D., Curran, H. V., Dockrell, M., Foulds, J., Fagerstrom, K., Letlape, K., Milton, A., Polosa, R., Ramsey, J., & Sweanor, D. (2014).

Estimating the harms of nicotine-containing products using the MCDA approach. *European Addiction Research, 20*(5), 218–225. https://doi.org/10.1159/000360220.

Royal College of Physicians. (2016, April 28). Nicotine without smoke: Tobacco harm reduction. RCP London. https://www.rcplondon.ac.uk/projects/outputs/nicotine-without-smoke-tobacco-harm-reduction-0.

Soneji, S., Barrington-Trimis, J. L., Wills, T. A., Leventhal, A. M., Unger, J. B., Gibson, L. A., Yang, J., Primack, B. A., Andrews, J. A., Miech, R. A., Spindle, T. R., Dick, D. M., Eissenberg, T., Hornik, R. C., Dang, R., & Sargent, J. D. (2017). Association between initial use of e-cigarettes and subsequent cigarette smoking among adolescents and young adults: A systematic review and meta-analysis. *JAMA Pediatrics, 171*(8), 788–797. https://doi.org/10.1001/jamapediatrics.2017.1488.

Wang, J. B., Olgin, J. E., Nah, G., Vittinghoff, E., Cataldo, J. K., Pletcher, M. J., & Marcus, G. M. (2018). Cigarette and e-cigarette dual use and risk of cardiopulmonary symptoms in the Health eHeart Study. *PLOS One, 13*(7), e0198681. https://doi.org/10.1371/journal.pone.0198681.

Wang, R. J., Bhadriraju, S., & Glantz, S. A. (2021). E-cigarette use and adult cigarette smoking cessation: A meta-analysis. *American Journal of Public Health, 111*(2), 230–246. https://doi.org/10.2105/AJPH.2020.305999.

Wang, T. W., Gentzke, A. S., Creamer, M. R., Cullen, K. A., Holder-Hayes, E., Sawdey, M. D., Anic, G. M., Portnoy, D. B., Hu, S., Homa, D. M., Jamal, A., & Neff, L. J. (2019). Tobacco product use and associated factors among middle and high school students—United States, 2019. *MMWR Surveillance Summaries, 68*(12), 1–22. https://doi.org/10.15585/mmwr.ss6812a1.

Wolff, R. K. (2015). Toxicology studies for inhaled and nasal delivery. *Molecular Pharmaceutics, 12*(8), 2688–2696. https://doi.org/10.1021/acs.molpharmaceut.5b00146.

Xie, W., Kathuria, H., Galiatsatos, P., Blaha, M. J., Hamburg, N. M., Robertson, R. M., Bhatnagar, A., Benjamin, E. J., & Stokes, A. C. (2020). Association of electronic cigarette use with incident respiratory conditions among US adults from 2013 to 2018. *JAMA Network Open, 3*(11), e2020816–e2020816. https://doi.org/10.1001/jamanetworkopen.2020.20816.

Nicotine Nasal Spray

Blondal, T., Franzon, M., & Westin, A. (1997). A double-blind randomized trial of nicotine nasal spray as an aid in smoking cessation. *European Respiratory Journal, 10*(7), 1585–1590.

Croghan, G. A., Sloan, J. A., Croghan, I. T., Novotny, P., Hurt, R. D., DeKrey, W. L., Walsh, D. J., Mailliard, J. A., Ebbert, L. P., Swan, D. K., Walsh, D. J., Wiesenfeld, M., Levitt, R., Stella, P., Johnson, P. A., Tschetter, L. K., & Loprinzi, C. (2003). Comparison of nicotine patch alone versus nicotine nasal spray alone versus a combination for treating smokers: A minimal intervention, randomized multicenter trial in a nonspecialized setting. *Nicotine & Tobacco Research, 5*(2), 181–187. https://doi.org/10.1080/1462220031000073252.

Fishbein, L., O'Brien, P., Hutson, A., Theriaque, D., Stacpoole, P., & Flotte, T. (2000). Pharmacokinetics and pharmacodynamic effects of nicotine nasal spray devices on cardiovascular and pulmonary function. *Journal of Investigative Medicine, 48*(6), 435–440.

Hajek, P., West, R., Foulds, J., Nilsson, F., Burrows, S., & Meadow, A. (1999). Randomized comparative trial of nicotine polacrilex, a transdermal patch, nasal spray, and an inhaler. *Archives of Internal Medicine*, 159(17), 2033–2038. https://doi.org/10.1001/archinte.159.17.2033.

Hjalmarson, A., Franzon, M., Westin, A., & Wiklund, O. (1994). Effect of nicotine nasal spray on smoking cessation: A randomized, placebo-controlled, double-blind study. *Archives of Internal Medicine*, 154(22), 2567–2572. https://doi.org/10.1001/archinte.1994.00420220059007.

Hurt, R. D., Dale, L. C., Croghan, G. A., Croghan, I. T., Gomez-Dahl, L. C., & Offord, K. P. (1998). Nicotine nasal spray for smoking cessation: Pattern of use, side effects, relief of withdrawal symptoms, and cotinine levels. *Mayo Clinic Proceedings*, 73(2), 118–125. https://doi.org/10.1016/S0025-6196(11)63642-2.

Hurt, R. D., Offord, K. P., Croghan, I. T., Croghan, G. A., Gomez-Dahl, L. C., Wolter, T. D., Dale, L. C., & Moyer, T. P. (1998). Temporal effects of nicotine nasal spray and gum on nicotine withdrawal symptoms. *Psychopharmacology*, 140(1), 98–104. https://doi.org/10.1007/s002130050744.

Jones, R. L., Nguyen, A., & Man, S. F. P. (1998). Nicotine and cotinine replacement when nicotine nasal spray is used to quit smoking. *Psychopharmacology*, 137(4), 345–350. https://doi.org/10.1007/s002130050629.

Schneider, N. G. (1994). Nicotine nasal spray. *Health Values: The Journal of Health Behavior, Education & Promotion*, 18(3), 10–14.

Schneider, N. G., Lunell, E., Olmstead, R. E., & Fagerström, K.-O. (1996). Clinical pharmacokinetics of nasal nicotine delivery. *Clinical Pharmacokinetics*, 31(1), 65–80. https://doi.org/10.2165/00003088-199631010-00005.

Schneider, N. G., Olmstead, R., Mody, F. V., Doan, K., Franzon, M., Jarvik, M. E., & Steinberg, C. (1995). Efficacy of a nicotine nasal spray in smoking cessation: A placebo-controlled, double-blind trial. *Addiction*, 90(12), 1671–1682. https://doi.org/10.1046/j.1360-0443.1995.901216719.x.

Schuh, K. J., Schuh, L. M., Henningfield, J. E., & Stitzer, M. L. (1997). Nicotine nasal spray and vapor inhaler: Abuse liability assessment. *Psychopharmacology*, 130(4), 352–361. https://doi.org/10.1007/s002130050250.

Stapleton, J. A., & Sutherland, G. (2011). Treating heavy smokers in primary care with the nicotine nasal spray: Randomized placebo-controlled trial. *Addiction*, 106(4), 824–832. https://doi.org/10.1111/j.1360-0443.2010.03274.x.

Sutherland, G., Stapleton, J. A., Russell, M. A. H., Jarvis, M. J., Hajek, P., Belcher, M., & Feyerabend, C. (1992). Randomised controlled trial of nasal nicotine spray in smoking cessation. *Lancet*, 340(8815), 324–329. https://doi.org/10.1016/0140-6736(92)91403-U.

Clinical Guidance Documents

American College of Obstetricians and Gynecologists. (2017). Tobacco and nicotine cessation during pregnancy. ACOG Committee on Obstetric Practice, opinion no. 807. https://www.acog.org/en/Clinical/Clinical Guidance/Committee Opinion/Articles/2020/05/Tobacco and Nicotine Cessation During Pregnancy.

Barua, R. S., Rigotti, N. A., Benowitz, N. L., Cummings, K. M., Jazayeri, M.-A., Morris, P. B., Ratchford, E. V., Sarna, L., Stecker, E. C., & Wiggins, B. S. (2018). 2018 ACC expert consensus decision pathway on tobacco cessation treatment: A report of the American College of Cardiology Task Force on Clinical Expert Consensus Documents. *Journal of the American College of Cardiology, 72*(25), 3332–3365. https://doi.org/10.1016/j.jacc.2018.10.027.

European Network for Smoking and Tobacco Prevention. (2021). Guidelines for treating tobacco dependence. https://ensp.network/ensp-tdt-guidelines/.

Fiore, M., Jaén, C., Baker, T., & et al. (2008). *Treating tobacco use and dependence: 2008 update.* Clinical practice guideline. U.S. Department of Health and Human Services, Public Health Service. https://www.ncbi.nlm.nih.gov/books/NBK63952/.

Leone, F. T., Evers-Casey, S., Toll, B. A., & Vachani, A. (2013). Treatment of tobacco use in lung cancer: Diagnosis and management of lung cancer (3rd ed.)—American College of Chest Physicians Evidence-Based Clinical Practice Guidelines. *Chest, 143*(Suppl. 5), e61S–77S. https://doi.org/10.1378/chest.12-2349.

Leone, F. T., Zhang, Y., Evers-Casey, S., Evins, A. E., Eakin, M. N., Fathi, J., Fennig, K., Folan, P., Galiatsatos, P., Gogineni, H., Kantrow, S., Kathuria, H., Lamphere, T., Neptune, E., Pacheco, M. C., Pakhale, S., Prezant, D., Sachs, D. P. L., Toll, B., . . . Farber, H. J. (2020). Initiating pharmacologic treatment in tobacco-dependent adults: An official American Thoracic Society Clinical Practice Guideline. *American Journal of Respiratory and Critical Care Medicine, 202*(2), e5–e31. https://doi.org/10.1164/rccm.202005-1982ST.

Patnode, C. D., Henderson, J. T., Melnikow, J., Coppola, E. L., Durbin, S., & Thomas, R. (2021). *Interventions for tobacco cessation in adults, including pregnant women: An evidence update for the U.S. Preventive Services Task Force.* Agency for Healthcare Research and Quality (US). http://www.ncbi.nlm.nih.gov/books/NBK567066/.

Richter, K. P., & Arnsten, J. H. (2006). A rationale and model for addressing tobacco dependence in substance abuse treatment. *Substance Abuse Treatment, Prevention, and Policy, 1*(1), 23. https://doi.org/10.1186/1747-597X-1-23.

Shields, P. G., Herbst, R. S., Arenberg, D., Benowitz, N. L., Bierut, L., Luckart, J. B., Cinciripini, P., Collins, B., David, S., Davis, J., Hitsman, B., Hyland, A., Lang, M., Leischow, S., Park, E. R., Purcell, W. T., Selzle, J., Silber, A., Spencer, S., . . . Scavone, J. (2016). Smoking cessation, version 1.2016, NCCN Clinical Practice Guidelines in Oncology. *Journal of the National Comprehensive Cancer Network, 14*(11), 1430–1468. https://doi.org/10.6004/jnccn.2016.0152.

U.S. Preventive Services Task Force. (2016). Behavioral and pharmacotherapy interventions for tobacco smoking cessation in adults, including pregnant women: Recommendation statement. *American Family Physician, 93*(10). https://www.aafp.org/afp/2016/0515/od1.html.

Chapter 10. Management

Adherence

Battaglioli-DeNero, A. M. (2007). Strategies for improving patient adherence to therapy and long-term patient outcomes. *Journal of the Association of Nurses in AIDS Care, 18*(Suppl. 1), S17–S22. https://doi.org/10.1016/j.jana.2006.11.020.

DiMatteo, M. R., Haskard-Zolnierek, K. B., & Martin, L. R. (2012). Improving patient adherence: A three-factor model to guide practice. *Health Psychology Review, 6*(1), 74–91. https://doi.org/10.1080/17437199.2010.537592.

Gadkari, A. S., & McHorney, C. A. (2012). Unintentional non-adherence to chronic prescription medications: How unintentional is it really? *BMC Health Services Research, 12*(1), 98. https://doi.org/10.1186/1472-6963-12-98.

Goldsmith, L. J., Kolhatkar, A., Popowich, D., Holbrook, A. M., Morgan, S. G., & Law, M. R. (2017). Understanding the patient experience of cost-related non-adherence to prescription medications through typology development and application. *Social Science & Medicine, 194*, 51–59. https://doi.org/10.1016/j.socscimed.2017.10.007.

Gross, R., Bellamy, S. L., Chapman, J., Han, X., O'Duor, J., Palmer, S. C., Houts, P. S., Coyne, J. C., & Strom, B. L. (2013). Managed problem solving for antiretroviral therapy adherence: A randomized trial. *JAMA Internal Medicine, 173*(4), 300–306. https://doi.org/10.1001/jamainternmed.2013.2152.

Maciel, E. M. G. de S., Amancio, J. de S., Castro, D. B. de, & Braga, J. U. (2018). Social determinants of pulmonary tuberculosis treatment non-adherence in Rio de Janeiro, Brazil. *PLOS One, 13*(1), e0190578. https://doi.org/10.1371/journal.pone.0190578.

Rogliani, P., Ora, J., Puxeddu, E., Matera, M. G., & Cazzola, M. (2017). Adherence to COPD treatment: Myth and reality. *Respiratory Medicine, 129*, 117–123. https://doi.org/10.1016/j.rmed.2017.06.007.

Ruppar, T. M., Dobbels, F., Lewek, P., Matyjaszczyk, M., Siebens, K., & De Geest, S. M. (2015). Systematic review of clinical practice guidelines for the improvement of medication adherence. *International Journal of Behavioral Medicine, 22*(6), 699–708. https://doi.org/10.1007/s12529-015-9479-x.

Shah, N. D., Dunlay, S. M., Ting, H. H., Montori, V. M., Thomas, R. J., Wagie, A. E., & Roger, V. L. (2009). Long-term medication adherence after myocardial infarction: Experience of a community. *American Journal of Medicine, 122*(10), 961.e7–961. e13. https://doi.org/10.1016/j.amjmed.2008.12.021.

Smith, A. L., Carter, S. M., Chapman, S., Dunlop, S. M., & Freeman, B. (2015). Why do smokers try to quit without medication or counselling? A qualitative study with ex-smokers. *BMJ Open, 5*(4), e007301. https://doi.org/10.1136/bmjopen-2014-007301.

Ulrik, C. S., Backer, V., Søes-Petersen, U., Lange, P., Harving, H., & Plaschke, P. P. (2006). The patient's perspective: Adherence or non-adherence to asthma controller therapy? *Journal of Asthma, 43*(9), 701–704. https://doi.org/10.1080/02770900600925569.

Unni, E. J., & Farris, K. B. (2011). Unintentional non-adherence and belief in medicines in older adults. *Patient Education and Counseling, 83*(2), 265–268. https://doi.org/10.1016/j.pec.2010.05.006.

World Health Organization. (2003). *Adherence to long-term therapies: Evidence for action.* World Health Organization. https://apps.who.int/iris/bitstream/handle/10665/42682/9241545992.pdf;jsessionid=4007BCCCE84B70182BBB889D6B-C06CE0?sequence=1.

Phenotypes

Batra, V., Patkar, A. A., Berrettini, W. H., Weinstein, S. P., & Leone, F. T. (2003). The genetic determinants of smoking. *Chest, 123*(5), 1730–1739.

Bough, K. J., Lerman, C., Rose, J. E., McClernon, F. J., Kenny, P. J., Tyndale, R. F., David, S. P., Stein, E. A., Uhl, G. R., Conti, D. V., Green, C., & Amur, S. (2013). Biomarkers for smoking cessation. *Clinical Pharmacology & Therapeutics, 93*(6), 526–538. https://doi.org/10.1038/clpt.2013.57.

Flory, J. D., & Manuck, S. B. (2009). Impulsiveness and cigarette smoking. *Psychosomatic Medicine, 71*(4), 431–437. https://doi.org/10.1097/PSY.0b013e3181988c2d.

Munafò, M. R., & Johnstone, E. C. (2008). Genes and cigarette smoking. *Addiction, 103*(6), 893–904. https://doi.org/10.1111/j.1360-0443.2007.02071.x.

O'Loughlin, J., Sylvestre, M.-P., Labbe, A., Low, N. C., Roy-Gagnon, M.-H., Dugas, E. N., Karp, I., & Engert, J. C. (2014). Genetic variants and early cigarette smoking and nicotine dependence phenotypes in adolescents. *PLOS One, 9*(12), e115716. https://doi.org/10.1371/journal.pone.0115716.

Pomerleau, O. F., Pomerleau, C. S., Mehringer, A. M., Snedecor, S. M., Ninowski, R., & Sen, A. (2005). Nicotine dependence, depression, and gender: Characterizing phenotypes based on withdrawal discomfort, response to smoking, and ability to abstain. *Nicotine & Tobacco Research, 7*(1), 91–102. https://doi.org/10.1080/14622 200412331328466.

Schnoll, R. A., & Leone, F. T. (2011). Biomarkers to optimize the treatment of nicotine dependence. *Biomarkers in Medicine, 5*(6), 745–761. https://doi.org/10.2217/bmm.11.91.

Strasser, A. A., Souprountchouk, V., Kaufmann, A., Blazekovic, S., Leone, F., Benowitz, N. L., & Schnoll, R. A. (2016). Nicotine replacement, topography, and smoking phenotypes of e-cigarettes. *Tobacco Regulatory Science, 2*(4), 352–362. https://doi.org/10.18001/TRS.2.4.7.

Wang, J., & Li, M. D. (2010). Common and unique biological pathways associated with smoking initiation/progression, nicotine dependence, and smoking cessation. *Neuropsychopharmacology, 35*(3), 702–719. https://doi.org/10.1038/npp.2009.178.

Nicotine Metabolite Ratio

Allenby, C. E., Boylan, K. A., Lerman, C., & Falcone, M. (2016). Precision medicine for tobacco dependence: Development and validation of the nicotine metabolite ratio. *Journal of Neuroimmune Pharmacology, 11*(3), 471–483. https://doi.org/10.1007/s11481-016-9656-y.

Arger, C. A., Taghavi, T., Heil, S. H., Skelly, J., Tyndale, R. F., & Higgins, S. T. (2019). Pregnancy-induced increases in the nicotine metabolite ratio: Examining changes during antepartum and postpartum. *Nicotine & Tobacco Research, 21*(12), 1706–1710. https://doi.org/10.1093/ntr/nty172.

Benowitz, N. L., Pomerleau, O. F., Pomerleau, C. S., & Jacob, P., III. (2003). Nicotine metabolite ratio as a predictor of cigarette consumption. *Nicotine & Tobacco Research, 5*(5), 621–624. https://doi.org/10.1080/1462220031000158717.

Carroll, D. M., Murphy, S. E., Benowitz, N. L., Strasser, A. A., Kotlyar, M., Hecht, S. S., Carmella, S. G., McClernon, F. J., Pacek, L. R., Dermody, S. S., Vandrey, R. G., Donny, E. C., & Hatsukami, D. K. (2020). Relationships between the nicotine metabolite ratio and a panel of exposure and effect biomarkers: Findings from two studies of U.S. commercial cigarette smokers. *Cancer Epidemiology and Prevention Biomarkers, 29*(4), 871–879. https://doi.org/10.1158/1055-9965.EPI-19-0644.

Chen, A., Krebs, N. M., Zhu, J., & Muscat, J. E. (2018). Nicotine metabolite ratio predicts smoking topography: The Pennsylvania Adult Smoking Study. *Drug and Alcohol Dependence, 190*, 89–93. https://doi.org/10.1016/j.drugalcdep.2018.06.003.

Chenoweth, M. J., Novalen, M., Hawk, L. W., Schnoll, R. A., George, T. P., Cinciripini, P. M., Lerman, C., & Tyndale, R. F. (2014). Known and novel sources of variability in the nicotine metabolite ratio in a large sample of treatment-seeking smokers. *Cancer Epidemiology and Prevention Biomarkers, 23*(9), 1773–1782. https://doi.org/10.1158/1055-9965.EPI-14-0427.

Chenoweth, M. J., Schnoll, R. A., Novalen, M., Hawk, L. W., George, T. P., Cinciripini, P. M., Lerman, C., & Tyndale, R. F. (2016). The nicotine metabolite ratio is associated with early smoking abstinence even after controlling for factors that influence the nicotine metabolite ratio. *Nicotine & Tobacco Research, 18*(4), 491–495. https://doi.org/10.1093/ntr/ntv125.

Fix, B. V., O'Connor, R. J., Benowitz, N., Heckman, B. W., Cummings, K. M., Fong, G. T., & Thrasher, J. F. (2017). Nicotine metabolite ratio (NMR) prospectively predicts smoking relapse: Longitudinal findings from ITC surveys in five countries. *Nicotine & Tobacco Research, 19*(9), 1040–1047. https://doi.org/10.1093/ntr/ntx083.

Jao, N. C., Veluz-Wilkins, A. K., Smith, M. J., Carroll, A. J., Blazekovic, S., Leone, F. T., Tyndale, R. F., Schnoll, R. A., & Hitsman, B. (2017). Does menthol cigarette use moderate the effect of nicotine metabolism on short-term smoking cessation? *Experimental and Clinical Psychopharmacology, 25*(3), 216–222. https://doi.org/10.1037/pha0000124.

Leone, F. T., Baldassarri, S. R., Galiatsatos, P., & Schnoll, R. (2018). Nicotine dependence: Future opportunities and emerging clinical challenges. *Annals of the American Thoracic Society, 15*(10), 1127–1130. https://doi.org/10.1513/AnnalsATS.201802-099PS.

Lerman, C., Tyndale, R., Patterson, F., Wileyto, E. P., Shields, P. G., Pinto, A., & Benowitz, N. (2006). Nicotine metabolite ratio predicts efficacy of transdermal nicotine for smoking cessation. *Clinical Pharmacology & Therapeutics, 79*(6), 600–608. https://doi.org/10.1016/j.clpt.2006.02.006.

Schnoll, R., Wileyto, E. P., Bauer, A.-M., Fox, E., Leone, F., Lerman, C., Tyndale, R. F., George, T. P., Hawk, L., Cinciripini, P., Quinn, M., Purnell, J., Hatzell, J., & Hitsman, B. (2021). Comparing the rate of nicotine metabolism among smokers with current or past major depressive disorder. *American Journal on Addictions, 30*(4), 382–388. https://doi.org/10.1111/ajad.13155.

Schnoll, R. A., Wileyto, E. P., Leone, F. T., Tyndale, R. F., & Benowitz, N. L. (2012). High dose transdermal nicotine for fast metabolizers of nicotine: A proof of concept placebo-controlled trial. *Nicotine & Tobacco Research, 15*(2), 348–354. https://doi.org/10.1093/ntr/nts129.

Siegel, S. D., Lerman, C., Flitter, A., & Schnoll, R. A. (2020). The use of the nicotine metabolite ratio as a biomarker to personalize smoking cessation treatment: Current evidence and future directions. *Cancer Prevention Research, 13*(3), 261–272. https://doi.org/10.1158/1940-6207.CAPR-19-0259.

St. Helen, G., Novalen, M., Heitjan, D. F., Dempsey, D., Jacob, P., Aziziyeh, A., Wing, V. C., George, T. P., Tyndale, R. F., & Benowitz, N. L. (2012). Reproducibility of the nicotine metabolite ratio in cigarette smokers. *Cancer Epidemiology and Prevention Biomarkers, 21*(7), 1105–1114. https://doi.org/10.1158/1055-9965.EPI-12-0236.

Strasser, A. A., Benowitz, N. L., Pinto, A. G., Tang, K. Z., Hecht, S. S., Carmella, S. G., Tyndale, R. F., & Lerman, C. E. (2011). Nicotine metabolite ratio predicts smoking topography and carcinogen biomarker level. *Cancer Epidemiology and Prevention Biomarkers, 20*(2), 234–238. https://doi.org/10.1158/1055-9965.EPI-10-0674.

Behavioral Health

Anthenelli, R. M., Benowitz, N. L., West, R., St Aubin, L., McRae, T., Lawrence, D., Ascher, J., Russ, C., Krishen, A., & Evins, A. E. (2016). Neuropsychiatric safety and efficacy of varenicline, bupropion, and nicotine patch in smokers with and without psychiatric disorders (EAGLES): A double-blind, randomised, placebo-controlled clinical trial. *Lancet, 387*(10037), 2507–2520. https://doi.org/10.1016/S0140-6736(16)30272-0.

Colleen E. McKay MA, C., & Faith Dickerson PhD, M. (2012). Peer supports for tobacco cessation for adults with serious mental illness: A review of the literature. *Journal of Dual Diagnosis, 8*(2), 104–112. https://doi.org/10.1080/15504263.2012.670847.

Evins, A. E., Cather, C., Pratt, S. A., Pachas, G. N., Hoeppner, S. S., Goff, D. C., Achtyes, E. D., Ayer, D., & Schoenfeld, D. A. (2014). Maintenance treatment with varenicline for smoking cessation in patients with schizophrenia and bipolar disorder: A randomized clinical trial. *Journal of the American Medical Association, 311*(2), 145–154. https://doi.org/10.1001/jama.2013.285113.

Evins, A. E., Mays, V. K., Cather, C., Goff, D. C., Rigotti, N. A., & Tisdale, T. (2001). A pilot trial of bupropion added to cognitive behavioral therapy for smoking cessation in schizophrenia. *Nicotine & Tobacco Research, 3*(4), 397–403. https://doi.org/10.1080/14622200110073920.

Fagerström, K., & Aubin, H.-J. (2009). Management of smoking cessation in patients with psychiatric disorders. *Current Medical Research and Opinion, 25*(2), 511–518. https://doi.org/10.1185/03007990802707568.

Hitsman, B., Moss, T. G., Montoya, I. D., & George, T. P. (2009). Treatment of tobacco dependence in mental health and addictive disorders. *Canadian Journal of Psychiatry, 54*(6), 368–378. https://doi.org/10.1177/070674370905400604.

Keizer, I., Gex-Fabry, M., Croquette, P., Humair, J.-P., & Khan, A. N. (2019). Tobacco craving and withdrawal symptoms in psychiatric patients during a motivational enhancement intervention based on a 26-hour smoking abstinence period. *Tobacco Prevention & Cessation, 5*(June). https://doi.org/10.18332/tpc/109785.

McFall, M., Saxon, A. J., Malte, C. A., Chow, B., Bailey, S., Baker, D. G., Beckham, J. C., Boardman, K. D., Carmody, T. P., Joseph, A. M., Smith, M. W., Shih, M.-C., Lu, J., Holodniy, M., Lavori, P. W., & CSP 519 Study Team. (2010). Integrating tobacco cessation into mental health care for posttraumatic stress disorder: A randomized controlled trial. *Journal of the American Medical Association, 304*(22), 2485–2493. https://doi.org/10.1001/jama.2010.1769.

Peterson, A. L., Hryshko-Mullen, A. S., & Cortez, Y. (2003). Assessment and diagnosis of nicotine dependence in mental health settings. *American Journal on Addictions, 12*(3), 192–197. https://doi.org/10.1080/10550490390201795.

Prochaska, J. J. (2010a). Failure to treat tobacco use in mental health and addiction treatment settings: A form of harm reduction? *Drug and Alcohol Dependence, 110*(3), 177–182. https://doi.org/10.1016/j.drugalcdep.2010.03.002.

Prochaska, J. J. (2010b). Integrating tobacco treatment into mental health settings. *Journal of the American Medical Association, 304*(22), 2534–2535. https://doi.org/10.1001/jama.2010.1759.

Prochaska, J. J., Fletcher, L., Hall, S. E., & Hall, S. M. (2006). Return to smoking following a smoke-free psychiatric hospitalization. *American Journal on Addictions, 15*(1), 15–22. https://doi.org/10.1080/10550490500419011.

Prochaska, J. J., Fromont, S. C., Wa, C., Matlow, R., Ramo, D. E., & Hall, S. M. (2013). Tobacco use and its treatment among young people in mental health settings: A qualitative analysis. *Nicotine & Tobacco Research, 15*(8), 1427–1435. https://doi.org/10.1093/ntr/nts343.

Schroeder, S. A. (2016). Smoking cessation should be an integral part of serious mental illness treatment. *World Psychiatry, 15*(2), 175–176. https://doi.org/10.1002/wps.20332.

Schroeder, S. A., & Morris, C. D. (2010). Confronting a neglected epidemic: Tobacco cessation for persons with mental illnesses and substance abuse problems. *Annual Review of Public Health, 31*(1), 297–314. https://doi.org/10.1146/annurev.publhealth.012809.103701.

Thorndike, A. N., Stafford, R. S., & Rigotti, N. A. (2001). US physicians' treatment of smoking in outpatients with psychiatric diagnoses. *Nicotine & Tobacco Research, 3*(1), 85–91. https://doi.org/10.1080/14622200020032132.

Thornicroft, G. (2011). Physical health disparities and mental illness: The scandal of premature mortality. *British Journal of Psychiatry, 199*(6), 441–442. https://doi.org/10.1192/bjp.bp.111.092718.

Williams, J. M., Anthenelli, R. M., Morris, C. D., Treadow, J., Thompson, J. R., Yunis, C., & George, T. P. (2012). A randomized, double-blind, placebo-controlled study evaluating the safety and efficacy of varenicline for smoking cessation in patients with schizophrenia or schizoaffective disorder. *Journal of Clinical Psychiatry, 73*(5), 654–660. https://doi.org/10.4088/JCP.11m07522.

Williams, J. M., & Foulds, J. (2007). Successful tobacco dependence treatment in schizophrenia. *American Journal of Psychiatry, 164*(2), 222–227; quiz 373. https://doi.org/10.1176/appi.ajp.164.2.222.

Williams, J. M., Steinberg, M. L., Griffiths, K. G., & Cooperman, N. (2013). Smokers with behavioral health comorbidity should be designated a tobacco use disparity group. *American Journal of Public Health, 103*(9), 1549–1555. https://doi.org/10.2105/AJPH.2013.301232.

Williams, J. M., Stroup, T. S., Brunette, M. F., & Raney, L. E. (2014). Integrated care: Tobacco use and mental illness—a wake-up call for psychiatrists. *Psychiatric Services, 65*(12), 1406–1408. https://doi.org/10.1176/appi.ps.201400235.

Ziedonis, D., Hitsman, B., Beckham, J. C., Zvolensky, M., Adler, L. E., Audrain-McGovern, J., Breslau, N., Brown, R. A., George, T. P., Williams, J., Calhoun, P. S., & Riley, W. T. (2008). Tobacco use and cessation in psychiatric disorders: National Institute of Mental Health report. *Nicotine & Tobacco Research, 10*(12), 1691–1715. https://doi.org/10.1080/14622200802443569.

Ziedonis, D. M., & George, T. P. (1997). Schizophrenia and nicotine use: Report of a pilot smoking cessation program and review of neurobiological and clinical issues. *Schizophrenia Bulletin, 23*(2), 247–254. https://doi.org/10.1093/schbul/23.2.247.

Ziedonis, D. M., & Williams, J. M. (2003). Management of smoking in people with psychiatric disorders. *Current Opinion in Psychiatry, 16*(3), 305–315. https://doi. org/10.1097/01.yco.0000069086.26384.5f.

Cardiovascular Disease

Benowitz, N. L., & Gourlay, S. (1997). Cardiovascular toxicity of nicotine: Implications for nicotine replacement therapy 1. *Journal of the American College of Cardiology, 29*(7), 1422–1431. https://doi.org/10.1016/S0735-1097(97)00079-X.

Benowitz, N. L., & Prochaska, J. J. (2013). Smoking cessation after acute myocardial infarction. *Journal of the American College of Cardiology, 61*(5), 533–535. https:// doi.org/10.1016/j.jacc.2012.11.017.

Eisenberg, M. J., Grandi, S. M., Gervais, A., O'Loughlin, J., Paradis, G., Rinfret, S., Sarrafzadegan, N., Sharma, S., Lauzon, C., Yadav, R., Pilote, L., & ZESCA Investigators. (2013). Bupropion for smoking cessation in patients hospitalized with acute myocardial infarction. *Journal of the American College of Cardiology, 61*(5), 524–532. https://doi.org/10.1016/j.jacc.2012.08.1030.

Eisenberg, M. J., Windle, S. B., Roy, N., Old, W., Grondin, F. R., Bata, I., Iskander, A., Lauzon, C., Srivastava, N., Clarke, A., Cassavar, D., Dion, D., Haught, H., Mehta, S. R., Baril, J.-F., Lambert, C., Madan, M., Abramson, B. L., Dehghani, P., & EVITA Investigators. (2016). Varenicline for smoking cessation in hospitalized patients with acute coronary syndrome. *Circulation, 133*(1), 21–30. https://doi.org/10.1161/ CIRCULATIONAHA.115.019634.

Ford, C. L., & Zlabek, J. A. (2005). Nicotine replacement therapy and cardiovascular disease. *Mayo Clinic Proceedings, 80*(5), 652–656. https://doi.org/10.4065/80.5.652.

Joseph, A. M., Norman, S. M., Ferry, L. H., Prochazka, A. V., Westman, E. C., Steele, B. G., Sherman, S. E., Cleveland, M., Antonuccio, D. O., Hartman, N., & McGovern, P. G. (1996). The safety of transdermal nicotine as an aid to smoking cessation in patients with cardiac disease. *New England Journal of Medicine, 335*(24), 1792–1798. https://doi.org/10.1056/NEJM199612123352402.

Kimmel, S. E., Berlin, J. A., Miles, C., Jaskowiak, J., Carson, J. L., & Strom, B. L. (2001). Risk of acute first myocardial infarction and use of nicotine patches in a general population. *Journal of the American College of Cardiology, 37*(5), 1297–1302. https://doi.org/10.1016/S0735-1097(01)01124-X.

Kondo, T., Osugi, S., Shimokata, K., Honjo, H., Morita, Y., Maeda, K., Yamashita, K., Muramatsu, T., Shintani, S., Matsushita, K., & Murohara, T. (2011). Smoking and smoking cessation in relation to all-cause mortality and cardiovascular events in 25,464 healthy male Japanese workers. *Circulation Journal, 75*(12), 2885–2892. https://doi.org/10.1253/circj.cj-11-0416.

Meine, T. J., Patel, M. R., Washam, J. B., Pappas, P. A., & Jollis, J. G. (2005). Safety and effectiveness of transdermal nicotine patch in smokers admitted with acute coronary syndromes. *American Journal of Cardiology, 95*(8), 976–978. https://doi. org/10.1016/j.amjcard.2004.12.039.

Mohiuddin, S. M., Mooss, A. N., Hunter, C. B., Grollmes, T. L., Cloutier, D. A., & Hilleman, D. E. (2007). Intensive smoking cessation intervention reduces mortality in high-risk smokers with cardiovascular disease. *Chest, 131*(2), 446–452. https://doi. org/10.1378/chest.06-1587.

Pack, Q. R., Priya, A., Lagu, T. C., Pekow, P. S., Atreya, A., Rigotti, N. A., & Lindenauer, P. K. (2018). Short-term safety of nicotine replacement in smokers hospitalized with coronary heart disease. *Journal of the American Heart Association, 7*(18), e009424. https://doi.org/10.1161/JAHA.118.009424.

Rea, T. D., Heckbert, S. R., Kaplan, R. C., Smith, N. L., Lemaitre, R. N., & Psaty, B. M. (2002). Smoking status and risk for recurrent coronary events after myocardial infarction. *Annals of Internal Medicine, 137*(6), 494–500. https://doi.org/10.7326/0003-4819-137-6-200209170-00009.

Reid, R., Pipe, A., Higginson, L., Johnson, K., D'Angelo, M. S., Cooke, D., & Dafoe, W. (2003). Stepped care approach to smoking cessation in patients hospitalized for coronary artery disease. *Journal of Cardiopulmonary Rehabilitation, 23*(3), 176–182. https://doi.org/10.1097/00008483-200305000-00003.

Rigotti, N. A., Pipe, A. L., Benowitz, N. L., Arteaga, C., Garza, D., & Tonstad, S. (2010). Efficacy and safety of varenicline for smoking cessation in patients with cardiovascular disease: A randomized trial. *Circulation, 121*(2), 221–229. https://doi.org/10.1161/CIRCULATIONAHA.109.869008.

Rigotti, N. A., Thorndike, A. N., Regan, S., McKool, K., Pasternak, R. C., Chang, Y., Swartz, S., Torres-Finnerty, N., Emmons, K. M., & Singer, D. E. (2006). Bupropion for smokers hospitalized with acute cardiovascular disease. *American Journal of Medicine, 119*(12), 1080–1087. https://doi.org/10.1016/j.amjmed.2006.04.024.

Tonstad, S., Farsang, C., Klaene, G., Lewis, K., Manolis, A., Perruchoud, A. P., Silagy, C., van Spiegel, P. I., Astbury, C., Hider, A., & Sweet, R. (2003). Bupropion SR for smoking cessation in smokers with cardiovascular disease: A multicentre, randomised study. *European Heart Journal, 24*(10), 946–955. https://doi.org/10.1016/s0195-668x(03)00003-4.

Twardella, D., Küpper-Nybelen, J., Rothenbacher, D., Hahmann, H., Wüsten, B., & Brenner, H. (2004). Short-term benefit of smoking cessation in patients with coronary heart disease: Estimates based on self-reported smoking data and serum cotinine measurements. *European Heart Journal, 25*(23), 2101–2108. https://doi.org/10.1016/j.ehj.2004.08.017.

Woolf, K. J., Zabad, M. N., Post, J. M., McNitt, S., Williams, G. C., & Bisognano, J. D. (2012). Effect of nicotine replacement therapy on cardiovascular outcomes after acute coronary syndromes. *American Journal of Cardiology, 110*(7), 968–970. https://doi.org/10.1016/j.amjcard.2012.05.028.

Pregnancy

American College of Obstetricians and Gynecologists. (2017). Tobacco and nicotine cessation during pregnancy. ACOG Committee on Obstetric Practice, opinion no. 807. https://www.acog.org/en/Clinical/Clinical Guidance/Committee Opinion/Articles/2020/05/Tobacco and Nicotine Cessation During Pregnancy.

Bar-Zeev, Y., Lim, L. L., Bonevski, B., Gruppetta, M., & Gould, G. S. (2018). Nicotine replacement therapy for smoking cessation during pregnancy. *Medical Journal of Australia, 208*(1), 46–51.

Bérard, A., Zhao, J.-P., & Sheehy, O. (2016). Success of smoking cessation interventions during pregnancy. *American Journal of Obstetrics and Gynecology, 215*(5), 611. e1–611.e8. https://doi.org/10.1016/j.ajog.2016.06.059.

Coleman, T., Chamberlain, C., Davey, M.-A., Cooper, S. E., & Leonardi-Bee, J. (2012). Pharmacological interventions for promoting smoking cessation during pregnancy. *Cochrane Database of Systematic Reviews, 9*, CD010078. https://doi.org/10.1002/14651858.CD010078.

Coleman, T., Cooper, S., Thornton, J. G., Grainge, M. J., Watts, K., Britton, J., & Lewis, S. (2012). A randomized trial of nicotine-replacement therapy patches in pregnancy. *New England Journal of Medicine, 366*(9), 808–818. https://doi.org/10.1056/NEJMoa1109582.

Gould, G. S., Havard, A., Lim, L. L., PSANZ Smoking in Pregnancy Expert Group, & Kumar, R. (2020). Exposure to tobacco, environmental tobacco smoke and nicotine in pregnancy: A pragmatic overview of reviews of maternal and child outcomes, effectiveness of interventions and barriers and facilitators to quitting. *International Journal of Environmental Research and Public Health, 17*(6), 2034. https://doi.org/10.3390/ijerph17062034.

Kapur, B., Hackman, R., Selby, P., Klein, J., & Koren, G. (2001). Randomized, double-blind, placebo-controlled trial of nicotine replacement therapy in pregnancy. *Current Therapeutic Research, 62*(4), 274–278. https://doi.org/10.1016/S0011-393X(01)80011-4.

Myung, S.-K., Ju, W., Jung, H.-S., Park, C.-H., Oh, S.-W., Seo, H. G., & Kim, H. S. (2012). Efficacy and safety of pharmacotherapy for smoking cessation among pregnant smokers: A meta-analysis. *BJOG: An International Journal of Obstetrics & Gynaecology, 119*(9), 1029–1039. https://doi.org/10.1111/j.1471-0528.2012.03408.x.

Oaks, L. (2001). *Smoking and pregnancy: The politics of fetal protection*. Rutgers University Press.

Oncken, C., Dornelas, E. A., Kuo, C.-L., Sankey, H. Z., Kranzler, H. R., Mead, E. L., & Thurlow, S. D. (2019). Randomized trial of nicotine inhaler for pregnant smokers. *American Journal of Obstetrics & Gynecology, 1*(1), 10–18. https://doi.org/10.1016/j.ajogmf.2019.03.006.

Richardson, J. L., Stephens, S., Yates, L. M., Diav-Citrin, O., Arnon, J., Beghin, D., Kayser, A., Kennedy, D., Cupitt, D., te Winkel, B., Peltonen, M., Kaplan, Y. C., & Thomas, S. H. L. (2017). Pregnancy outcomes after maternal varenicline use; analysis of surveillance data collected by the European Network of Teratology Information Services. *Reproductive Toxicology, 67*, 26–34. https://doi.org/10.1016/j.reprotox.2016.11.010.

Turner, E., Jones, M., Vaz, L. R., & Coleman, T. (2019). Systematic review and meta-analysis to assess the safety of bupropion and varenicline in pregnancy. *Nicotine & Tobacco Research, 21*(8), 1001–1010. https://doi.org/10.1093/ntr/nty055.

Wigginton, B., & Lee, C. (2013). Stigma and hostility towards pregnant smokers: Does individuating information reduce the effect? *Psychology & Health, 28*(8), 862–873. https://doi.org/10.1080/08870446.2012.762101.

Wisborg, K., Henriksen, T. B., Jespersen, L. B., & Secher, N. J. (2000). Nicotine patches for pregnant smokers: A randomized controlled study. *Obstetrics & Gynecology, 96*(6), 967–971. https://doi.org/10.1016/S0029-7844(00)01071-1.

Chapter 11. Routines

Defining the Problem and Making It Cognitive

Beyer, B. (1984). Improving thinking skills: Defining the problem. *Phi Delta Kappan,* 65(7), 486–490. https://www.jstor.org/stable/20387092.

Dewey, J. (1922). An analysis of reflective thought. *Journal of Philosophy, 19*(2), 29–38. https://doi.org/10.2307/2939444.

Farra, H. (1988). The reflective thought process: John Dewey re-visited. *Journal of Creative Behavior, 22*(1), 1–8.

Ham, S. H. (2007). Can interpretation really make a difference? Answers to four questions from cognitive and behavioral psychology. In P. Caputo (Ed.), *Proceedings, Interpreting World Heritage Conference* (pp. 42–52). March 25–29, Vancouver, Canada. National Association for Interpretation.

Kaasbøll, J. J. (1998). Teaching critical thinking and problem defining skills. *Education and Information Technologies, 3*(2), 101–117. https://doi.org/10.1023/A:1009682924511.

León, F. R. (2014). About the reflective thought also known as the critical thinking. *Journal of Educational Psychology—Propositos y Representaciones, 2*(1), 189–214. https://pdfs.semanticscholar.org/a236/1be088af034053b891234a0d60de4475f49e.pdf.

Lydon-Staley, D. M., Kuehner, C., Zamoscik, V., Huffziger, S., Kirsch, P., & Bassett, D. S. (2019). Repetitive negative thinking in daily life and functional connectivity among default mode, fronto-parietal, and salience networks. *Translational Psychiatry, 9*(1), 234. https://doi.org/10.1038/s41398-019-0560-0.

Mamede, S., & Schmidt, H. G. (2004). The structure of reflective practice in medicine. *Medical Education, 38*(12), 1302–1308. https://doi.org/10.1111/j.1365-2929.2004.01917.x.

Miettinen, R. (2000). The concept of experiential learning and John Dewey's theory of reflective thought and action. *International Journal of Lifelong Education, 19*(1), 54–72. https://doi.org/10.1080/026013700293458.

Millar, M. G., & Tesser, A. (1986). Effects of affective and cognitive focus on the attitude–behavior relation. *Journal of Personality and Social Psychology, 51*(2), 270–276. https://doi.org/10.1037/0022-3514.51.2.270.

Risku, H. (2010). A cognitive scientific view on technical communication and translation: Do embodiment and situatedness really make a difference? *Target: International Journal of Translation Studies, 22*(1), 94–111. https://doi.org/10.1075/target.22.1.06ris.

Strohm, S. M., & Baukus, R. A. (1995). Strategies for fostering critical-thinking skills. *Journalism & Mass Communication Educator, 50*(1), 55–62. https://doi.org/10.1177/107769589505000107.

Forecasting Error

Baron, J. (1992). The effect of normative beliefs on anticipated emotions. *Journal of Personality and Social Psychology, 63*(2), 320–330. https://doi.org/10.1037//0022-3514.63.2.320.

Buehler, R., & McFarland, C. (2001). Intensity bias in affective forecasting: The role of temporal focus. *Personality and Social Psychology Bulletin, 27*(11), 1480–1493. https://doi.org/10.1177/01461672012711009.

Carstensen, L. L., Pasupathi, M., Mayr, U., & Nesselroade, J. R. (2000). Emotional experience in everyday life across the adult life span. *Journal of Personality and Social Psychology, 79*(4), 644–655.

Cox, B. J., & Swinson, R. P. (1994). Overprediction of fear in panic disorder with agoraphobia. *Behaviour Research and Therapy, 32*(7), 735–739. https://doi.org/10.1016/0005-7967(94)90030-2.

Crawford, M. T., McConnell, A. R., Lewis, A. C., & Sherman, S. J. (2002). Reactance, compliance, and anticipated regret. *Journal of Experimental Social Psychology, 38*(1), 56–63. https://doi.org/10.1006/jesp.2001.1481.

Easterbrook, J. A. (1959). The effect of emotion on cue utilization and the organization of behavior. *Psychological Review, 66*(3), 183–201. https://doi.org/10.1037/h0047707.

Gilbert, D. T., & Ebert, J. E. J. (2002). Decisions and revisions: The affective forecasting of changeable outcomes. *Journal of Personality and Social Psychology, 82*(4), 503–514.

Isen, A. M. (1984). The influence of positive affect on decision making and cognitive organization. In T. C. Kinnear (Ed.), *NA—Advances in consumer research* (Vol. 11, pp. 534–537). Association for Consumer Research. https://www.acrwebsite.org/volumes/6302/volumes/v11/NA-11/full.

Isen, A. M. (1993). Positive affect and decision making. In *Handbook of emotions* (pp. 261–277). Guilford Press.

Klaaren, K. J., Hodges, S. D., & Wilson, T. D. (1994). The role of affective expectations in subjective experience and decision-making. *Social Cognition, 12*(2), 77–101. https://doi.org/10.1521/soco.1994.12.2.77.

Rachman, S. (1994). The overprediction of fear: A review. *Behaviour Research and Therapy, 32*(7), 683–690. https://doi.org/10.1016/0005-7967(94)90025-6.

Wilson, T. D., & Gilbert, D. T. (2003). Affective forecasting. In *Advances in experimental social psychology* (Vol. 35, pp. 345–411). Academic Press. https://doi.org/10.1016/S0065-2601(03)01006-2.

Depletion

Baumeister, R. F. (2002). Ego depletion and self-control failure: An energy model of the self's executive function. *Self and Identity, 1*(2), 129–136. https://doi.org/10.1080/152988602317319302.

Baumeister, R. F. (2003). Ego depletion and self-regulation failure: A resource model of self-control. *Alcoholism: Clinical and Experimental Research, 27*(2), 281–284. https://doi.org/10.1097/01.ALC.0000060879.61384.A4.

Baumeister, R. F., Sparks, E. A., Stillman, T. F., & Vohs, K. D. (2008). Free will in consumer behavior: Self-control, ego depletion, and choice. *Journal of Consumer Psychology, 18*(1), 4–13. https://doi.org/10.1016/j.jcps.2007.10.002.

Fischer, P., Kastenmüller, A., & Asal, K. (2012). Ego depletion increases risk-taking. *Journal of Social Psychology, 152*(5), 623–638. https://doi.org/10.1080/00224545.2012.683894.

Furley, P., Bertrams, A., Englert, C., & Delphia, A. (2013). Ego depletion, attentional control, and decision making in sport. *Psychology of Sport and Exercise, 14*(6), 900–904. https://doi.org/10.1016/j.psychsport.2013.08.006.

Muraven, M. (2012). Ego depletion: Theory and evidence. In *The Oxford handbook of human motivation* (pp. 111–126). Oxford University Press.

Unger, A., & Stahlberg, D. (2011). Ego-depletion and risk behavior. *Social Psychology, 42*(1), 28–38. https://doi.org/10.1027/1864-9335/a000040.

Decatastrophizing

Akkoyunlu, S., & Türkçapar, M. H. (2013). A technique: Generating alternative thoughts. *Journal of Cognitive-Behavioral Psychotherapy and Research, 2*(1), 53–59.

Dattilio, F. M., & Freeman, A. (1992). Introduction to cognitive therapy. In A. Freeman & F. M. Dattilio (Eds.), *Comprehensive casebook of cognitive therapy* (pp. 3–11). Springer US. https://doi.org/10.1007/978-1-4757-9777-0_1.

Hoodin, F., & Gillis, M. (2007). Applications of exposure techniques in behavioral medicine. In D. C. S. Richard & D. Lauterbach (Eds.), *Handbook of exposure therapies* (pp. 271–298). Academic Press. https://doi.org/10.1016/B978-012587421-2/50013-2.

Mashal, N. M., Beaudreau, S. A., Hernandez, M. A., Duller, R. C., Romaniak, H., Shin, K. E., Paller, K. A., & Zinbarg, R. E. (2020). A brief worry reappraisal paradigm (REAP) increases coping with worries. *Cognitive Therapy and Research, 44*(1), 216–228. https://doi.org/10.1007/s10608-019-10053-8.

Otto, M. W., Safren, S. A., & Pollack, M. H. (2004). Internal cue exposure and the treatment of substance use disorders: Lessons from the treatment of panic disorder. *Journal of Anxiety Disorders, 18*(1), 69–87. https://doi.org/10.1016/j.janxdis.2003.07.007.

Otto, M. W., Smits, J. A. J., Fitzgerald, H. E., Powers, M. B., & Baird, S. O. (2019). Anxiety sensitivity and your clinical practice. In J. A. J. Smits, M. W. Otto, M. B. Powers, & S. O. Baird (Eds.), *The clinician's guide to anxiety sensitivity treatment and assessment* (pp. 179–193). Academic Press. https://doi.org/10.1016/B978-0-12-813495-5.00009-7.

Vasey, M. W., & Borkovec, T. D. (1992). A catastrophizing assessment of worrisome thoughts. *Cognitive Therapy and Research, 16*(5), 505–520. https://doi.org/10.1007/BF01175138.

Warner, M. J., & Studwell, R. W. (1991). Humor: A powerful counseling tool. *Journal of College Student Psychotherapy, 5*(2), 59–70. https://doi.org/10.1300/J035v05n02_06.

Worden, B. L., Genova, M., & Tolin, D. F. (2017). Randomized pilot of an anxiety sensitivity-based intervention for individuals in a substance use day program. *Journal of Psychoactive Drugs, 49*(4), 333–343. https://doi.org/10.1080/02791072.2017.1329570.

Implementation Orientation

Brandstätter, V., Lengfelder, A., & Gollwitzer, P. M. (2001). Implementation intentions and efficient action initiation. *Journal of Personality and Social Psychology, 81*(5), 946–960. https://doi.org/10.1037/0022-3514.81.5.946.

Gollwitzer, P. M. (1999). Implementation intentions: Strong effects of simple plans.

American Psychologist, 54(7), 493–503. https://doi.org/10.1037/0003-066X.54.7.493.

Gollwitzer, P. M., & Brandstätter, V. (1997). Implementation intentions and effective goal pursuit. *Journal of Personality and Social Psychology, 73*(1), 186–199. https://doi.org/10.1037/0022-3514.73.1.186.

Gollwitzer, P. M., & Schaal, B. (1998). Metacognition in action: The importance of implementation intentions. *Personality and Social Psychology Review, 2*(2), 124–136. https://doi.org/10.1207/s15327957pspr0202_5.

Gollwitzer, P. M., & Sheeran, P. (2006). Implementation intentions and goal achievement: A meta-analysis of effects and processes. In *Advances in experimental social psychology* (Vol. 38, pp. 69–119). Academic Press. https://doi.org/10.1016/S0065-2601(06)38002-1.

Orbell, S., Hodgkins, S., & Sheeran, P. (1997). Implementation intentions and the theory of planned behavior. *Personality and Social Psychology Bulletin, 23*(9), 945–954. https://doi.org/10.1177/0146167297239004.

Rogers, T., & Bazerman, M. H. (2008). Future lock-in: Future implementation increases selection of "should" choices. *Organizational Behavior and Human Decision Processes, 106*(1), 1–20. https://doi.org/10.1016/j.obhdp.2007.08.001.

Sheeran, P., Webb, T. L., & Gollwitzer, P. M. (2005). The interplay between goal intentions and implementation intentions. *Personality & Social Psychology Bulletin, 31*(1), 87–98. https://doi.org/10.1177/0146167204271308.

General Cognitive Behavioral Therapy (CBT)

Brown, R. A., Kahler, C. W., Niaura, R., Abrams, D. B., Sales, S. D., Ramsey, S. E., Goldstein, M. G., Burgess, E. S., & Miller, I. W. (2001). Cognitive–behavioral treatment for depression in smoking cessation. *Journal of Consulting and Clinical Psychology, 69*(3), 471–480. https://doi.org/10.1037/0022-006X.69.3.471.

Brown, R. A., Niaura, R., Lloyd-Richardson, E. E., Strong, D. R., Kahler, C. W., Abrantes, A. M., Abrams, D., & Miller, I. W. (2007). Bupropion and cognitive–behavioral treatment for depression in smoking cessation. *Nicotine & Tobacco Research, 9*(7), 721–730. https://doi.org/10.1080/14622200701416955.

Hernández-López, M., Luciano, M. C., Bricker, J. B., Roales-Nieto, J. G., & Montesinos, F. (2009). Acceptance and commitment therapy for smoking cessation: A preliminary study of its effectiveness in comparison with cognitive behavioral therapy. *Psychology of Addictive Behaviors, 23*(4), 723–730. https://doi.org/10.1037/a0017632.

Killen, J. D., Fortmann, S. P., Schatzberg, A. F., Arredondo, C., Murphy, G., Hayward, C., Celio, M., Cromp, D., Fong, D., & Pandurangi, M. (2008). Extended cognitive behavior therapy for cigarette smoking cessation. *Addiction, 103*(8), 1381–1390. https://doi.org/10.1111/j.1360-0443.2008.02273.x.

Perkins, K. A., Conklin, C. A., & Levine, M. D. (2008). *Cognitive-behavioral therapy for smoking cessation: A practical guidebook to the most effective treatments* (pp. xxii, 258). Routledge/Taylor & Francis Group.

Perkins, K. A., Marcus, M. D., Levine, M. D., D'Amico, D., Miller, A., Broge, M., Ashcom, J., & Shiffman, S. (2001). Cognitive–behavioral therapy to reduce weight concerns improves smoking cessation outcome in weight-concerned women. *Journal of Consulting and Clinical Psychology, 69*(4), 604–613. https://doi.org/10.1037/0022-006X.69.4.604.

Webb, M. S., de Ybarra, D. R., Baker, E. A., Reis, I. M., & Carey, M. P. (2010). Cognitive–behavioral therapy to promote smoking cessation among African American smokers: A randomized clinical trial. *Journal of Consulting and Clinical Psychology, 78*(1), 24–33. https://doi.org/10.1037/a0017669.

Chapter 12. Influence

Soft Skills and Emotional Intelligence

Beauvais, A., Andreychik, M., & Henkel, L. A. (2017). The role of emotional intelligence and empathy in compassionate nursing care. *Mindfulness & Compassion, 2*(2), 92–100. https://doi.org/10.1016/j.mincom.2017.09.001.

Coelho, K. R. (2012). Bridging the divide for better health: Harnessing the power of emotional intelligence to foster an enhanced clinician-patient relationship. *International Journal of Collaborative Research on Internal Medicine & Public Health, 4*(3). https://escholarship.org/uc/item/6sn117v8.

Hess, J. D., & Bacigalupo, A. C. (2011). Enhancing decisions and decision-making processes through the application of emotional intelligence skills. *Management Decision, 49*(5), 710–721. https://doi.org/10.1108/00251741111130805.

Mintz, L. J., & Stoller, J. K. (2014). A systematic review of physician leadership and emotional intelligence. *Journal of Graduate Medical Education, 6*(1), 21–31. https://doi.org/10.4300/JGME-D-13-00012.1.

Stoller, J. K. (2020). Leadership essentials for the chest physician: Emotional intelligence. *Chest 159*(5), 1942–1948. https://doi.org/10.1016/j.chest.2020.09.093.

Stoller, J. K., Taylor, C. A., & Farver, C. F. (2013). Emotional intelligence competencies provide a developmental curriculum for medical training. *Medical Teacher, 35*(3), 243–247. https://doi.org/10.3109/0142159X.2012.737964.

Wagner, P. J., Moseley, G. C., Grant, M. M., Gore, J. R., & Owens, C. (2002). Physicians' emotional intelligence and patient satisfaction. *Family Medicine, 34*(10), 750–754.

Weng, H.-C. (2008). Does the physician's emotional intelligence matter? Impacts of the physician's emotional intelligence on the trust, patient-physician relationship, and satisfaction. *Health Care Management Review, 33*(4), 280–288. https://doi.org/10.1097/01.HCM.0000318765.52148.b3.

Zhou, K. (2016). Non-cognitive skills: Definitions, measurement and malleability. UNESCO Digital Library. https://unesdoc.unesco.org/ark:/48223/pf0000245576.

Homophily

Berry, D. L., Blonquist, T. M., Pozzar, R., & Nayak, M. M. (2018). Understanding health decision making: An exploration of homophily. *Social Science & Medicine, 214*, 118–124. https://doi.org/10.1016/j.socscimed.2018.08.026.

Brechwald, W. A., & Prinstein, M. J. (2011). Beyond homophily: A decade of advances in understanding peer influence processes. *Journal of Research on Adolescence, 21*(1), 166–179. https://doi.org/10.1111/j.1532-7795.2010.00721.x.

Centola, D. (2011). An experimental study of homophily in the adoption of health behavior. *Science, 334*(6060), 1269–1272. https://doi.org/10.1126/science.1207055.

Currarini, S., & Mengel, F. (2016). Identity, homophily and in-group bias. *European*

Economic Review, 90, 40–55. https://doi.org/10.1016/j.euroecorev.2016.02.015.

Lawrence, B. S., & Shah, N. P. (2020). Homophily: Measures and meaning. *Academy of Management Annals, 14*(2), 513–597. https://doi.org/10.5465/annals.2018.0147.

Mccroskey, J. C., Richmond, V. P., & Daly, J. A. (1975). The development of a measure of perceived homophily in interpersonal communication. *Human Communication Research, 1*(4), 323–332. https://doi.org/10.1111/j.1468-2958.1975.tb00281.x.

McPherson, J. M., & Smith-Lovin, L. (1987). Homophily in voluntary organizations: Status distance and the composition of face-to-face groups. *American Sociological Review, 52*(3), 370–379. https://doi.org/10.2307/2095356.

Tang, J., Gao, H., Hu, X., & Liu, H. (2013). Exploiting homophily effect for trust prediction. In *Proceedings of the Sixth ACM International Conference on Web Search and Data Mining* (pp. 53–62). Association for Computing Machinery. https://doi.org/10.1145/2433396.2433405.

Warren, K., Campbell, B., Cranmer, S., De Leon, G., Doogan, N., Weiler, M., & Doherty, F. (2020). Building the community: Endogenous network formation, homophily and prosocial sorting among therapeutic community residents. *Drug and Alcohol Dependence, 207,* 107773. https://doi.org/10.1016/j.drugalcdep.2019.107773.

Cognitive Bias

Bhatti, A. (2018). Cognitive bias in clinical practice: Nurturing healthy skepticism among medical students. *Advances in Medical Education and Practice, 9,* 235–237. https://doi.org/10.2147/AMEP.S149558.

Campbell, S. G., Croskerry, P., & Petrie, D. A. (2017). Cognitive bias in health leaders. *Healthcare Management Forum, 30*(5), 257–261. https://doi.org/10.1177/0840470417716949.

Edwards, W. (1954). The theory of decision making. *Psychological Bulletin, 51*(4), 380–417.

Hershberger, P. J., Markert, R. J., Part, H. M., Cohen, S. M., & Finger, W. W. (1996). Understanding and addressing cognitive bias in medical education. *Advances in Health Sciences Education, 1*(3), 221–226. https://doi.org/10.1007/BF00162919.

Kahneman, D., & Tversky, A. (1979). Prospect theory: An analysis of decision under risk. *Econometrica, 47*(2), 263–292.

Leone, F. T., Evers-Casey, S., Graden, S., & Schnoll, R. (2015). Behavioral economic insights into physician tobacco treatment decision-making. *Annals of the American Thoracic Society, 12*(3), 364–369. https://doi.org/10.1513/AnnalsATS.201410-467BC.

Manoogian, J., & Benson, B. (2016). Cognitive bias codex [graphic]. https://cdn-images-1.medium.com/max/2000/1*71TzKnr7bzXU_l_pU6DCNA.jpeg.

McIlvain, H. E., Backer, E. L., Crabtree, B. F., & Lacy, N. (2002). Physician attitudes and the use of office-based activities for tobacco control. *Family Medicine, 34*(2), 114–119.

O'Sullivan, E. D., & Schofield, S. (2018). Cognitive bias in clinical medicine. *Journal of the Royal College of Physicians of Edinburgh, 48*(3), 225–231. https://doi.org/10.4997/JRCPE.2018.306.

Phillips-Wren, G., Jefferson, T., & McKniff, S. (2019). Cognitive bias and decision aid use under stressful conditions. *Journal of Decision Systems, 28*(2), 162–184. https://doi.org/10.1080/12460125.2019.1643695.

Reilly, J. B., Ogdie, A. R., Feldt, J. M. V., & Myers, J. S. (2013). Teaching about how doctors think: A longitudinal curriculum in cognitive bias and diagnostic error for residents. *BMJ Quality & Safety, 22*(12), 1044–1050. https://doi.org/10.1136/bmjqs-2013-001987.

Saposnik, G., Redelmeier, D., Ruff, C. C., & Tobler, P. N. (2016). Cognitive biases associated with medical decisions: A systematic review. *BMC Medical Informatics and Decision Making, 16*(1), 138. https://doi.org/10.1186/s12911-016-0377-1.

Slovic, P. (1995). The construction of preference. *American Psychologist, 50*(5), 364–371.

Tversky, Amos, & Kahneman, D. (1974). Judgment under uncertainty: Heuristics and biases. *Science, 185*, 1124–1131.

Tversky, A, & Kahneman, D. (1981). The framing of decisions and the psychology of choice. *Science, 211*(4481), 453–458.

Yuen, T., Derenge, D., & Kalman, N. (2018). Cognitive bias: Its influence on clinical diagnosis. *Journal of Family Practice, 67*(6), 366, 368, 370, 372.

Stigma

Bayer, R., & Stuber, J. (2006). Tobacco control, stigma, and public health: Rethinking the relations. *American Journal of Public Health, 96*(1), 47–50. https://doi.org/10.2105/AJPH.2005.071886.

Bell, K., McCullough, L., Salmon, A., & Bell, J. (2010). 'Every space is claimed': Smokers' experiences of tobacco denormalisation. *Sociology of Health & Illness, 32*(6), 914–929. https://doi.org/10.1111/j.1467-9566.2010.01251.x.

Bell, K., Salmon, A., Bowers, M., Bell, J., & McCullough, L. (2010). Smoking, stigma and tobacco "denormalization": Further reflections on the use of stigma as a public health tool—a commentary on *Social Science & Medicine*'s Stigma, Prejudice, Discrimination and Health Special Issue (67:3). *Social Science & Medicine, 70*(6), 795–799. https://doi.org/10.1016/j.socscimed.2009.09.060.

Bresnahan, M. J., Silk, K., & Zhuang, J. (2013). You did this to yourself! Stigma and blame in lung cancer. *Journal of Applied Social Psychology, 43*(Suppl. 1), E132–E140. https://doi.org/10.1111/jasp.12030.

Brown Johnson, C. G., Brodsky, J. L., & Cataldo, J. K. (2014). Lung cancer stigma, anxiety, depression, and quality of life. *Journal of Psychosocial Oncology, 32*(1), 59–73. https://doi.org/10.1080/07347332.2013.855963.

Burgess, D., Widome, R., Ryn, M. van, Phelan, S., & Fu, S. (2012). Self-stigma, stress, and smoking among African American and American Indian female smokers: An exploratory qualitative study. *Journal of Health Disparities Research and Practice, 5*(1). https://digitalscholarship.unlv.edu/jhdrp/vol5/iss1/2.

Castaldelli-Maia, J. M., Ventriglio, A., & Bhugra, D. (2016). Tobacco smoking: From "glamour" to "stigma": A comprehensive review. *Psychiatry and Clinical Neurosciences, 70*(1), 24–33. https://doi.org/10.1111/pcn.12365.

Cataldo, J. K., Jahan, T. M., & Pongquan, V. L. (2012). Lung cancer stigma, depression, and quality of life among ever and never smokers. *European Journal of Oncology Nursing, 16*(3), 264–269. https://doi.org/10.1016/j.ejon.2011.06.008.

Evans-Polce, R. J., Castaldelli-Maia, J. M., Schomerus, G., & Evans-Lacko, S. E. (2015). The downside of tobacco control? Smoking and self-stigma: A systematic review. *Social Science & Medicine, 145*, 26–34. https://doi.org/10.1016/j.socscimed.2015.09.026.

Gamarel, K. E., Finer, Z., Resnicow, K., Green-Jones, M., Kelley, E., Jadwin-Cakmak, L., & Outlaw, A. (2020). Associations between internalized HIV stigma and tobacco smoking among adolescents and young adults living with HIV: The moderating role of future orientations. *AIDS and Behavior, 24*(1), 165–172. https://doi.org/10.1007/s10461-019-02567-9.

Graham, H. (2012). Smoking, stigma and social class. *Journal of Social Policy, 41*(1), 83–99. http://dx.doi.org/10.1017/S004727941100033X.

Hatzenbuehler, M. L., Jun, H.-J., Corliss, H. L., & Austin, S. B. (2014). Structural stigma and cigarette smoking in a prospective cohort study of sexual minority and heterosexual youth. *Annals of Behavioral Medicine, 47*(1), 48–56. https://doi.org/10.1007/s12160-013-9548-9.

Hatzenbuehler, M. L., Phelan, J. C., & Link, B. G. (2013). Stigma as a fundamental cause of population health inequalities. *American Journal of Public Health, 103*(5), 813–821. https://doi.org/10.2105/AJPH.2012.301069.

Helweg-Larsen, M., Sorgen, L. J., & Pisinger, C. (2019). Does it help smokers if we stigmatize them? A test of the stigma-induced identity threat model among U.S. and Danish smokers. *Social Cognition, 37*(3), 294–313. https://doi.org/10.1521/soco.2019.37.3.294.

McCool, J., Hoek, J., Edwards, R., Thomson, G., & Gifford, H. (2013). Crossing the smoking divide for young adults: Expressions of stigma and identity among smokers and nonsmokers. *Nicotine & Tobacco Research, 15*(2), 552–556. https://doi.org/10.1093/ntr/nts136.

McGinty, E. E., & Barry, C. L. (2020). Stigma reduction to combat the addiction crisis: Developing an evidence base. *New England Journal of Medicine, 382*(14), 1291–1292. https://doi.org/10.1056/NEJMp2000227.

Nolan, L. J., & Eshleman, A. (2016). Paved with good intentions: Paradoxical eating responses to weight stigma. *Appetite, 102*, 15–24. https://doi.org/10.1016/j.appet.2016.01.027.

Ritchie, D., Amos, A., & Martin, C. (2010). "But it just has that sort of feel about it, a leper": Stigma, smoke-free legislation and public health. *Nicotine & Tobacco Research, 12*(6), 622–629. https://doi.org/10.1093/ntr/ntq058.

Scheffels, J. (2009). Stigma, or sort of cool: Young adults' accounts of smoking and identity. *European Journal of Cultural Studies, 12*(4), 469–486. https://doi.org/10.1177/1367549409342513.

Stuber, J., & Galea, S. (2009). Who conceals their smoking status from their health care provider? *Nicotine & Tobacco Research, 11*(3), 303–307. https://doi.org/10.1093/ntr/ntn024.

Stuber, J., Galea, S., & Link, B. G. (2008). Smoking and the emergence of a stigmatized social status. *Social Science & Medicine, 67*(3), 420–430. https://doi.org/10.1016/j.socscimed.2008.03.010.

Stuber, J., Galea, S., & Link, B. G. (2009). Stigma and smoking: The consequences of our good intentions. *Social Service Review, 83*(4), 585–609. https://doi.org/10.1086/650349.

Stuber, J., Meyer, I., & Link, B. (2008). Stigma, prejudice, discrimination and health. *Social Science & Medicine, 67*(3), 351–357. https://doi.org/10.1016/j.socscimed.2008.03.023.

Volkow, N. D. (2020). Stigma and the toll of addiction. *New England Journal of*

Medicine, 382(14), 1289–1290. https://doi.org/10.1056/NEJMp1917360.

Weiner, B., Perry, R. P., & Magnusson, J. (1988). An attributional analysis of reactions to stigmas. *Journal of Personality and Social Psychology, 55*(5), 738–748.

Weiss, J., Yang, H., Weiss, S., Rigney, M., Copeland, A., King, J. C., & Deal, A. M. (2017). Stigma, self-blame, and satisfaction with care among patients with lung cancer. *Journal of Psychosocial Oncology, 35*(2), 166–179. https://doi.org/10.1080/0734733 2.2016.1228095.

Wigginton, B., & Lee, C. (2013). A story of stigma: Australian women's accounts of smoking during pregnancy. *Critical Public Health, 23*(4), 466–481. https://doi.org/1 0.1080/09581596.2012.753408.

Culpability and Sin or Sickness

Barnes, R. D., Ickes, W., & Kidd, R. F. (1979). Effects of the perceived intentionality and stability of another's dependency on helping behavior. *Personality and Social Psychology Bulletin, 5*(3), 367–372. https://doi.org/10.1177/014616727900500320.

Bass, B., Lake, E., Elvy, C., Fodemesi, S., Iacoe, M., Mazik, E., Brooks, D., & Lee, A. (2018). Smoking-related stigma expressed by physiotherapists toward individuals with lung disease. *Physiotherapy Canada, 70*(1), 65–71. https://doi.org/10.3138/ptc.2016-98.

Betancourt, H. (1990). An attribution-empathy model of helping behavior: Behavioral intentions and judgments of help-giving. *Personality and Social Psychology Bulletin, 16*(3), 573–591. https://doi.org/10.1177/0146167290163015.

Bhargava, M. (2019, January 11). What happens when the doctor blames you for your own cancer? *Washington Post.* Retrieved January 19, 2019, from https://www.washingtonpost.com/outlook/what-happens-when-the-doctor-blames-you-for-your-own-cancer/2019/01/11/2791611e-14ff-11e9-90a8-136fa44b80ba_story.html?utm_term=.b0de3ebb611a.

Blair, I. V., Steiner, J. F., & Havranek, E. P. (2011). Unconscious (implicit) bias and health disparities: Where do we go from here? *Permanente Journal, 15*(2), 71–78.

Brewin, C. R. (1984). Perceived controllability of life-events and willingness to pre-scribe psychotropic drugs. *British Journal of Social Psychology, 23*(Pt. 3), 285–287.

Clark, C. J., Chen, E. E., & Ditto, P. H. (2015). Moral coherence processes: Constructing culpability and consequences. *Current Opinion in Psychology, 6*, 123–128. https://doi.org/10.1016/j.copsyc.2015.07.016.

DeJong, W. (1980). The stigma of obesity: The consequences of naive assumptions concerning the causes of physical deviance. *Journal of Health and Social Behavior, 21*(1), 75–87. https://doi.org/10.2307/2136696.

Evers-Casey, S., Schnoll, R., Jenssen, B. P., & Leone, F. T. (2019). Implicit attribution of culpability and impact on experience of treating tobacco dependence. *Health Psychology, 38*(12), 1069–1074. https://doi.org/10.1037/hea0000784.

Finchilescu, G. (2002). HIV/AIDS versus smoking-induced cancer: A comparison of South African students' attributions of culpability, and risk-taking behaviour. *Social Dynamics, 28*(1), 109–131. https://doi.org/10.1080/02533950208458725.

Galiatsatos, P., Brigham, E., Krasnoff, R., Rice, J., Van Wyck, L., Sherry, M., Rand, C. S., Hansel, N. N., & McCormack, M. C. (2020). Association between neighborhood socioeconomic status, tobacco store density and smoking status in pregnant women in an urban area. *Preventive Medicine, 136,* 106107. https://doi.org/10.1016/j. ypmed.2020.106107.

Meyer, J. P., & Mulherin, A. (1980). From attribution to helping: An analysis of the mediating effects of affect and expectancy. *Journal of Personality and Social Psychology, 39*(2), 201–210. https://doi.org/10.1037/0022-3514.39.2.201.

Miller, D. P., Spangler, J. G., Vitolins, M. Z., Davis, S. W., Ip, E. H., Marion, G. S., & Crandall, S. J. (2013). Are medical students aware of their anti-obesity bias? *Academic Medicine, 88*(7), 978–982. https://doi.org/10.1097/ACM.0b013e318294f817.

Schmidt, G., & Weiner, B. (1988). An attribution-affect-action theory of behavior: Replications of judgments of help-giving. *Personality and Social Psychology Bulletin, 14*(3), 610–621. https://doi.org/10.1177/0146167288143021.

Weiner, B. (1985). An attributional theory of achievement motivation and emotion. *Psychological Review, 92*(4), 548–573.

Weiner, B. (1993). On sin versus sickness: A theory of perceived responsibility and social motivation. *American Psychologist, 48*(9), 957–965.

Weiner, B., Perry, R. P., & Magnusson, J. (1988). An attributional analysis of reactions to stigmas. *Journal of Personality and Social Psychology, 55*(5), 738–748.

Persuasion

Barilan, Y. M., & Weintraub, M. (2001). Persuasion as respect for persons: An alternative view of autonomy and of the limits of discourse. *Journal of Medicine and Philosophy, 26*(1), 13–34. https://doi.org/10.1076/jmep.26.1.13.3033.

Biener, L., Wakefield, M., Shiner, C. M., & Siegel, M. (2008). How broadcast volume and emotional content affect youth recall of anti-tobacco advertising. *American Journal of Preventive Medicine, 35*(1), 14–19. https://doi.org/10.1016/j.amepre.2008.03.018.

Cacioppo, J. T., Pett, R. E., & Stoltenberg, C. D. (1985). Processes of social influence: The elaboration likelihood model of persuasion. In *Advances in cognitive-behavioral research and therapy* (Vol. 4, pp. 215–274). Academic Press. https://doi.org/10.1016/B978-0-12-010604-2.50012-4.

Goldman, L. K., & Glantz, S. A. (1998). Evaluation of antismoking advertising campaigns. *Journal of the American Medical Association, 279*(10), 772–777.

Jotterand, F., Amodio, A., & Elger, B. S. (2016). Patient education as empowerment and self-rebiasing. *Medicine, Health Care and Philosophy, 19*(4), 553–561. https://doi.org/10.1007/s11019-016-9702-9.

Leshner, G., Bolls, P., & Wise, K. (2011). Motivated processing of fear appeal and disgust images in televised anti-tobacco ads. *Journal of Media Psychology, 23*(2), 77–89. https://doi.org/10.1027/1864-1105/a000037.

Meisel, Z. F., & Karlawish, J. (2011). Narrative vs evidence-based medicine—and, not or. *Journal of the American Medical Association, 306*(18), 2022–2023. https://doi.org/10.1001/jama.2011.1648.

Petty, R. E., Barden, J., & Wheeler, S. C. (2009). The elaboration likelihood model of persuasion: Developing health promotions for sustained behavioral change. In *Emerging theories in health promotion practice and research* (2nd ed., pp. 185–214). Jossey-Bass/Wiley.

Petty, R. E., & Cacioppo, J. T. (1984). Source factors and the elaboration likelihood model of persuasion. *Advances in Consumer Research, 11,* 668–672.

Rimer, B. K., & Kreuter, M. W. (2006). Advancing tailored health communication: A persuasion and message effects perspective. *Journal of Communication, 56*(Suppl. 1), S184–S201. https://doi.org/10.1111/j.1460-2466.2006.00289.x.

Shen, L. (2011). The effectiveness of empathy- versus fear-arousing antismoking PSAs. *Health Communication, 26*(5), 404–415. https://doi.org/10.1080/10410236.2011.55 2480.

Swindell, J. S., McGuire, A. L., & Halpern, S. D. (2010). Beneficent persuasion: Techniques and ethical guidelines to improve patients' decisions. *Annals of Family Medicine, 8*(3), 260–264. https://doi.org/10.1370/afm.1118.

Wagner, B. C., & Petty, R. E. (2011). The elaboration likelihood model of persuasion: Thoughtful and non-thoughtful social influence. In *Theories in social psychology* (pp. 96–116). Wiley Blackwell.

Chapter 13. Organization

Fifth Vital Sign

Ahluwalia, J. S., Gibson, C. A., Kenney, R. E., Wallace, D. D., & Resnicow, K. (1999). Smoking status as a vital sign. *Journal of General Internal Medicine, 14*(7), 402–408. https://doi.org/10.1046/j.1525-1497.1999.09078.x.

Andrews, J. O., Tingen, M. S., Waller, J. L., & Harper, R. J. (2001). Provider feedback improves adherence with AHCPR smoking cessation guideline. *Preventive Medicine, 33*(5), 415–421. https://doi.org/10.1006/pmed.2001.0907.

Fiore, M. (1996). Smoking cessation. Clinical Practice Guideline, Number 18. Department of Health and Human Services, Public Health Service, Agency for Healthcare Policy and Research.

Katz, D. A., Muehlenbruch, D. R., Brown, R. L., Fiore, M. C., Baker, T. B., & for the AHRQ Smoking Cessation Guideline Study Group. (2004). Effectiveness of implementing the Agency for Healthcare Research and Quality Smoking Cessation Clinical Practice Guideline: A randomized, controlled trial. *Journal of the National Cancer Institute, 96*(8), 594–603. https://doi.org/10.1093/jnci/djh103.

Leone, F., Evers-Casey, S., Halenar, M., & O'Connell, K. (2013). Potential social, environmental, and regulatory threats to the effectiveness of EHR-supported tobacco treatment in healthcare. *Journal of Smoking Cessation, 15*, 1–9.

Lindell, K. O., & Reinke, L. F. (1999). Nursing strategies for smoking cessation. *Heart & Lung, 28*(4), 295–302. https://doi.org/10.1016/S0147-9563(99)70077-4.

McCullough, A., Fisher, M., Goldstein, A. O., Kramer, K. D., & Ripley-Moffitt, C. (2009). Smoking as a vital sign: Prompts to ask and assess increase cessation counseling. *Journal of the American Board of Family Medicine, 22*(6), 625–632. https://doi.org/10.3122/jabfm.2009.06.080211.

Papadakis, S., McDonald, P., Mullen, K.-A., Reid, R., Skulsky, K., & Pipe, A. (2010). Strategies to increase the delivery of smoking cessation treatments in primary care settings: A systematic review and meta-analysis. *Preventive Medicine, 51*(3), 199–213. https://doi.org/10.1016/j.ypmed.2010.06.007.

Piper, M. E., Fiore, M. C., Smith, S. S., Jorenby, D. E., Wilson, J. R., Zehner, M. E., & Baker, T. B. (2003). Use of the vital sign stamp as a systematic screening tool to promote smoking cessation. *Mayo Clinic Proceedings, 78*(6), 716–722. https://doi. org/10.4065/78.6.716.

Rothemich, S. F., Woolf, S. H., Johnson, R. E., Burgett, A. E., Flores, S. K., Marsland, D. W., & Ahluwalia, J. S. (2008). Effect on cessation counseling of documenting smoking status as a routine vital sign: An ACORN study. *Annals of Family Medicine, 6*(1), 60–68. https://doi.org/10.1370/afm.750.

Solberg, L. I., Maciosek, M. V., Edwards, N. M., Khanchandani, H. S., & Goodman, M. J. (2006). Repeated tobacco-use screening and intervention in clinical practice: Health impact and cost effectiveness. *American Journal of Preventive Medicine, 31*(1), 62–71. https://doi.org/10.1016/j.amepre.2006.03.013.

Zwar, N. A., Mendelsohn, C. P., & Richmond, R. L. (2014). Supporting smoking cessation. *British Medical Journal, 348*, f7535. https://doi.org/10.1136/bmj.f7535.

Responsibility

Clark, J. M., Rowe, K., & Jones, K. (1993). Evaluating the effectiveness of the coronary care nurses' role in smoking cessation. *Journal of Clinical Nursing, 2*(5), 313–322. https://doi.org/10.1111/j.1365-2702.1993.tb00184.x.

Curry, S. J., Keller, P. A., Orleans, C. T., & Fiore, M. C. (2008). The role of health care systems in increased tobacco cessation. *Annual Review of Public Health, 29*(1), 411–428. https://doi.org/10.1146/annurev.publhealth.29.020907.090934.

Fiore, M. C., & Baker, T. B. (1995). Smoking cessation treatment and the good doctor club. *American Journal of Public Health, 85*(2), 161–163.

Jackson, G., Bobak, A., Chorlton, I., Fowler, G., Hall, R., Khimji, H., Matthews, H., Stapleton, J., Steele, C., Stillman, P., Sutherland, G., & Swanton, R. (2001). Smoking cessation: A consensus statement with special reference to primary care. *International Journal of Clinical Practice, 55*(6), 385–392.

Johnson, J. L., Malchy, L. A., Ratner, P. A., Hossain, S., Procyshyn, R. M., Bottorff, J. L., Groening, M., Gibson, P., Osborne, M., & Schultz, A. (2009). Community mental healthcare providers' attitudes and practices related to smoking cessation interventions for people living with severe mental illness. *Patient Education and Counseling, 77*(2), 289–295. https://doi.org/10.1016/j.pec.2009.02.013.

Lally, R. M., Chalmers, K. I., Johnson, J., Kojima, M., Endo, E., Suzuki, S., Lai, Y.-H., Yang, Y.-H., Degner, L., Anderson, E., & Molassiotis, A. (2008). Smoking behavior and patient education practices of oncology nurses in six countries. *European Journal of Oncology Nursing, 12*(4), 372–379. https://doi.org/10.1016/j.ejon.2008.04.008.

Leone, F. T., & Evers-Casey, S. (2015). Examining the role of the health care professional in controlling the tobacco epidemic: Individual, organizational and institutional responsibilities. In R. Loddenkemper and M. Kreuter (Eds.), *The tobacco epidemic* (2nd ed., Vol. 42, pp. 219–228). Karger.

Matouq, A., Khader, Y., Khader, A., Al-Rabadi, A., Al Omari, M., Iblan, I., & Al-sheyab, N. (2018). Knowledge, attitude, and behaviors of health professionals towards smoking cessation in primary healthcare settings. *Translational Behavioral Medicine, 8*(6), 938–943. https://doi.org/10.1093/tbm/ibx045.

Meijer, E., Van der Kleij, R. M. J. J., & Chavannes, N. H. (2019). Facilitating smoking cessation in patients who smoke: A large-scale cross-sectional comparison of fourteen groups of healthcare providers. *BMC Health Services Research, 19*(1), 750. https://doi.org/10.1186/s12913-019-4527-x.

Raw, M., McNeill, A., & West, R. (1999). Smoking cessation: Evidence based recommendations for the healthcare system. *British Medical Journal, 318*(7177), 182–185. https://doi.org/10.1136/bmj.318.7177.182.

Rossem, C. van, Spigt, M. G., Kleijsen, J. R., Hendricx, M., Schayck, C. P. van, & Kotz, D. (2015). Smoking cessation in primary care: Exploration of barriers and solutions in current daily practice from the perspective of smokers and healthcare professionals. *European Journal of General Practice, 21*(2), 1–7. https://doi.org/10.3109/1 3814788.2014.990881.

Stead, L. F., Buitrago, D., Preciado, N., Sanchez, G., Hartmann-Boyce, J., & Lancaster, T. (2013). Physician advice for smoking cessation. *Cochrane Database of Systematic Reviews, 2*, CD000165. https://doi.org/10.1002/14651858.CD000165.pub4.

Youdan, B., & Queally, B. (2005). Nurses' role in promoting and supporting smoking cessation. *Nursing Times, 101*(10), 26–27.

Building a Better System and Constructionism

Benton, J. Z., Lodh, A., Watson, A. M., Tingen, M. S., Terris, M. K., Wallis, C. J. D., & Klaassen, Z. (2020). The association between physician trust and smoking cessation: Implications for motivational interviewing. *Preventive Medicine, 135*, 106075. https://doi.org/10.1016/j.ypmed.2020.106075.

Bentz, C. J. (2000). Implementing tobacco tracking codes in an individual practice association or a network model health maintenance organisation. *Tobacco Control, 9*(Suppl. 1), i42–i45. https://doi.org/10.1136/tc.9.suppl_1.i42.

Evans, J. M., Baker, R. G., Berta, W., & Jan, B. (2014). The evolution of integrated health care strategies. In *Annual review of health care management: Revisiting the evolution of health systems organization* (Vol. 15, pp. 125–161). Emerald Group Publishing. https://doi.org/10.1108/S1474-8231(2013)0000015011.

Gröne, O., & Garcia-Barbero, M. (2001). Integrated care. *International Journal of Integrated Care, 1*, e21. https://www.ncbi.nlm.nih.gov/pmc/articles/PMC1525335/.

Herie, M., Connolly, H., Voci, S., Dragonetti, R., & Selby, P. (2012). Changing practitioner behavior and building capacity in tobacco cessation treatment: The TEACH project. *Patient Education and Counseling, 86*(1), 49–56. https://doi.org/10.1016/j.pec.2011.04.018.

Hudmon, K. S., Corelli, R. L., Chung, E., Gundersen, B., Kroon, L. A., Sakamoto, L. M., Hemberger, K. K., Fenlon, C., & Prokhorov, A. V. (2003). Development and implementation of a tobacco cessation training program for students in the health professions. *Journal of Cancer Education, 18*(3), 142–149. https://doi.org/10.1207/ S15430154JCE1803_07.

Jackson, S. F., Perkins, F., Khandor, E., Cordwell, L., Hamann, S., & Buasai, S. (2006). Integrated health promotion strategies: A contribution to tackling current and future health challenges. *Health Promotion International, 21*(Suppl. 1), 75–83. https://doi.org/10.1093/heapro/dal054.

Leone, F. T., Evers-Casey, S., Mulholland, M. A., & Sachs, D. P. L. (2016). Integrating tobacco use treatment into practice: Billing and documentation. *Chest, 149*(2), 568–575. https://doi.org/10.1378/chest.15-0441.

Lieu, T. A., & Madvig, P. R. (2019). Strategies for building delivery science in an integrated health care system. *Journal of General Internal Medicine, 34*(6), 1043–1047. https://doi.org/10.1007/s11606-018-4797-8.

Mayhew, S. H., Hopkins, J., & Warren, C. E. (2017). Building integrated health systems: Lessons from HIV, sexual and reproductive health integration. *Health Policy and Planning, 32*(Suppl. 4), iv1–iv5. https://doi.org/10.1093/heapol/czx142.

Montenegro, H., Holder, R., Ramagem, C., Urrutia, S., Fabrega, R., Tasca, R., Alfaro, G., Salgado, O., & Angelica Gomes, M. (2011). Combating health care fragmentation through integrated health service delivery networks in the Americas: Lessons learned. *Journal of Integrated Care, 19*(5), 5–16. https://doi.org/10.1108/14769011111176707.

Norman, C. D., & Huerta, T. (2006). Knowledge transfer and exchange through social networks: Building foundations for a community of practice within tobacco control. *Implementation Science, 1*(1), 20. https://doi.org/10.1186/1748-5908-1-20.

Orleans, C. T., Woolf, S. H., Rothemich, S. F., Marks, J. S., & Isham, G. J. (2006). The top priority: Building a better system for tobacco-cessation counseling. *American Journal of Preventive Medicine, 31*(1), 103–106. https://doi.org/10.1016/j.amepre.2006.03.015.

Pbert, L. (2003). Healthcare provider training in tobacco treatment: Building competency. *American Journal of the Medical Sciences, 326*(4), 242–247. https://doi.org/10.1097/00000441-200310000-00018.

Pbert, L., Ockene, J. K., Ewy, B. M., Leicher, E. S., & Warner, D. (2000). Development of a state wide tobacco treatment specialist training and certification programme for Massachusetts. *Tobacco Control, 9*(4), 372–381. https://doi.org/10.1136/tc.9.4.372.

Sheffer, C. E., Al-Zalabani, A., Aubrey, A., Bader, R., Beltrez, C., Bennett, S., Carl, E., Cranos, C., Darville, A., Greyber, J., Karam-Hage, M., Hawari, F., Hutcheson, T., Hynes, V., Kotsen, C., Leone, F., McConaha, J., McCary, H., Meade, C., . . . Wendling, A. (2021). The emerging global tobacco treatment workforce: Characteristics of tobacco treatment specialists trained in council-accredited training programs from 2017 to 2019. *International Journal of Environmental Research and Public Health, 18*(5), 2416. https://doi.org/10.3390/ijerph18052416.

Walsh, S. E., Singleton, J. A., Worth, C. T., Krugler, J., Moore, R., Wesley, G. C., & Mitchell, C. K. (2007). Tobacco cessation counseling training with standardized patients. *Journal of Dental Education, 71*(9), 1171–1178. https://doi.org/10.1002/j.0022-0337.2007.71.9.tb04381.x.

Index

Figures and tables are indicated by page numbers followed by fig. and tab. respectively.

Acknowledgments

The list of people who have helped us—in ways big and small—as we've worked to come to this understanding of the tobacco-dependence problem is too long to fit in print. However, there are a few folks who were particularly influential for us and without whom this book would never have been possible. To them, we'd like to send a special word of gratitude.

In the introduction, we briefly mentioned the contribution of the thousands of patients and research subjects with whom we have interacted over the years. While they know who they are, they may not know how much our time with them has meant to us. Their willingness to share of themselves and to teach us, in the hope of someday helping others, was a gift for which we can't say thanks enough.

We have hundreds of earnest and dedicated colleagues with whom we have often shared ideas and debated controversial topics. Without such a wonderful and committed academic community, so generous with their insights and perspectives, it would have been very hard for us to see the forest for the trees.

We have had the honor of working with a number of brilliant partners and team members over the years. Finding true working partnerships that lead to system change and discovery can be difficult, but we've been lucky to be abundantly surrounded. In particular, Dr. Robert Schnoll of Penn Psychiatry has been a treasured colleague and a friend. Tierney Fisher and Jody Nicoloso deserve special thanks for their boundless commitment to our patients' well-being and their dedication to making a difference in healthcare.

Printed and bound by CPI Group (UK) Ltd, Croydon, CR0 4YY

19/10/2023

08153113-0001